NEUROLOGICAL DISABILITIES

Assessment and Treatment

NEUROLOGICAL DISABILITIES

Assessment and Treatment

Susan E. Bennett, PT, EdD

Associate Professor, Department of Physical Therapy
D'Youville College
Buffalo, New York

James L. Karnes, PhD, PT

Associate Professor, Department of Physical Therapy
D'Youville College
Buffalo, New York

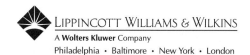

LIPPINCOTT WILLIAMS & WILKINS
A **Wolters Kluwer** Company
Philadelphia · Baltimore · New York · London
Buenos Aires · Hong Kong · Sydney · Tokyo

Acquisitions Editor: Margaret Biblis
Project Editor: Tom Gibbons
Senior Production Manager: Helen Ewan
Production Coordinator: Mike Carcel
Assistant Art Director: Kathy Kelley-Luedtke
Indexer: Victoria Boyle

ISBN 0-397-55151-7

Care has been taken to confirm the accuracy of the information presented and to describe generally accepted practices. However, the authors, editors, and publisher are not responsible for errors or omissions or for any consequences from application of the information in this book and make no warranty, express or implied, with respect to the contents of the publication.

The authors, editors and publisher have exerted every effort to ensure that drug selection and dosage set forth in this text are in accordance with current recommendations and practice at the time of publication. However, in view of ongoing research, changes in government regulations, and the constant flow of information relating to drug therapy and drug reactions, the reader is urged to check the package insert for each drug for any change in indications and dosage and for added warnings and precautions. This is particularly important when the recommended agent is a new or infrequently employed drug.

Some drugs and medical devices presented in this publication have Food and Drug Administration (FDA) clearance for limited use in restricted research settings. It is the responsibility of the health care provider to ascertain the FDA status of each drug or device planned for use in their clinical practice.

9 8 7 6 5 4 3

This textbook is dedicated to our patients and students.

Treating patients who have sustained damage to the nervous system is a rewarding and often challenging experience. Teaching entry-level students how to examine, assess, and treat patients with a neurological disability is equally rewarding and challenging. *Neurological Disabilities: Assessment and Treatment* was written to provide entry-level students with a framework for assessment and treatment of adults with neurological disabilities to enable their development as movement scientists.

This textbook is very different from other neuro-rehabilitative textbooks in that emphasis is placed on identifying disabilities and underlying impairments, rather than the disease process. Disabilities are limitations in the performance of functional mobility or tasks. Impairments are problems or signs and symptoms that result from pathological conditions or trauma. In other neuro-rehabilitative textbooks chapters are organized by diagnosis (e.g., stroke, multiple sclerosis, Parkinson's disease, etc.), with assessment and treatment addressing the problems related to the specific diagnosis. This text is focused on the examination of functional mobility and four commonly occurring impairments (weakness, sensory/perceptual dysfunction, incoordination, and balance dysfunction) that may produce disabilities.

To facilitate entry-level students' understanding of very complex neurological adult patients, a simplified framework is provided to examine functional mobility and discern the four commonly occurring impairments that

may produce disabilities. To some extent, then, the text is limited in its scope since we do not address impairments or disabilities in children, nor do we discuss problems associated with cognition, motivation, or behavior. Readers are referred to Cohen, *Neuroscience for Rehabilitation,* and Shumway-Cook and Woollacott, *Motor Control, Theory and Practical Applications,* for additional information on cognition. This text addresses patients' ability to make decisions related to movement, primarily based on their physical abilities and the environment in which they are functioning.

Organization of the Text

This textbook falls into two major sections. Chapters 1 through 4 provide the groundwork for understanding disabilities and impairments, the anatomy of movement, a model for the assessment of disabilities and impairments, and theoretical perspectives on treatment. Chapters 5 through 8 describe the four impairments (weakness, sensory/perceptual dysfunction, incoordination, and balance dysfunction) that are commonly found in a variety of neurological diagnoses. For example, a person who has suffered a stroke may have weakness, problems with balance, and sensory dysfunction. These same impairments may be seen in patients with multiple sclerosis or in those who have suffered traumatic brain injury. The disabilities that result from these three neurological diagnoses may be similar if they all share common impairments.

There are many more impairments that are associated with neurological diagnoses beyond the four discussed in this text. However, it is our intent to limit discussion for the entry-level student to the four commonly occurring impairments seen with lesions of the motor pathways. For each of the four impairments, an overview is presented, followed by anatomical locations of lesions that may produce the impairment, examination of functional mobility, standardized assessment procedures for the impairment, and treatment that emphasizes task-oriented activities. Readers should understand that just as there are several impairments beyond those four described in this text, there are also other disabilities that may be displayed (e.g., dressing, hygiene activities, eating).

Neurological Disabilities is primarily focused on the assessment and treatment provided by physical therapists to achieve adequate functional mobility needed for discharge to home from an in-patient facility (acute care hospital, medical rehabilitation unit, or subacute unit). The focus of treatment on functional mobility should also be incorporated in therapy provided in the home or in an outpatient setting, with the understanding that treatment in these environments should incorporate reintegration to the community and/or work environment. Treatment techniques described emphasize incorporating activities or tasks that patients are unable to perform safely and efficiently into treatment sessions. Treatment of impairments alone, without application and practice of tasks associated with functional mobility, is discouraged. Empirical data support the use of contemporary task-oriented treatment as effective in relearning functional activities. In some patients it may be appropriate to incorporate traditional ther-apeutic techniques when practicing task-oriented postures or movements. For this reason, several traditional therapeutic techniques (e.g., tapping, joint compression, proprioceptive neuromuscular facilitation) have been described. We advocate the incorporation of some of the traditional techniques as components of the task-oriented activity for patients who are low functioning. For example, a patient who is unable to activate the triceps brachii muscle may benefit from the therapist tapping the muscle belly while the patient reaches for a cup of water. The task-oriented activity is the focus of the treatment; however, tapping is incorporated to assist in the initial activation of the muscle. It is the therapist's prerogative to utilize traditional therapeutic techniques if deemed appropriate.

Neurological Disabilities is intended for physical therapists, but occupational therapists would also benefit from it, although examples of functional mobility are limited to those movements required for daily mobility. Examples of dressing activities or hygiene care frequently addressed by occupational therapists are not provided in this text. It would be an excellent reference source for physical therapist assistants seeking to understand how movement occurs and refining a task-oriented treatment approach.

Functional mobility items described in this text were identified based on the frequency with which they occur on standardized functional assessment scales (e.g., Functional Independence Measure, Barthel). Certainly the role of the therapist in rehabilitation is beyond patient function within the home; however, the purpose of this text is to establish a base of knowledge on which we hope entry-level students will build to understand their role in diminishing or eliminating handicapping conditions within the community and work environment. Readers are referred to Wade; *Measurement in Neuro-Rehabilitation,* for additional information on measuring disabilities and/or handicaps.

•••••••••••••••••••••••••••••••••••
Features of This Text

Style Notes

In this text, the individual who has a neurological condition is referred to as a patient. *Patient* is defined by *Webster's New World Dictionary* as "1. bearing or enduring pain, trouble, . . . a person receiving care or treatment." The focus of this book is on individuals who have disabilities from neurological lesions and receive treatment to reduce or eliminate the disability—hence, a patient. Whenever possible the plural form (e.g., patients, individuals, their) has been used to avoid the use of pronouns (he or she). At times, a patient may be referred to in the singular when referring to a specific case study or to photographs presented in the text.

The subheading "Disability", which appears in Chapters 5 through 8, reviews how functional mobility may be altered when weakness, sensory/perceptual loss, incoordination, or balance dysfunction is present. This material is initially described in Chapter 3 and therefore may appear redundant to the reader. However, the intent is to emphasize how disabilities may result from impairments.

Adult functional rehabilitation is the focus of this text. Children who have neurological conditions present with different problems since they have not developed a mature, intact nervous system. Addressing disabilities of children with neurological dysfunction requires a different approach from what is presented here. This text is not all inclusive in presenting disabling conditions of adults with neurological diagnoses, nor are pathological states described. Readers are referred to Rubin and Farber, *Essential Pathology,* for a description of pathological conditions of the nervous system.

Learning Objectives

At the beginning of each chapter is a set of learning objectives to assist the reader in the focus of each chapter. The learning objectives highlight the major concepts presented and draw attention to key points that will be summarized at the conclusion of each chapter.

Summary

Each chapter concludes with a summary that reinforces the learning objectives established for each chapter and summarizes the main concepts presented.

Appendices

Appendix A consists of a description of three standardized measures of disability and two instruments to assess quality of life. The use of standardized functional assessment tools is encouraged to provide uniform measurement and documentation of functional mobility. The measures of disability include the Functional Independence Measure (FIM), the Barthel, and the Rivermead Mobility Index. The tools to assess quality of life are the SF-36 and the Health Status Questionnaire 12 (HSQ-12).

Appendix B contains a table of the standardized instruments presented in Chapters 5 through 8. The table contains the reference(s) for the reliability and validity of the instruments and the chapter in this text in which the instrument is discussed.

ACKNOWLEDGMENTS

Our course in neurological rehabilitation has been taught for several years in the format presented in this text. Providing this context for students to develop skills as movement scientists has resulted in competent, knowledgeable entry-level practitioners who can examine and treat any patient with a neurological lesion. Converting the lecture material and laboratory activity into a textbook has been a long, tedious, grueling, and at times painful event. However, it has also been challenging, exciting, and well worth the effort. It could not have been done without the hard work and commitment of the following people: Dr. Andrew Allen, previously of Lippincott-Raven Publishers, who nurtured us in the formative stages of the text and encouraged us through the many difficult times; Crystal Norris, for her helpful editorial and organizational comments; Margaret Biblis, for her assistance and kind suggestions; and Margaret Frye, MA, OTR, for her expertise and contributions to the chapter on Sensory and Perceptual Dysfunction.

We could not have completed this text without the assistance of Tim Heiman and David Weimer, both of whom helped with literature searches and photographs. We would also like to thank Rosemary Bennett and Leon Cowan for their assistance with photographs. Finally, we are indebted to the therapists and staff at DeGraff Memorial Hospital for allowing us to utilize their facility for patient recruitment and photography settings.

On a personal note, we would like to thank Tamara Owen, Michele Karnes, Margaret Karnes, Kim Bennett, and Rosemary Bennett for their patience, support, understanding, and kind and frequent words of encouragement throughout the production of this text.

CONTENTS

CHAPTER 4

Theoretical Approach to Treatment   69

CHAPTER 5

Weakness   85

CHAPTER 6
Sensory and Perceptual Dysfunction   *131*

CHAPTER 7

Incoordination   157

Conceptual Models of Disability

LEARNING OBJECTIVES

After reading this chapter, you should be able to:

1. Compare and contrast the Nagi and the International Classification of Impairment, Disability, and Handicap (ICIDH) models of disability.
2. Apply the ICIDH model of disability in a clinical situation.
3. Conceptualize the major differences between traditional and task-oriented treatment approaches.
4. Discuss the role quality-of-life issues play in neurological assessment and treatment.
5. Analyze use of standardized tests in treatment approaches.

As movement scientists, physical therapists constantly analyze how patients move. This analysis is performed to determine if movement is effective, efficient, and safe. The primary goal of the physical therapist's interaction with patients should be to enhance functional mobility within a variety of environments. Simply stated, **functional mobility** is the ability to perform a set of useful tasks.* These *tasks* amount to the common movements needed for daily activity. The list includes but is not limited to:

- Bed mobility (eg, rolling from side to side)
- Moving from the supine to a sitting posture
- Moving from sitting to a standing posture
- Transferring from one surface to another (eg, moving from a bed to a wheelchair)
- Ambulating
- Climbing stairs

A **disability** is any limitation in functional mobility. In other words, a disability is the *inabil-*

---

* Terms in bold appear in the glossary at the end of the book.

ity to perform a task. It is not to be confused with an **impairment,** which is a problem or symptom that a patient presents as a result of the abnormal structure or function of organs or tissues. Pain, edema, and weakness are all examples of common impairments.

Accurate analysis of functional mobility assists the physical therapist in determining if specific impairments exist that contribute to a patient's inability to move. Historically, therapists have concentrated on assessing and treating impairments, with the expectation that the disabilities incurred from impairments would be reduced or eliminated. The emphasis on impairments may have derived from the viewpoint of workers' compensation that prevailed in the late 1950s. Because impairments could be measured objectively, the authors of workers' compensation legislation viewed them as the real criteria by which an individual's disability could be assessed (Nagi, 1991).

Physical therapists who limit their assessment and treatment to impairments alone fail to set functional goals for their patients to achieve. There is thus no verifiable means of assessing the patient's progress along the continuum from disability to full function. This failure to establish functional goals is deceptively dangerous for another reason: It allows the physical therapist to consider impairments and disabilities as discrete elements in the patient's physical repertoire. Unless connections are drawn between impairments and disabilities, assessment will be incomplete and treatment will never be specific enough to improve the patient's abilities.

Traditional, impairment-oriented approaches are generally seen as less effective for rehabilitating patients precisely because they fail to set functional goals for the patients. In the task-oriented approach, which is promoted in this text, the rehabilitative effort is on getting patients to relearn and practice the ordinary activities they will need to get through the day. An impairment-oriented therapist might concen-

trate on relieving a patient's weakness with weight training. Task-oriented therapists might well use this traditional strengthening regimen, but they would also help their patients reorganize any movement strategies due to weakness so that they can sit, stand, and dress themselves with minimal or no assistance.

CONCEPTUAL MODELS

In the field of disability, there are two major conceptual models: the model developed by Saad Nagi, and the World Health Organization (WHO) International Classification of Impairments, Disabilities, and Handicaps (ICIDH). This text uses the concepts of impairment and disability derived from the WHO model. Because the conceptual model of disability developed by Nagi provided the groundwork for the ICIDH model, it, too, is discussed in detail.

Nagi Model

The Nagi model, developed in 1965, was the first to examine the health status of a patient vis-á-vis the disease state (Fig. 1-1). Previously, all models of health had been based on the medical model of disease (Fig. 1-2). The etiology of a particular disease was understood to lead to pathology, followed by the manifestation of the disease. Medical intervention applied at this stage either led to a cure or resulted in death.

Nagi's work followed the tumultuous 1950s, when differing concepts of disability and lack of clarity of terminology led to heavy reliance on the impairment classification. Decisions on vocational roles and earning potential after disabling conditions were based on which impairment(s) the individual had suffered. The American Medical Association's Committee on

PATHOLOGY	→	IMPAIRMENT	→	FUNCTIONAL LIMITATION	→	DISABILITY
Interruption or interference of normal bodily processes or structures		Loss and/or abnormality of mental, emotional, physiological, or anatomical structure or function; includes all losses or abnormalities, not just those attributable to active pathology; also includes pain		Restriction or lack of ability to perform an action or activity in the manner or within the range considered normal that results from impairment		Inability or limitation in performing socially defined activities and roles expected of individuals within a social and physical environment
Example						
Loss of innervation to iliopsoas muscle, resulting in atrophy of muscle		Cannot flex hip		Problems with gait, may contribute to circumducted gait		Problems ascending curbs or walking up stairs or a ramp

FIGURE 1-1. The Nagi model.

Medical Rating of Mental and Physical Impairment (1958), and the House Ways and Means Subcommittee (1959), concluded that impairment measures were the only criteria of permanent disability (Nagi, 1991). A uniform definition of disability and a criterion for determining varying levels of disability were needed.

Building on the work of the Social Security Disability Insurance program in the early 1960s,

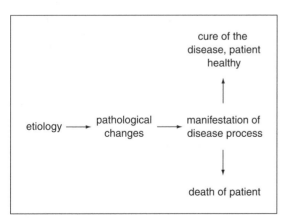

FIGURE 1-2. The medical model of disease developed for the International Classification of Disease (ICD).

Nagi used existing knowledge to establish his model. Nagi's model is comprised of four concepts: pathology, impairment, functional limitation, and disability. Nagi (1991) defines *pathology* as an interruption of or interference in the body's normal processes, with a simultaneous effort for return to the normal state. In his model, pathology is forever linked with the body's fight to regain health.

Pathology has many possible etiologies, including infection, trauma, degenerative conditions, or disease processes. Nagi's expanded definition of *impairment* includes loss or abnormality of an anatomic, physiologic, mental, or emotional nature (Nagi, 1991). According to his model, every pathology necessarily has an impairment because every pathology either damages the anatomy or interrupts the physiology of the system in some way. Impairments may, however, exist in the absence of pathology. Such is the case when the impairment is due to a congenital formation, such as a malformed upper limb, spina bifida, or a cleft palate (Nagi, 1991).

It is often helpful to think of impairments and functional limitations as occupying different levels in the physical hierarchy of the human body. Impairments occur at the organ level (eg, soft tissue adhesion, muscular weakness), whereas functional limitations are visible only at the level of the whole organism. A person may have a completely invisible impairment, such as a soft tissue adhesion in the shoulder. Should that same person lose the ability to dress independently, he or she would be said to suffer a **functional limitation** (inability to perform a functional task) as a result of the underlying impairment.

Nagi particularized the definition of disability to describe a person's inability or limitation in performing socially defined roles, such as those demanded by work, family responsibilities, or recreational activities. A *disability*, as described by Nagi (1991), is labeled as such because it prevents those afflicted from rising to the challenges of the physical environment and fulfilling sociocultural expectations. Wheelchair-bound persons who have decided to go out to a restaurant have to contend with several obstacles, all of which conspire to get them labeled ''disabled.'' They are expected to go to the restaurant whether or not it is handicapped accessible. In this case, the wheelchair, which was originally designed to *enable* the nonambulatory person, is insufficient to allow the person to answer the demands of the physical environment. The person is thus saddled with the double burden of being physically unable to complete a certain task, and socially incapacitated as well.

The personal costs of being labeled disabled can run much higher, depending on the circumstances. For example, a parent who is confined to a wheelchair may be deemed inadequate to the socially defined role of parenting. The unspoken logic may unfold as follows: How, people may wonder, can this person who is incapable of self-care take care of a child? This example alone offers proof that words, and the perceptions they help shape, can have a serious impact on the individual.

The ICIDH Model

The WHO developed the International Classification of Impairment, Disabilities, and Handicaps (ICIDH) model in the mid-1970s (Fig. 1-3) to begin to narrow the gap between ''what health care systems can do and what they might do ''(WHO, 1980, p. 7). Health care systems had previously focused on disease, as evidenced by the use of the International Classification of Disease (ICD), which has been in existence since 1893 (see Fig. 1-2). This conceptualization of disease, or pathology, is fairly simple: Once disease manifests itself, it can be cured, or it can progress until the organism dies.

Advances in medical technology have radically altered the potential outcomes of pathologic conditions beyond measuring morbidity and mortality. Today, treatment of pathology is more likely than ever before to result in manageable conditions that are chronic or disabling in nature. It is in these conditions that impairments and disabilities figure prominently. Because health problems that were chronic or disabling in nature could not be assessed with the ICD model, there was a demand for a new model that would make assessment more meaningful.

The ICIDH was established for this purpose. This complement to the ICD examines the consequences of nonfatal disease to the individual, as well as on the interaction between the individual and society.

The ICIDH model has four components related to the state of health: disease, impairment, disability, and handicap. **Disease** represents changes that occur at the level of the organ (eg, infection, inflammation, fractured bones). This is similar, if not identical, to how Nagi characterizes pathology. Disease represents changes in body structure or function (WHO, 1980). *Impairment*, as defined by ICIDH and Nagi, are synonymous.

Disability occurs at the person level and is a restriction in or lack of ability to perform

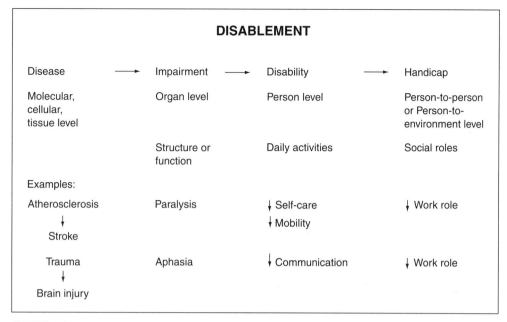

FIGURE 1-3. The International Classification of Impairment, Disabilities, and Handicaps (ICIDH) model.

common activities in the manner or within the range considered normal (WHO, 1980). Disability in the ICIDH model is similar to the concept of functional limitations in the Nagi model. The inability to transfer between surfaces, ambulate, or climb stairs would all qualify as disabilities according to the ICIDH model. Any limitations in movement that result from impairments would be categorized as disabilities. Also included within the concept of disability are psychological responses to illness, such as sick-role behavior.

The impact of a handicap registers on the social rather than the personal scale. The inability to hold a job may be viewed as a **handicap,** a societal limitation placed on a person who is physically unable to navigate the environment without assistive devices. Social isolation or a feeling of being devalued (WHO, 1980) may well be the social price paid by the handicapped individual. The ICIDH definition of handicap

is similar to Nagi's concept of disability in that both address limitations imposed by society and the physical environment.

It is important to note that the ICIDH is not a linear model, that is, a causal mode does not exist between the three planes of impairment, disability, and handicap; nor does this model represent change over time. A handicap should not be considered to be directly related to disability or impairment. In fact, it has been suggested that arrows be added to the model represented in Figure 1-3 to show the reciprocal relationship between handicap and disability, and handicap and impairments.

An individual with **hemiplegia** (an impairment involving paralysis of one side of the body) and disability in walking may not have a significant handicap given appropriate equipment and a supportive physical and social environment. A nonsupportive environment, however, would contribute to a significant handicap for this individual. If the individual with hemiplegia is unable to return to a previous job because of physical and social barriers, the situation may lead to depression and **deconditioning** (progression of impairments) and diminished activities of daily living. In this example, the handicap can lead to the development of additional impairments and diminished abilities (Peters, 1995).

The ICIDH is a more useful model for conceptualizing disability than the Nagi model for a variety of reasons:

- It can be applied to a wide range of activities.
- It can be used to examine the prevalence of disability.
- It is instrumental in formulating health care policies and for planning and staffing health care facilities.
- It allows for delivery of care through appropriate diagnosis and treatment, evaluation of treatment results, and assessment for work.
- It serves as a uniform system for clarifying information in curricula for the training of health professionals.
- It allows for the collection of data that can be used for research activities (Halbertsma, 1995).

Because the ICIDH is so versatile and universally used, this text embraces it as the foundational model of disability.

Criticisms of the ICIDH Model

The ICIDH model is not, however, without its shortcomings. The most noteworthy is its use of the term "handicap," which implies limitation in performance and is perceived as a negative term (Pope & Tarlov, 1991). The definition of handicap has been a problematic area for the ICIDH model because it makes no reference to environmental and social factors. In the foreword to the 1993 reprinting of the ICIDH, the WHO grappled with the issue:

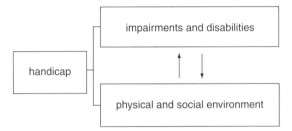

FIGURE 1-4. The interaction of impairments and disabilities with the physical and social environments.

Handicap is more problematical. . . . The items are not classified according to individuals or their attributes, but rather according to the circumstances in which people with disabilities are likely to find themselves, circumstances that can be expected to place such individuals at a disadvantage in relation to their peers when viewed from the norms of society. (WHO, 1980; reprinted with revised foreword, WHO, 1993)

Another criticism of the model cites its failure to make a clear distinction between the disability and handicap planes (Pope & Tarlov, 1991).*

As depicted in Figure 1-4, Badley (1987) and Chaime (1990) have suggested that handicaps result from the interaction of an individual's impairments and disabilities with external environmental factors.

Comparison of the Two Models

Jette (1994) compared the ICIDH model to the Nagi scheme and concluded that the two models differ in how they define and interpret the last two stages. The ICIDH definition of handi-

---

* The ICIDH was drafted in 1980 with the intention of having it revised based on feedback from those who use the model. The proposed publication date of the revised version is 1998.

cap sets up a clear distinction between limitations in societal performance caused by the environment and those that result from the disabled person's interaction with the environment. According to Nagi (1991), the two factors, environment and interaction in the environment, should not be separated. Nagi's model accounts for the interrelatedness of the variety of difficulties a handicapped person might have with something as mundane as visiting the restroom on a coffee break. It poses and then answers in the affirmative the following questions:

- Is the bathroom handicapped accessible?
- Is the handicapped employee given a long enough break to take care of hygienic needs?

Although differences exist in the interpretation of the Nagi and ICIDH models, both agree that the physical therapist is there to minimize or eliminate *disability* (as defined by the ICIDH) or *functional limitations* (as defined by Nagi), to promote the patient's integration into normal social roles.

Table 1-1 summarizes the similarities and differences between the Nagi and ICIDH models, with illustrative examples.

Application of the ICIDH Model

To better understand the ICIDH model, the following clinical example is provided:

A 32-year-old woman developed multiple sclerosis (MS) 5 years ago, after the delivery of her first child. She has had three exacerbations of her symptoms since the onset of the disease. She is now in an acute care hospital recovering from the third exacerbation. Physical therapy evaluation indicates the following:

- Poor bilateral lower extremity muscle strength
- Normal bilateral upper extremity muscle strength
- Intact cortical sensation
- Intact proprioception (perception of movements and position of the body)
- Coordination in both lower extremities successful in 6 of 10 trials
- Independent in rolling from side to side in bed
- Minimal assistance required when moving from a supine position to sitting
- Minimal assistance required to maintain sitting
- Moderate assistance required to move into standing
- Presently nonambulatory, but was walking with a wide base quad cane before admission
- Balance dysfunction (inability to maintain balance in a static sitting or standing)

Discharge plans are for her to return to her one-floor home with her husband and two preschool-age children.

According to the ICIDH model, this patient's clinical status can be separated into the four previously defined categories of *disease, impairment, disability,* and *handicap:*

Disease: MS, a demyelinating disease of the central nervous system (CNS). The etiology of MS is unknown but is suspected to be viral. Pathologically, the disease is predominantly one of inflammation of *myelin* (a fatlike sheath covering the axons of certain neurons; also known as CNS white matter). This inflammation results in *demyelination,* or loss of myelin.

TABLE 1-1   The Nagi and ICIDH Models Compared

Nagi Model*	ICIDH Model†	Level of Reference	Examples	Differences
Pathology	Disease	*Cells and tissues †Molecules, cells, and tissues	*Denervated muscle in arm due to trauma †Atherosclerosis → Stroke → Trauma → Brain injury	Synonymous
Impairment	Impairment	*Organs and organ systems †Organs	*Atrophy of muscle †Paralysis, aphasia	Synonymous
Functional limitation	Disability	*Organism †Person	*Unable to dress using the involved arm †Incapable of self-care and unassisted mobility; difficulty communicating	Similar
Disability	Handicap	*Society †Person to environment	*Loss of job; inability to engage in usual recreational activities †Change in work role	*The environment and the person's interaction with the environment are not distinct factors. †There is a clear distinction between limitations imposed by the environment and those that result from the handicapped person's interaction in the environment.

*Indicates aspects of Nagi model.
†Indicates aspects of ICIDH model.

Impairment: Problems associated with MS can vary depending on which myelinated area in the CNS is involved. Common impairments include weakness, **spasticity** (increased tone or contraction of antigravity muscles), **incoordination** (inability to produce smooth, rhythmic motion that is not due to weakness), sensory loss, balance dysfunction, and visual abnormalities. (Each of these common impairments is the subject of a chapter in Section II, where they will be given expanded discussion.)

In the clinical case depicted above, the impairments are weakness, incoordination, and balance dysfunction.

Disability: Like impairments, disabilities associated with MS can vary based on the anatomic site(s) of demyelination. In this case, the patient showed the following problems with functional mobility:

- Required minimal assistance with moving from a supine position to sitting
- Was unable to maintain sitting without minimal assistance
- Required moderate assistance to move into standing position
- Was nonambulatory

Handicap: Because this patient was evaluated in an acute care hospital, it is impossible to determine which functional difficulties she may encounter in her home and community. It is known that she resides in a one-floor home with her husband and two young children. A home assessment by a physical therapist is indicated to determine home, environment, and community accessibility.

ANALYSIS AND TREATMENT

Physical therapists have traditionally focused on treating impairments such as muscle weakness or dyscoordination with therapeutic exercise in nonfunctional patterns. The assumption was that strengthening muscles while the patient was supine or prone would lead to improved function in upright postures (eg, transfers or ambulation). It was also assumed that benefits gained in gait training on smooth, flat surfaces would be transferable to ambulation on any surface in any environment. However, experience proved that strengthening the muscles of hip flexion in the supine position did not necessarily improve the swing phase of the gait cycle. Likewise, independent ambulation on a smooth, hard surface that is free of any obstacles does not ensure safe, independent ambulation on carpeting and around furniture.

Light (1995) was the first to provide evidence that treating impairments in nonfunctional patterns may not carry over into improved func-

tion. She described a case study in which a neurologically impaired woman with poor standing balance control was provided with a balance training program that included both static postures and dynamic actions performed while kneeling. Results of her aggressive training program showed vast improvement in the patient's kneeling balance, but no significant improvement in her standing balance control. Light (1995) concluded that "physical therapists need to consider specific task demands and the specificity of training in order to design efficient treatment programs" (p. 11). Although much more research is needed in this area, task-oriented training appears to be more efficient than traditional impairment-oriented treatment programs.

Furthermore, according to Rothstein (1994), "We can no longer seek to merely affect the impairments of patients–we must do so in a way that matters" (p. 376). Analysis and treatment must be refocused on disabilities that patients present and the environmental barriers that limit patients' full integration into society. As the reader will see, this text focuses on task-oriented activities based on functional mobility.

QUALITY OF LIFE

Quality of life has been defined as generally corresponding to total well-being, in that it encompasses both physical and psychological determinants (Wenger, Mattson, Furberg, & Elinson, 1984), such as emotional well-being, behavioral competence, sleep and rest, energy and vitality, and general life satisfaction. The ability of the patient to function without limitation in role performance is an important aspect of quality of life. Health care providers must consider whether their patient's physical state or the treatment provided causes dependency on the therapist or depression related to the disability, which may then limit role performance (Pope & Tarlov, 1991).

As physical therapists address their patient's functional outcomes, quality of life becomes an important consideration in the development of treatment plans and goals. Jette (1993) suggests that quality of life comprises the last two stages of the Nagi model (*functional limitation* and *disability*). Individuals limited in functional mobility and the ability to interact within their environment and society will most likely perceive their quality of life to be poor. Figure 1-5 depicts Jette's conception of the relationship of *disablement* (disability) to quality of life.

If quality of life depends on functional abilities and interaction with the environment and society, then these areas must be addressed in rehabilitation. The example used earlier of the individual with hemiplegia suggests that a disability or handicap can have an effect on an individual's mental state, potentially causing depression. The perception of quality of life can have a tremendous influence on motivation and compliance as well. Many therapists include quality-of- life measures as part of their assessment and discharge procedures.

● ●
STANDARDIZED MEASURES OF DISABILITY

Appendix A describes three standardized measures of disability and two instruments to assess quality of life. Use of standardized functional assessment tools to measure and document functional activities is encouraged. Functional assessment tools can be incorporated into movement analysis for documentation of patients' functional abilities.

The Barthel, the Functional Independence Measure (FIM), and the Rivermead Mobility Index all assess some aspect of function. The Barthel and FIM assess the activities of daily living, including the patients' abilities to transfer from one surface to another, ambulate, and climb stairs. The Rivermead Mobility Index is a measure of mobility that examines all the tasks of functional mobility identified in this chapter as well as a few others, such as getting into and out of the bathtub, walking outside, picking up objects off the floor, and running.

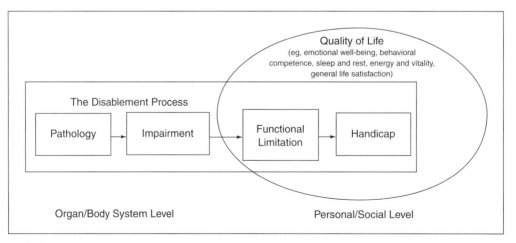

FIGURE 1-5. The relationship of quality of life to the disablement concept. (Jette A.M. [1994]. *Physical Therapy, 74,* 380–386.)

The instruments to assess quality of life are the SF-36 and the 12-Item Health Status Questionnaire (HSQ-12). These self-report questionnaires are focused on functional or societal limitations experienced and the impact they have on the perceptions of one's quality of life. The reliability and validity of each scale are discussed in the appendix. (It is a good idea to review these scales before beginning Section II.)

Standardized measurement and documentation of movement in functional activities will enhance communication and reporting of outcomes within the profession and across disciplines. At present, the FIM is the most widely used functional assessment scale, with a uniform data base representingnearly 700 inpatient medical rehabilitation facilities in the United States and Canada. All facilities participating in the FIM have access to national and international data on diagnostic-related functional outcomes. Not only is communication enhanced within one facility by having all rehabilitation personnel use the same instrument, but communication to other rehabilitation centers regarding patient status and progress is now possible.

SUMMARY

- The Nagi and the International Classification of Impairments, Disabilities, and Handicaps (ICIDH) models of disability are the two major conceptual frameworks that dominate the field of rehabilitation.
- Although the Nagi model was the first to address the patient's health status with respect to the disease state, the ICIDH model is more comprehensive in its conceptualization of the consequences of nonfatal disease. As such, it is the ideal point of reference for this textbook on neurological rehabilitation.
- Both the Nagi and the ICIDH models are built on four concepts each. The building blocks of the Nagi model are *pathology, impairment, functional limitations,* and *disability.* The ICIDH model rests on the four basic components of *disease, impairment, disability,* and *handicap.*
- A comparative analysis of the two models reveals certain equivalences:

Nagi	*ICIDH*
- Pathology	- Disease
- Impairment	- Impairment
- Functional limitation	- Disability
- Disability	- Handicap

- Although the first two stages are synonymous across models, the last two differ in their conceptualizations of disabled individuals and their relationship to the environment.
- Quality of life and the interaction of individuals with society and their environment are the driving forces of rehabilitative health care today. Physical therapists assess their patients' abilities to function in varied environments as a measure of their quality of life, and they provide the most effective treatments to help their patients achieve the desired functional outcomes.
- The use of standardized assessment tools helps physical therapists to establish a uniform language for outcome measures in rehabilitation. This, in turn, assists with goal setting, treatment planning, program evaluation, treatment efficacy, and quality assurance for all of rehabilitation.

REFERENCES

Badley, E. M. (1987). The ICIDH format, application in different settings, and distinction between disability and handicap: A critique of papers on the application of the International Classification of Impairments, Disabilities, and Handicaps. *International Disability Studies, 9,* 122–125.

Chaime, M. (1990). The status and use of the International Classification of Impairments, Disabilities, and Handicaps (ICIDH). *World Health Statistics Quarterly, 43,* 273–280.

Halbertsma, J. (1995). The ICIDH; health problems in a medical and social perspective. *Disability and Rehabilitation, 17*(3/4), 128–134.

Jette, A. M. (1993). Using health related quality of life measures in physical therapy outcomes research. *Physical Therapy, 8,* 528–537.

Jette, A. M. (1994). Physical disablement concepts or physical therapy research and practice. *Physical Therapy, 74,* 380–386.

Light, C. M. (1995). The effect of tall-kneeling practice on upright balance control: A case study. *Neurology Report, 15*(4), 10–11.

Nagi, S. A. (1991). Disability concepts revisited. In A. Pope & A. Tarlov (Eds.). *Disability in America: Toward a national agenda for prevention.* Washington, DC: National Academy Press.

Peters, D. J. (1995). Human experience in disablement: The imperative of the ICIDH. *Disability and Rehabilitation, 17*(3/4), 135–144

Pope, A., & Tarlov, A. (Eds.). (1991). *Disability in America: Toward a national agenda for prevention.* Washington, DC: National Academy Press.

Rothstein, J. M. (1994). [Editor's Note]. Disability and our identity. *Physical Therapy, 74,* 375–378.

Wenger, N. K., Mattson, M. E., Furberg, C. D., & Elinson, J. (Eds.). (1984). *Assessment of quality of life in clinical trials of cardiovascular therapies.* New York: LeJacq.

World Health Organization. (1980). *International Classification of Impairments, Disabilities and Handicaps: A manual of classification relating to the consequences of disease.* Geneva, Switzerland: Author.

SUGGESTED READINGS

Agency for Health Care Policy and Research. (1995). *Post-stroke rehabilitation, clinical practice guidelines.* Washington, DC: U.S. Department of Health and Human Services.

> The proceedings of a panel of experts representing medical and rehabilitation specialists in stroke rehabilitation produced the clinical guidelines. The guidelines are comprehensive and include the epidemiology and natural history of stroke, assessment methods, rehabilitation during acute care, screening for rehabilitation settings, managing rehabilitation, and transition to the community.

Physical Therapy 8. (1993)

> This issue of *Physical Therapy* is devoted to the assessment of disabilities. The Nagi and the ICIDH models are contrasted with a new model from the National Center for Medical Rehabilitation Research (NCMRR). Various authors contributed to this volume and address the assessment of disability in a variety of disease states.

Pope, A., & Tarlov, A. (Eds.). (1991). *Disability in America: Toward a national agenda for prevention.* Washington, DC: National Academy Press.

> This book provides an historical perspective on the development of the Nagi and ICIDH models, as well as some discussion on the need for them to address outcomes beyond morbidity and mortality. The ICD medical model is also discussed.

Wade, D. (1992). *Measurement in neurological rehabilitation.* New York: Oxford Medical Publications.

> This is an in-depth review of measurement tools associated with neurological rehabilitation. The early chapters provide an overview of the ICIDH. Tools to measure quality of life are also provided.

CHAPTER 2

Anatomy of Movement: Why Movement Problems Exist

LEARNING OBJECTIVES

After reading this chapter, you should be able to:

1. Understand functional neuroanatomy and the anatomic structures involved in movement.
2. Describe the differences between upper and lower motor neurons and how lesions of each affect function.
3. Understand the integration of sensory information.
4. Identify the role of neuroplasticity in the assignment of control for specific motor functions in the presence of a neurological impairment.
5. Analyze the four impairments that result from lesions of the movement pathways.

Movement involves the interaction of multiple systems. The simple task of moving from sitting to standing requires interaction between the peripheral and central nervous systems, muscles, joints, and tendons. The interaction of these multiple systems results in motor control, which is exerted over the muscles by the central nervous system (CNS) (Shepherd, 1994). Adequate numbers of motor units must be recruited to generate force in extensor muscles to enable movement of any kind. Once recruited, these motor units must fire at a well-timed rate and in an appropriately sequenced pattern to ensure smooth execution of the movement.

In addition to this internal exchange of information, the nervous system perceives information regarding the external environment. Examples of perceivable variables in the external environment include seat heights, chair surfaces, presence of arm rests, and the stability of the surface on which one is standing. Information about these properties allows the CNS to adjust the rate and direction of movement, or indeed, to decide whether or not movement is initiated at all.

FUNCTIONAL NEUROANATOMY

Movement Pathways

Although it is clear that information on motor control is continually evolving, it is known that the CNS, the peripheral nervous system (PNS), and the musculoskeletal system are all involved in the successful completion of movement. The CNS components involved in motor function include the primary motor cortex, sensory cortex, premotor area, supplemental motor area, basal ganglia, and cerebellum (Fig. 2-1). All connections within the cortex are **reciprocal,** meaning that information transmitted from the sensory cortex to the motor cortex is then relayed back to the sensory cortex via association fibers. Descending tracts and pathways from the CNS transmit impulses to peripheral components (ie, cranial nerve nuclei or motor neuron

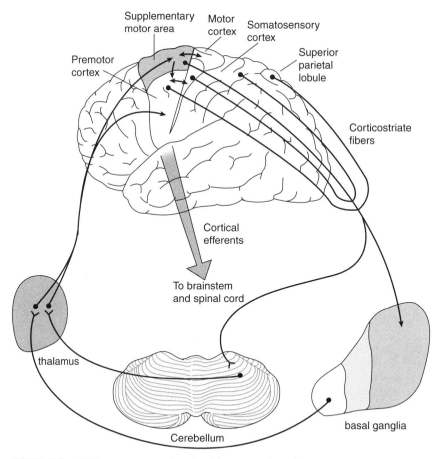

FIGURE 2-1.   CNS components involved in motor functions.

cell bodies in the spinal cord). Cranial nerves and spinal motor neurons shuttle these messages to the **effector organs,** muscles or glands that contract or secrete in direct response to nerve impulses.

The proper functioning of motor control depends on continuous input from sensory systems. Vision, hearing, and sensory receptors on the body surface inform the CNS where objects are in space and what the body's position is relative to these objects. Receptors in muscles, joints, and the **vestibular apparatus** (composed of receptors in the inner ear and their connections with nuclei and concerned with equilibrium) inform the motor system about the length and tension of muscles, joint angles, and the body's position in space. This information is required for planning movements and altering movements already in progress (Kandel, Schwartz, & Jessel, 1991). The cerebellum and basal ganglia play important roles in proper motor functioning. Both receive and use sensory information to modulate the timing and the trajectory of movement. The cerebellum and basal ganglia are essential for proper and smoothly executed movements (Kandel et al., 1991).

Anatomy Overview

This text presupposes the reader's prior exposure to basic neuroanatomy. Even so, this chapter includes a number of tools designed to help refresh the reader's memory of previously learned information. Table 2-1 summarizes the cortical lobes, the location of functional regions, and Brodmann's designations of the regions in each lobe.

The following sections outline important aspects of motor anatomy: the association cortices, descending tracts, and upper and lower motor neurons; sensory anatomy; and the ascending tracts.

Display 2-1 lists terms used to describe the location and orientation of various anatomic structures, as well as the conventions for naming the various tracts and pathways that connect neuroanatomic structures.

Motor Anatomy

The **motor cortex** is the center of activity for all voluntary movement. It is found in the frontal lobe, the largest of all the brain's lobes. Somatic motor projections to the body surface and muscle are arranged in the cortex in **somatotopic** order, to show the correspondence between a given area of the brain and a specific part of the body.

Figure 2-2 illustrates the **motor homunculus.** The word *homunculus* means ''little man'' and is used to refer to a hypothetical creature that controls the human being. This figure (and other similar figures) is derived from movement studies produced by surface stimulation of the brain of man and other animals.

The motor homunculus is an oversimplification because it does not consider any overlap of body segments, nor does it represent dual representation of motor function in the motor cortex. However, it does provide us with a map of the motor cortex responsible for motor activity in different regions of the body. Some parts of the body take up a greater proportion of the motor cortex, indicating differences in innervation density in different areas of the body. The hand, for example, occupies more cortical space than the leg because it is more densely innervated to allow it to execute the many intricate movements involved in fine motor coordination.

The three principal motor areas in the motor cortex are the:

- Primary motor cortex
- Premotor area
- Supplementary motor area

TABLE 2-1.   Major Sensory, Association, and Motor Cortices

Functional Designation	Lobe	Location in Lobe	Brodmann's Area
Primary sensory cortex			
Somatic sensory	Parietal	Postcentral gyrus	1, 2, 3
Visual	Occipital	Calcarine fissure	17
Auditory	Temporal	Heschl's gyrus	41, 42
Higher-order sensory cortex			
Somatic sensory II	Parietal	Dorsal bank of Sylvian fissure	2 (opercular portion)
Visual II	Occipital	Occipital gyri	18
Visual III, IIIa, IV, V	Occipital, temporal	Occipital gyri and superior temporal sulcus	19 and area rostral to 19
Visual inferotemporal area	Temporal	Anterior and inferior temporal cortex	21, 20
Posterior parietal cortex (somatic sensation, vision)	Parietal	Superior parietal lobule	5 (somatic) 7 (visual)
Auditory	Temporal	Superior temporal gyrus	22
Association cortex			
Parietal–temporal–occipital (polymodal sensory, language)	Parietal, temporal, and occipital	Junction between lobes	39, 40 and portions of 19, 21, 22, 37
Prefrontal (cognitive behavior) and motor planning)	Frontal	Rostral portion of dorsal and lateral surface	Area rostral to 6
Limbic (emotion and memory)	Temporal, parietal, and frontal	Cingulate and parahippocampal gyri, temporal pole, and orbital surface of frontal lobe	23, 24, 38, 28, 11
Higher-order motor cortex			
Premotor (including supplementary motor area)	Frontal	Rostral to postcentral gyrus	6, 8
Primary motor cortex	Frontal	Precentral gyrus	4

From Kandel, ER, Schwartz, JH, and Jessel, TM. (1995). *Essentials of neural science and behavior* (3rd ed.). Appleton & Lange, p. 324.

Primary Motor Cortex.   The primary motor cortex, also known as area 4 of Brodmann, is found within the precentral gyrus and concerned with contralateral voluntary movement. Approximately one-third of the one million motor neurons that make up the corticospinal tract arise from the primary motor cortex. Large axons from specific neurons called Betz cells are found in area 4. However, only a small percent-age of these large axons comprise the corticospinal tract; the majority of the tract is made up of smaller pyramidal cells in the primary motor cortex.

Motor neurons found in the primary motor cortex become active, or *fire*, during initiation of movement. The frequency with which these motor neurons fire dictates the force of muscle contraction. That is, low firing frequencies oc-

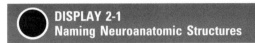

DISPLAY 2-1
Naming Neuroanatomic Structures

The names of many neuroanatomic structures are composed of terms that provide information on where the structures are located within the brain or nervous system. In may cases, this information makes it relatively easy to picture both the position and the orientation of the structures under discussion. Many of the major orienting terms (including prefixes, suffixes, and root words) are presented below for ease of reference.

anterior/antero- (prefix):	Before; in front of. Opposed to *posterior*
caudal:	Occupying an inferior position; resembling or pertaining to the tail or tail end. Opposed to *rostral*
collateral:	Accompanying; refers to side branches of blood vessels and nerves
contra- (prefix):	Opposite or against. Opposed to *ipsi-*
dorsal/dorso- (prefix):	A position toward the back or rear. Opposed to *ventral*
extra- (prefix):	Beyond, outside of
inferior/infero- (prefix):	Referring to the underside of an organ or structure. Opposed to *superior*
ipsi- (prefix):	Same side. Opposed to *contra-*
lateral:	Relating to the side
medial:	Pertaining to the middle
posterior:	Dorsal. Opposed to *anterior*
rostral:	Toward the front, or face, of a structure. Opposed to *caudal*
sub- (prefix):	Beneath, under, below normal
super- (prefix):	Above, superior
supra- (prefixes):	Above, superior, on the top
ventral/ventro- (prefix):	Pertaining to the belly or the anterior surface. Opposed to *dorsal*

You will note that many neuroanatomic structures are named with a combination of the above-mentioned terms. When this occurs, just incorporate the various meanings of the constituents to get the meaning of the term. For example, *ipsilateral* means *on the same side* or *affecting the same side*.

Neural Pathways and Tracts

Neural pathways and tracts, too, are named in a consistent fashion to show the path of the connection under consideration. These names are typically composed of at least two recognizable structures, as is the case in the term *corticospinal*. The first term indicates the origin of the pathway (in this case, the cortex) and the second term identifies the end point (the spine).

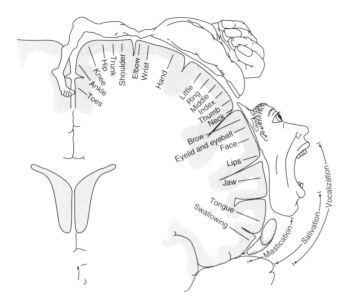

FIGURE 2-2. The somatotopic representation of the body in the sensorimotor cortex. Some parts of the body are drawn disproportionately large to indicate their relative importance in sensory perception (eg, the hand is large compared to the leg). This uneven representation indicates differences in innervation density in different areas of the body.

cur when little muscle force is needed, whereas increased loads requiring greater muscle forces cause higher firing rates of motor neurons located in area 4.

Interestingly, neurons in the primary motor cortex have peripheral receptive fields that provide them with information on the body's position and speed of movement. The primary motor cortex receives this information indirectly from the sensory cortex and directly from the thalamus.

Lesions of the primary motor cortex result in contralateral **paralysis** (loss or impairment of motor function in part due to decreased or absent muscular tone), **hypotonia** (diminished tone of skeletal muscle), and decreased reflexes, with distal musculature affected the most. For example, an individual suffering an acute thrombotic stroke involving the right middle cerebral artery (which provides blood to the primary motor cortex) may present with left upper extremity immobility; decreased muscle tone (possibly to the extent that if the limb were moved passively, it would feel like ''dead weight'' to the person moving the limb); and decreased or absent reflexes. The lower extremity may also be involved.

The involvement of the anterior cerebral artery would also result in ischemia to, among other areas, the paracentral lobule. This, in turn, would trigger the motor neurons that activate the lower extremity, thus making it possible to elicit the **Babinski reflex.** This reflex results in the dorsiflexion of the big toe on stimulation of the sole of the foot. Under these circumstances, **myotatic** (pertaining to the proprioceptive sense of muscles) reflexes would generally return, but they might be exaggerated. The upper extremity might show signs of involvement as well.

Premotor Area.   The premotor area, Brodmann area 6, is located rostral to the primary motor area. The premotor area is the most poorly understood cortical region. Major afferent fibers to the premotor area are from the posterior parietal cortex, a higher order sensory cortex involved in sensory and motor processing and the integration of the different sensory modalities necessary for perception. Thus, the premotor area is thought to be concerned with the initiation of voluntary movements that may result from sensory information.

Reciprocal communication occurs between the premotor and sensory cortices, especially those regions related to visual, auditory, and somatosensory stimuli. This communication enables sensory information to be used in planning movement. The axons of premotor area neurons also project to the primary motor cortex, subcortical structures, and spinal cord. Approximately one-third of the fibers that make up the corticospinal tract originate in area 6.

The constant exchange of information that occurs between the premotor area and the motor cortex allows information in the premotor area to reach targeted organs. Neurons in the premotor area anticipate complex motor actions. Activity in these premotor neurons appears to prepare motor neurons in the primary motor cortex for action.

Unlike lesions of the primary motor cortex, lesions of the premotor area do not result in **paresis** (slight or incomplete loss of motor function) or **hypertonia** (excessive tone of skeletal muscle). Rather, these lesions cause a slowing of movement due to an inability of the premotor area to facilitate the primary motor area in preparation for the anticipated motor commands. That is, lesions of the premotor area result in an inability to develop appropriate movement strategies or motor plans.

Supplemental Motor Area. Neurons in the supplemental motor area are found rostral to area 6, on the medial surface of the frontal lobe. They are responsible for programming, planning, and perhaps for initiating the bilateral motor functions of both proximal and distal musculature. Furthermore, the supplemental motor area is responsible for coordinating posture and voluntary movement.

The supplemental motor region possesses neurons that fire during different voluntary movements. Some neurons are activated only during proximal or distal movements; others are activated for the duration of a motor activity. Interestingly, the neurons in the supplemental motor area are active during bilateral motor activity (ie, the supplemental motor area is involved in bimanual tasks).

Neurons in the supplemental motor area have reciprocal ipsilateral projections to the primary motor and premotor cortices, and contralateral projections to the supplemental motor areas. Approximately 5% of the neurons in the supplemental motor area project bilaterally into the spinal cord. Further projections from the supplemental motor area include the basal ganglia (caudate and putamen) and the thalamic nuclei.

Unilateral lesions of the supplemental motor area usually do not result in deficits in the ability to maintain posture or in the capacity for movement. Lesions in this area result in motor **apraxia** (loss of the ability to perform movement in the absence of motor or sensory impairments) and problems coordinating complex motor tasks, such as sewing, typing, writing, lacing and tying shoes, and buttoning shirts.

Association Cortices. The largest part of the cerebrum is composed of association areas whose functions are twofold:

- To integrate diverse information for purposeful action
- To connect the sensory cortices to the motor cortices

The association areas are involved in sharing sensory perception, voluntary movement, cognition, emotional behavior, memory, and language. The following three association areas are involved with movement, either directly or indirectly.

Parietal–Temporal–Occipital Association Cortex

Several cortical areas make up this association cortex, which has reciprocal connections with higher order somatic areas, visual areas, and auditory areas. Because the parietal–temporal–occipital association cortex links information from several sensory modalities, it is important in processing sensory information such as perception and language.

Prefrontal Association Cortex

Located just rostral to the premotor area on the frontal lobe, the prefrontal association cortex is involved in planning responses to movement. **Afferent connections** (those that carry messages to the CNS) to this association cortex are from various higher order sensory cortices that are less directly connected to primary sensory areas. **Efferent fibers** (those that carry messages from the CNS to the periphery) from the prefrontal association cortex project to the premotor cortex, which in turn projects neurons to the primary motor cortex. This demonstrates how sensory information can influence motor behavior. One can trace the ''impulse'' to move back to its origin as actual neural impulses along the sensory projections to the prefrontal association cortex. From there, the impulses travel to the premotor cortex, which relays the message they encode to the primary motor cortex. It is in the motor cortex that these impulses are translated into action, or movement.

Limbic Association Cortex

This association cortex is located in portions of the parietal, frontal, and temporal lobes on the inferomedial surfaces of the cerebrum. It includes the orbitofrontal cortex, the cingulate region, and the parahippocampal area. The limbic association cortex is involved in motivation, emotion, and memory. Afferent fibers to this association area project from higher order sensory areas, whereas efferent fibers project to the prefrontal cortex, among other cortical regions. This limbic association cortex-to-prefrontal cortex connection may provide some insight into the anatomic basis of the possible influence of emotions on motor behavior.

Corticospinal Tract. The corticospinal tract is composed of approximately one million axons whose origins derive equally from area 4, area 6, and areas 3, 1, and 2 (the somatosensory cortex). Fibers from the corticospinal tract travel with corticobulbar fibers (which control cranial motor nerve nuclei) through the posterior limb of the internal capsule to reach the ventral part of the midbrain. (The **internal capsule** is a collection of myelinated fibers composed of sensory axons traveling from the thalamus to the cortex, and motor fibers originating in cortical regions and projecting to the brain stem and spinal cord.)

In the medulla, corticospinal fibers form pyramids, easily identifiable external landmarks on the ventral portion of the medulla. Just before the junction of the medulla and the spinal cord, about 75% of the corticospinal tract fibers **decussate,** or cross over, to the contralateral side in a process known as *pyramidal decussation.* From there, they continue their descent in the lateral funiculus of the spinal cord. These fibers are now referred to as the *lateral corticospinal tract.* Those corticospinal tract fibers that did not cross in the pyramidal decussation continue to descend in the ventral funiculus of the spinal cord and are now called the *anterior corticospinal tract.*

Lateral corticospinal tract fibers terminate directly and indirectly on cell bodies of anterior horn motor neurons (Fig. 2-3). These fibers are involved in highly skilled movements, especially in the distal upper and lower extremities. That is because lateral corticospinal tract fibers possess few **collateral** branches, thus allowing discrete control of single distal muscles.

Anterior corticospinal tract fibers terminate bilaterally in the spinal cord on motor neurons that innervate the axial muscles (see Fig. 2-3).

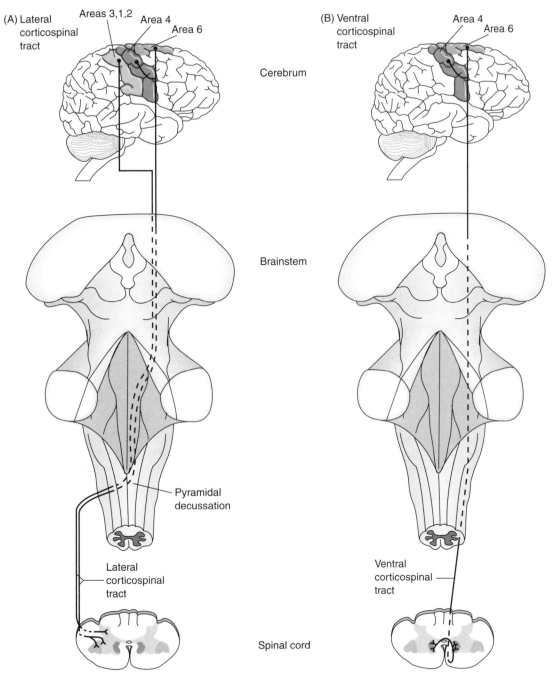

FIGURE 2-3. The descending cortical pathways to the spinal segments. (*A*) The crossed lateral corticospinal tract originates from Brodmann's areas 4 and 6, and sensory areas 3, 2, and 1. The tract then crosses at the pyramidal decussation, descends in the dorsolateral column, and terminates in the shaded area of spinal gray matter. (*B*) Uncrossed pathways (ventral corticospinal tract) originate principally in Brodmann's area 6 and in zones controlling the neck and trunk in area 4. Terminations are bilateral.

Overall, axial muscles perform less skilled movements than do the distal appendicular muscles. As a result, more collateral axons are present in the anterior corticospinal tract than in the lateral corticospinal tract.

Basal Ganglia

The basal ganglia consist of five subcortical nuclei that are indirectly involved in motor control and maintenance of muscle tone. The nuclei that form the basal ganglia include the caudate, the putamen, the globus pallidus, the subthalamic nucleus, and the substantia nigra. The caudate, putamen, and the globus pallidus are collectively referred to as the *corpus striatum;* the putamen and caudate are known as the *striatum* (or *neostriatum*). The globus pallidus is also referred to as the *pallidum* (or *paleostriatum*) and is anatomically divided into internal and external segments. The subthalamic nucleus is found inferior to the thalamus, where it meets the midbrain. The substantia nigra is found in the midbrain.

The putamen and caudate are the receptive components of the basal ganglia (ie, afferent fibers project to the striatum), while output is via the globus pallidus and the substantia nigra. The following discussion is broken down into two sections. The first focuses on the projection of the afferent fibers to the basal ganglia, and the second addresses efferent fibers traveling from the basal ganglia.

Input to the Striatum.   The striatum receives input from many regions of the cerebrum and from the intralaminar nuclei of the thalamus. All regions of the cerebral cortex (including the motor, sensory, and association areas) project excitatory messages to the striatum. Cortico-striate fibers arising from area 4 project bilaterally and topographically on the putamen (Fig. 2-4); fibers from area 6 project ipsilaterally to both the caudate and the putamen.

The substantia nigra also sends fibers to the striatum via the nigrostriatal pathway. Dopamine, an important neurotransmitter involved in diseases of the basal ganglia, is the neurotransmitter synthesized by afferent axons from the substantia nigra. Lack of or a decreased level of dopamine is associated with Parkinson's disease, a neurodegenerative disorder characterized by resting tremors, bradykinesia (slowness of movement), muscle **rigidity** of the extremities and trunk, and a masklike face (ie, lack of normal facial expressions). The gait patterns of patients with Parkinson's disease is one of short, rapid steps, stooped posture, and little upper extremity movement.

Information from the intralaminar nuclei of the thalamus to the striatum is topographically organized. This is important because the intralaminar nuclei receive information from the motor cortex and their projections to the striatum are the means by which the motor cortex may influence the basal ganglia.

Efferent fibers from the caudate and putamen project to the globus pallidus and the substantia nigra. That the motor cortex projects to the caudate and putamen, and efferent fibers from these nuclei project to the globus pallidus and the substantia nigra, offers proof that certain parts of the motor cortex act indirectly on the globus pallidus and the substantia nigra (Kandel et al., 1991).

Output From the Basal Ganglia.   The corpus striatum exerts its influences on motor activity via projections to the thalamus, not via direct projections to the spinal cord. Thalamocortical fibers containing information from the corpus striatum then project to the frontal lobe.

Efferent axons from the globus pallidus project to the ipsilateral thalamic nuclei, which in turn project to the motor cortex, the prefrontal cortex, the premotor cortex, and the supplementary motor area. This globus pallidus-to-thalamus-to-motor areas connec-

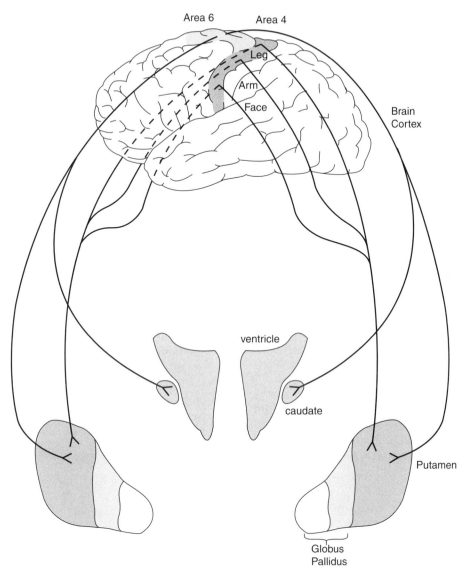

FIGURE 2-4. Schematic diagram of bilateral and ipsilateral somatotopic projections from areas 4 and 6, respectively.

tion shows how the basal ganglia influence motor behavior.

The striatum also has reciprocal connections with the substantia nigra. The impaired synthesis of and the failure to deploy the neurotransmitters involved in striatal functions are an im- portant feature of the metabolic disturbances associated with **dyskinesia** (defect of movement). Diseases of the basal ganglia may result in any of the following motor disturbances, either singly or in combination: tremor and other involuntary movements, postural changes, muscle tone changes, decreased movement, or decreased movement speed. For example, in Parkinson's disease, **akinesia** (loss of movement, either complete or partial), **bradykinesia** (slowness of movement), and impaired postural reflexes are a result of decreased amounts of dopamine in the striatum. Huntington's disease—characterized by **athetosis** (slow, irregular, twisting movements, especially of the hands and fingers), **chorea** (a condition marked by involuntary muscular twitching), and excessive movement—is a result of genetic abnormalities and is caused by the degeneration of the striatal neurons.

Cerebellum

The cerebellum consists of an external cerebellar cortex, an internal medullary layer, and four pairs of deep nuclei located in the medullary layer. The cortex has many transversely oriented folds, called **folia.** The cortex is divided into three layers: the granular, the Purkinje, and the molecular. The median portion of the cerebellum is referred to as the **vermis,** after its wormlike appearance. Laterally, the cerebellum possesses two lobes or hemispheres.

The cerebellum can be categorized into three functional areas: the archicerebellum, which is composed of the flocculonodular lobule; the paleocerebellum, which is made up of the anterior lobe; and the neocerebellum, which is composed of the posterior lobe. The archicerebellum is the oldest portion of the cerebellum, and it is associated with the vestibular system. The paleocerebellum receives sensory information via these spinocerebellar tracts; it is chiefly concerned with information from stretch receptors such as the muscle spindles and the Golgi tendon organs (GTOs). The neocerebellum coordinates voluntary motor function, as it receives information from the contralateral cerebrum via the pontine, or *bridgelike,* nuclei.

Afferent nerves that originate directly from the vestibular nuclei (ie, vestibulocerebellar) and muscle stretch receptors (ie, spinocerebellar, cuneocerebellar), and indirectly from the contralateral motor cortex (ie, pontocerebellar), travel to the cerebellar cortex via all three cerebellar peduncles, especially the inferior and the middle. The superior peduncle connects the cerebellum and the midbrain; the middle peduncle joins the cerebellum and the basilar area of the pons; and the inferior peduncle connects the medulla with the cerebellum.

Afferent axons bring information from these different anatomic sites and make either direct or indirect excitatory synapses on Purkinje cells in the cerebellar cortex. A **synapse** is the junction at which the axon of one neuron comes into contact with the body of another cell, or its dendrites, for the purpose of communicating neurochemical messages. Purkinje fibers are the only efferent fibers that exit from the cerebellar hemispheres. Efferent axons from Purkinje cells travel to deep cerebellar nuclei, such as the fastigial, globose, emboliform, and the dentate nuclei.

Axons from the fastigial nucleus leave the cerebellum and terminate bilaterally on the reticular formation and on the ipsilateral and medial vestibular nuclei. Efferent fibers from the emboliform and globose nuclei synapse on the contralateral red nucleus. Axons from the dentate nucleus terminate on the contralateral red nucleus and the ventrolateral nucleus of the thalamus.

Given this vast network of direct connections, it is easy to see how highly implicated the cerebellum is in motor control. The cerebellum may exert this control through the reticulospinal, vestibulospinal, and the rubrospinal tracts through its synapses on the reticular formation, the vestibular nuclei, and the red nucleus. Furthermore, the cerebellum may indirectly influence motor control through its connections with the motor cortex via the thalamus. Like basal ganglia projections to the thalamus, thalamocortical fibers containing information from the cerebellum project to the frontal lobe. Again, it is the frontal lobe that contains the motor cortex whose output regulates motor function.

Lower and Upper Motor Neurons

Lower Motor Neurons. Lower motor neurons, also known as the *final common pathway,* are simply those neurons whose cell bodies are found in the anterior horn of the spinal gray matter and in certain cranial nerve nuclei (eg, facial, oculomotor). Axons whose cell bodies lie in the anterior horn of the spinal gray matter exit the spinal cord via the ventral roots, and travel to and innervate effector organs such as skeletal muscle. Axons from the motor nuclei of certain cranial nerves exit through various *foramina* (openings or passageways; singular, **foramen**) in the skull to get to their target tissue. Aside from being the conduit for a reflex arc, anterior horn cells receive information from and are activated by the descending tracts in the spinal cord. The motor nuclei of certain cranial nerves are excited by the upper motor neurons that comprise the corticobulbar tract.

Lesions of the lower motor neurons, whether on their cell bodies or their axons, will result in what is known as a *lower motor neuron lesion.* Lesions may result from injury (eg, transection of the spinal nerve); inflammation (eg, facial nerve involvement in Bell's palsy); compression of nerves (eg, carpal tunnel syndrome); or disease (eg, amyotrophic lateral sclerosis, poliomyelitis, Guillain-Barré syndrome). Regardless of the cause, lower motor neuron lesions result in paralysis, loss of muscle tone, **areflexia** (complete loss of myotatic reflexes), and, in time, atrophy of the muscle(s) innervated by the lower motor neurons.

Upper Motor Neurons. A simple view of upper motor neurons holds that they are those neurons whose axons make up the corticospinal

and corticobulbar tracts. Many other descending motor tracts (eg, the vestibulospinal, reticulospinal, and rubrospinal tracts) also influence the activity of lower motor neurons and play a role in changes in tone or equilibrium reactions.

Lesions of upper motor neurons, such as those caused by a stroke, multiple sclerosis, spinal cord transection, Huntington's chorea, or a traumatic brain injury, result in paresis or paralysis depending on the severity of the lesion. (*Paresis* refers to weakness, which is a temporary or permanent loss of function.) In upper motor neuron lesions, there is initial loss of muscle tone. This is followed by *hypertonicity* (spasticity); increased *myotatic* (stretch) reflexes; and the presence of **Babinski's sign** (the actual loss or lessening of the Babinski reflex, commonly seen in patients with sciatica). Because innervation via the lower motor neurons and the reflex arc remains, muscle **atrophy** (wasting) is not seen in the short term with upper motor neuron lesions. However, disuse atrophy will be seen in the later stages.

Activation of Movement

The integration of information processed in the cerebrum is transmitted to the cranial and spinal nerves via the corticobulbar and the corticospinal tracts, respectively. Both tracts originate in the motor, sensory, and premotor cortices. These tracts provide direct linkage of motor information from the CNS to the cell bodies of the lower motor neurons in the brainstem and the spinal cord.

The synaptic activity between the descending tracts (ie, upper motor neurons) and the cell bodies of the cranial nerves and anterior horn cells (ie, lower motor neurons) produce impulses that result in muscle contractions. The lower motor neurons (which are efferent nerves) innervate muscle fibers, thus transmitting to them an **action potential** (a transient electrical signal) (Kandel et al., 1991). This action potential results in a chemical synapse at the motor unit. The activation of an electrical charge at the motor end plate of the muscle results in a muscle contraction.

Tracts that carry indirect motor information from higher centers to the spinal cord include the rubrospinal tract (which runs from the red nucleus to the spinal cord), the reticulospinal tract, and the vestibulospinal tract. These tracts are located subcortically and traditionally have been referred to as the extrapyramidal system because they provide information for the maintenance of muscular and postural tone.

Vestibular nuclei receive afferent fibers from the semicircular canals located in the inner ear that inform the CNS about the position of the head in space. Descending neurons that originate in the vestibular nuclei terminate in the spinal cord on motor neurons that control muscles of the neck, back, and proximal limbs.

The reticular formation is a diffuse collection of neuronal circuits located in the brain stem from the rostral midbrain to the caudal medulla. Neurons originating in the reticular formation that descend into the spinal cord synapse on those motor neurons that control axial and proximal limb muscles. Together, the vestibulospinal and reticulospinal tracts help maintain posture.

Projections from the red nucleus to the spinal cord only descend to cervical regions in humans. Rubrospinal tract fibers synapse on motor neurons that influence postural tone in arm muscles, especially flexor muscles.

Sensory Anatomy

This overview focuses on **somatosensation** (body sense), including different types of stimuli and receptors; peripheral nerve conduction; *synaptic transmission* (the ability of nerve cells to communicate with one another) (Kandel et al., 1991); and the integration of information within the CNS. Older sensory pathways, such as the spino-olivary and the spinoreticular pathways, are not included in this discussion because of their limited importance in humans. Rather, newer sensory systems (eg, the lemniscal, spinothalamic, trigeminal, and the spinocerebellar) are discussed because they are highly implicated in the discriminative tasks of somatosensation.

Sensory systems process all the sensations that have an impact on and within the body. Light, sound waves, pressure, noxious stimuli, touch, odor, taste, and autonomic activity communicate themselves to the human organism via sensory systems.

The somatosensory system can be divided into two separate systems, one **protopathic** and phylogenetically older, the other **epicritic** and phylogenetically newer. Anatomically, the older system is referred to as the *spinothalamic system,* which is further subdivided into its ventral and lateral portions. The newer system is called the *lemniscal system.* Head (1920) was the first to describe the functional differences between the two systems. The spinothalamic system is less specific than the lemniscal system and is organized to respond to stimuli for the purpose of initiating self-protective responses. The lemniscal system is more specific in function than the spinothalamic system in that it possesses the discriminative properties basic to somatosensation.

The spinothalamic and lemniscal systems are discussed separately. This should not lead readers to believe that these two systems do not work together. They do. In fact, most somatosensory stimuli can activate both systems at the same time. However, because these two systems are so distinct, discussing them separately should allow for better understanding. After this discussion, brief synopses of the other sensory tracts follow.

Lemniscal System. This "division" of the somatosensory system is involved with the transmission of touch, *proprioception,* and **kinesthesia** (the sense by which position, weight, and movement are perceived). The ability to sense the texture and movement of objects across the skin is referred to as the sense of **touch.** Proprioception is the sense of static limb position, and kinesthesia is the sense of limb movement.

The lemniscal system receptors are located in the skin, joints, and soft tissue, as well as in other body tissues. They transform mechanical energy into electrical energy. Each receptor is sensitive primarily to one form of physical energy. Table 2-2 summarizes receptor types and the sensory modalities with which they are associated. Lemniscal receptors are, for the most part, encapsulated, and may include the following types of receptors (defined by their functions):

- Merkel's disks: touch–pressure
- Meissner's corpuscles: two-point discrimination and **stereognosis** (the ability to recognize objects by touch)
- Pacinian corpuscles: deep pressure and quick stretch

- Ruffini's corpuscles: touch and spatial discrimination
- Muscle spindles: muscle length and changes in muscle length and the rate of such change (Scholz & Campbell, 1981)
- GTOs: muscle tension (Quillian & Ridley, 1971)

Muscle spindles and tendon organs are instrumental in allowing the unconscious awareness of limb position (Houk & Hennemou, 1967; Moor, 1974). When these receptors are initially stimulated, their cell membranes become either depolarized or hyperpolarized, depending on the type of stimulation. This is referred to as **stimulus transduction.** The neural signal produced by the initial stimulation causes an action potential in the receptor that is then transmitted to the axon of the peripheral nerve that relays information about the stimulus (eg, intensity and duration). This is referred to as **neural encoding.**

Sensory receptors in the somatosensory and olfactory systems are referred to as *primary sensory neurons.* The peripheral portion of the neuron acts as the receptor, that is, it transduces stimulus energy to its axon, which transmits

TABLE 2-2. Mammalian Sensory Systems

Modality	Stimulus	Receptor Type	Specific Receptor
Vision	Light	Photoreceptor	Rods, cones
Hearing	Air-pressure waves	Mechanoreceptor	Hair cells (cochlear)
Balance	Head motion	Mechanoreceptor	Hair cells (semicircular canals)
Touch	Mechanical, thermal, noxious (chemical)	Mechanoreceptor, thermoreceptor, nociceptor, chemoreceptor	Dorsal root ganglion neurons
Taste	Chemical	Chemoreceptor	Taste buds
Smell	Chemical	Chemoreceptor	Olfactory sensory neurons

From Kandel, ER, Schwartz, JH, Jessel, TM. (1995). *Essentials of neural science and behavior* (3rd ed.). Appleton & Lange, p. 324.

action potentials to the CNS. This differs from the other sensory systems (ie, the gustatory, visual, auditory, and vestibular) in that receptors in those systems are separate epithelial cells that communicate with the axons of sensory neurons in ways similar to synaptic transmission.

Generally, somatosensory information is transmitted along large, myelinated peripheral nerves (Table 2-3). These fibers possess high conduction speeds that allow for quick re-sponses to stimuli from both the external and internal environments. Touch, pressure, and changes in muscle length and tension are just a few of the responses which can be generated.

The cell bodies of these large, myelinated neurons are located in the dorsal root ganglia, with their central processes projecting through the dorsal roots into the spinal cord. Spinal reflexes notwithstanding, these central processes ascend in the dorsal columns of the spinal cord (ie, fasciculus gracilis and fasciculus

TABLE 2-3. Classifications of Peripheral Nerves According to Size

Gasser-Erlanger	Lloyd	Motor (Functional Component)	Sensory (Functional Component)
A fibers: large myelinated fibers with a high conduction rate			
Aα	Ia	Large, fast fibers of the alpha motor system (large cells of anterior horn to extrafusal motor fibers)	Muscle spindle: primary afferent endings, (primary stretch or low threshold stretch; Ia tonic responds to length. Ia phasic responds to rate)
	Ib		Golgi tendon organ for contraction: responds to tendon stretch or tension
Aβ	II		Muscle spindle: secondary afferent endings—tonic receptors responding to length
			Exteroceptive afferent endings from skin and joints: respond to light or low threshold stretch
Aγ 1 and 2	II	Gamma motor system (small cells of anterior horn to intrafusal motor fibers)	Bare nerve endings: joint receptors, mechanoreception of soft tissues— exteroceptors for pain, touch, and cold (low threshold)
AΔ	III		
B fibers: medium-sized myelinated fibers with a fairly rapid conduction rate			
Bβ		Preganglionic fibers of autonomic system (effective on glands and smooth muscle: motor branch of alpha): unknown function	
C fibers: small, poorly myelinated or unmyelinated fibers having the slowest conduction rate: augmentation and recruiting occur within the nervous system after stimulation of these fibers has ceased			
	IV	Postganglionic fibers of sympathetic system	Exteroceptors: pain, temperature, touch

From Umphred, DA. (1995). *Neurological rehabilitation* (3rd ed.). St. Louis: Mosby Year Book, p. 122.

cuneatus) until they synapse in the medulla on neurons in the gracile and cuneate nuclei. The axons of these second order neurons then cross the midline via the internal arcuate fibers and continue to ascend in the brain stem. They are referred to as the *medial lemniscus*. Fibers in the medial lemniscus ascend to the ventral posterior lateral nucleus of the thalamus, where they synapse on third order fibers, known generally as *thalamocortical fibers*. Third order fibers project to the primary somatosensory cortex via the posterior limb of the internal capsule. A characteristic of the dorsal column–medial lemniscus pathway is its somatotopic orientation. The primary somatosensory cortex is located in the postcentral gyrus of the parietal lobe. Here, different cortical regions represent different areas of the body (see Fig. 2-2).

Spinothalamic System.   The spinothalamic system includes the lateral and anterior spinothalamic tracts and is involved with the perception of pain, temperature, light touch, sexual sensations, and noxious stimuli. The spinothalamic system is also implicated in the generation of primitive self-protective responses. Spinothalamic system receptors are nonencapsulated or simply free nerve endings. Free nerve endings are found throughout the body, especially throughout connective tissue of the skin and in the viscera. **Nociceptors** detect pain and have either free nerve endings or free nerve endings are encapsulated.

Generally, information transmitted in the spinothalamic system via free nerve endings travels along small, unmyelinated A∆ or C fibers (see Table 2-3). These fibers have much slower conduction rates than the fibers involved in the lemniscal system.

Like those in the lemniscal system, the cell bodies of the primary neurons of the spinothalamic system are located in the dorsal root ganglia. Their central processes project through the dorsal roots into the spinal cord, where they synapse on second order neurons in the dorsal horn laminae. Second order neurons then decussate in the spinal cord and ascend contralaterally. These second order neurons make up what are known as the *lateral* and the *anterior spinothalamic tracts* and continue through the brain stem, where they synapse in the ventral posterior lateral nucleus of the thalamus. From the thalamus, the axons of third order neurons project through the posterior limb of the internal capsule to the postcentral gyrus in the parietal lobe of the cerebrum.

As in the lemniscal system, spinothalamic information is somatotopically arranged in the cerebral cortex. Interestingly, some information traveling in the spinothalamic tracts may not reach the thalamus, but rather terminates in the brain stem reticular formation, which regulates the autonomic nervous system, the limbic system, and the brain stem nuclei. Given an understanding of these collaterals, one can surmise the possible role of the spinothalamic system in arousal mechanisms to potentially harmful stimuli.

Dorsal Spinocerebellar Tract.   Not all the information from the muscle spindles, GTOs, and touch and pressure receptors ascends the spinal cord in dorsal columns. Some of it enters the spinal cord and synapses on large cell bodies in a distinct column called *Clarke's column,* or the nucleus dorsalis. Clarke's column is continuous in the thoracic and upper lumbar spinal cord regions. Information caudal to upper lumbar cord levels (eg, L2 or L3) travels in the dorsal columns to upper lumbar segments and then terminates on large cell bodies located in Clarke's column.

From Clarke's column, large axons ascend ipsilaterally in the posterolateral periphery of the spinal cord. This tract is called the dorsal spinocerebellar tract (DSCT). It reaches the ipsilateral cerebellum via the inferior cerebellar peduncle, where it terminates on the rostral and caudal portions of the vermis. The DSCT is somatotopically arranged in the spinal cord and cerebellum, and it carries information concerned with the fine coordination of posture and kinesthesia from muscles in the limbs. This information does not reach conscious levels.

Ventral Spinocerebellar Tract.   Fibers that make up the ventral spinocerebellar tract (VSCT) receive signals from the GTOs found in the lower extremities. These afferent fibers from tendon organs have their cell bodies located in the dorsal root ganglia. The cells of origin of the VSCT are found in laminae V, VI, and VII of the spinal cord and extend from the coccygeal levels to the upper lumbar levels.

The VSCT is a double crossing tract. When afferent fibers enter the spinal cord, they decussate and ascend contralaterally in the spinal cord, but when these fibers reach the cerebellar peduncles, they cross back and enter the cerebellum ipsilateral to their side of origin. The VSCT is concerned with coordinated movements and posture from the lower extremities. From laminae V, VI, and VII in the spinal cord, fibers decussate and ascend contralaterally in the spinal cord near the lateral spinothalamic tract. At the level of the pons, most fibers decussate through the superior cerebellar peduncle to terminate in the anterior vermis.

Cuneocerebellar Tract.   This tract is the upper extremity equivalent of the DSCT. Afferent fibers from muscle spindles and the GTOs travel in the fasciculus cuneatus and terminate at the level of the medulla in the lateral (accessory) cuneate nucleus rather than in the nucleus cuneatus. Fibers originating in the lateral cuneate nucleus make up the cuneocerebellar tract and travel through the inferior cerebellar peduncle and terminate ipsilaterally in the cerebellar cortex.

Integration of Sensory Information

A large component of motor control is the processing of information in the CNS to determine the effectiveness of a movement pattern. Within the muscle, two sensory receptors—the muscle spindle and the GTO—provide information regarding the length and tension of the muscle. In addition to these receptors in the muscle, **mechanoreceptors** in the surrounding joints provide information on joint position. These peripheral receptors send information into the spinal cord through the dorsal root ganglion. On entering the spinal cord, information can be transmitted immediately to the **alpha motor neuron** for a motor response. This information can also be transmitted via the dorsal column to the CNS for further processing.

The visual and tactile systems also contribute to the development of motor control. Visual information is transmitted along the optic nerves and tracts for integration in the occipital lobe. Association fibers transfer the information from the occipital lobe to the parietal and frontal lobes for the modification of motor output. Tactile information is carried along afferent fibers and the dorsal columns, in much the same way information on joint position is transmitted.

The ability of the CNS to influence motor control highly depends on the processing of sensory information. Reaching for and missing a glass of water is not an effective movement pattern. The CNS must analyze why the task was not successfully completed and then modify the movement pattern to increase its accuracy and effectiveness. This analysis must include the integration of information from vision, touch, joint position, and the length and tension of muscles.

Within the spinal cord there exist motor programs that can be activated for routine movement behavior without higher CNS processing. The existence of these **segmental programs** (central program generators) has been identified in experimental studies of cats with spinal cord lesions. When placed on a moving treadmill, the cats are able to activate a walking pattern (Grillner & Wallen, 1991). This type of motor behavior, which occurs in the absence of any cortical influence, demonstrates the existence of spinal cord motor programs.

Neuroplasticity

Plastic changes in the cerebral cortex were once thought to be impossible. However, recent animal research has shown that certain cortices, especially the sensory and visual cortices, have the ability to undergo change. Research involving recordings from the sensory cortices of monkeys months after amputation of certain digits has shown expansion of the cortical representation of existing digits. Similar plastic changes in the sensory cortex have been seen when monkeys have been trained to use a specific digit to perform a certain task. In this scenario, a functional expansion of the cortical representation for that particular digit is seen.

Research has demonstrated that focal lesions of the retinas of monkeys and cats cause temporary unresponsiveness of the neurons in the visual cortex that correspond to those retinal areas with lesions. However, after a short period of time, those once unresponsive neurons begin to respond to stimulation of the retinal areas adjacent to the lesions.

The mechanisms involved in these neuroplastic changes are not fully understood. It is likely that they result from either strengthening or weakening of already present synapses rather than from a ''rewiring'' of the cortex. It is further surmised that these observed changes in the neuroplasticity of the cerebral cortices of animals have their counterpart in humans.

Summary of Movement Pathways

The initiation, execution, and completion of a motor task involve at a minimum the muscles, afferent nerves, synapses within the spinal cord, and the efferent nerves that connect with the muscle fibers. As the complexity of the motor task increases, other components of the CNS are called on to assist in the planning and execution of the task.

Figure 2-5 is a simplified illustration that represents various components of the musculoskeletal and neuromuscular systems that are activated when performing a motor task. Excluded from Figure 2-5 is the environment's influence over the performance of a motor task and the individual's desire or motivation to move. These are two additional systems that should not be overlooked in the analysis of the movement of patients with neurological lesions.

IMPAIRMENTS RESULTING FROM LESIONS OF THE MOVEMENT PATHWAYS

Damage to the nervous system or the musculoskeletal system, whether caused by trauma or disease, may result in impairment. As discussed in Chapter 1, impairments are signs and symptoms that patients present (eg, weakness, pain, numbness, loss of vision, or limitations in the range of motion). Lesions along movement pathways may result in impairments that contribute to disability. Lesion sites may include the sensory receptors, afferent nerves, and ascending tracts; the spinal cord, sensory cortex, motor cortex, premotor cortex, supplementary

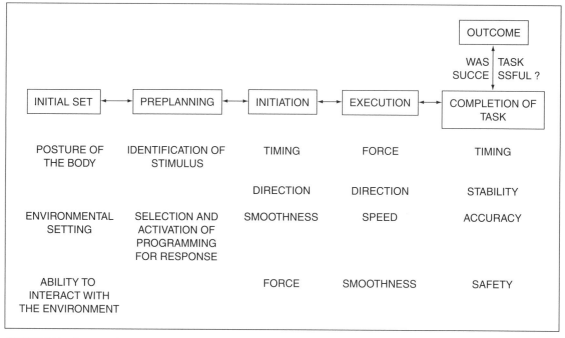

FIGURE 2-5. Stages of movement and associated parameters.

motor cortex, and the cerebellum; and the basal ganglia, the corticospinal and cortico-bulbar tracts, alpha motor neurons, motor units, and muscle fibers.

Table 2-4 lists the anatomic structures within the movement pathways described in this chapter, along with the associated impairments seen following lesions in each of the areas. It is important to recognize that lesions may extend over several regions or structures and that damage to one structure may have an impact on several other structures as a result of loss of neuronal and synaptic activity.

Table 2-4 is provided to demonstrate the association between impairments and anatomic structures. However, the reader is cautioned that a singular relationship does not exist between a lesion site and an impairment or between an impairment and a disability. For exam-

ple, a lesion of the left motor cortex may result in right-sided weakness that limits a patient's ability to ambulate on irregular surfaces without assistance. A similar lesion within the left motor cortex may result in right-sided weakness and additional problems in sensory awareness (due to synaptic inactivity between the motor and sensory cortices). The additional involvement of the sensory cortex may prevent the patient from ambulating on any surface. Other factors to consider in functional mobility, beyond the anatomic structures, are the cognitive state of the patient, other premorbid conditions, the environment in which the patient will function, and the presence or lack of a supportive network of family or friends.

It should be noted from Table 2-4 that lesions along the movement pathway generally result in the following impairments:

TABLE 2-4. Lesion Sites and Impairments

Anatomic Region	Impairment
Primary motor cortex	Weakness or paralysis, change in tone
Sensory cortex	Loss of sensation, perception, proprioception, problems with motor control
Premotor region	Weakness from disuse, difficulty with planning motor tasks, apraxia
Supplemental motor region	Weakness from disuse, difficulty with complex motor tasks
Basal ganglia	Absence of movement, weakness from disuse, abnormal movements (chorea, tremor), or abnormal tone (rigidity)
Cerebellum	Incoordination, weakness from disuse, balance problems, changes in tone
Corticospinal tract	Weakness
Alpha motor neuron	Weakness or atrophy
Muscle	Weakness
Afferent sensory input	Loss of sensory awareness, uncoordinated movements, balance problems

---

- Weakness
- Abnormal muscle tone
- Sensory and perceptual dysfunction
- Incoordination
- Balance dysfunction

For example, lesions within the motor cortex result in muscle weakness or paralysis. **Weakness** (see Chap. 5) is defined as the inability to generate normal levels of tension in muscle. It is related to a decrease in the rate of motor unit firing or the inability of motor units to respond to stimulation. Weakness is also seen with lesions in the premotor and supplemental motor regions, the cerebellum, the corticospinal tract, the alpha motor neuron, and in muscle. Weakness from disuse can occur with lesions of the basal ganglia, as well as of the sensory cortex.

Sensory and perceptual dysfunction is seen with lesions of the sensory cortex and the afferent sensory system. Incoordination can occur with lesions of the sensory cortex, the premotor and supplemental motor regions, the basal ganglia, the cerebellum, and the afferent sensory system. Balance dysfunction may be associated

with any lesion that results in weakness or sensory and perceptual loss. The overlap seen with impairments from various lesion sites demonstrates the complexity and intensity of the communication that exists within this system.

Abnormal tone (abnormal force with which a muscle resists being lengthened; abnormal stiffness) (Kandel et al., 1991) has been deemphasized in this text. Although abnormal tone is an impairment that can occur with lesions of the movement pathways, we have chosen to focus our attention on restoring muscle balance. To this end, this text presents treatment techniques to strengthen weak **agonist** muscles (those that are the prime movers) and weak **antagonist** muscles (those that counteract the action of other muscles).

Other impairments beyond these four can result from lesions within the movement pathways. However, from our clinical experience, the four that we have decided to focus on appear to be the most prevalent in primary neurological diagnoses. Other examples of impairments may include difficulty with motor planning, completing complex motor tasks, and excessive involuntary movement. Although impairments are frequently related to the development of disabilities, they do not always result in disabilities (eg, edema may be present in a finger without loss or limitation of hand function).

Other factors, such as cognitive state and premorbid status, may contribute to movement problems as well. Lack of attention, motivation, or musculoskeletal changes such as **bony blocks** or shortened connective tissue are just a few of the potential sources of movement difficulty. It should also be noted that the movement pathways described in this chapter have been discussed in isolation of the systems model (see Chap. 3). Functional mobility is not limited to the physiologic movement pathways, but also involves the attention and motivation of the patient, in addition to environmental factors and support systems.

SUMMARY

- The successful completion of movement depends on the integration of input from the CNS, the PNS, and the musculoskeletal system.
- Lesions of the upper and lower motor neurons result in distinct deficits, regardless of whether they are caused by injury, inflammation, or disease. Lower motor neuron lesions result in paralysis, loss of muscle tone, areflexia, and, eventually, muscle atrophy. Upper motor neuron lesions result in paresis or paralysis, depending on the severity of the lesion. Muscle atrophy is not seen in the short term with upper motor neuron lesions, although disuse atrophy is common in the later stages.

- Sensory feedback plays an important role in the proper planning and alteration of movement patterns. The two most important "divisions" in the somatosensory system are the lemniscal and the spinothalamic systems. The lemniscal system orchestrates touch, proprioception, and kinesthesia; the spinothalamic system is involved with the perception of pain, temperature, light touch, sexual sensations, and noxious stimuli.
- Animal research has provided convincing evidence that the sensory cortex can change in the aftermath of amputation and focal lesions to compensate for, at least in part, the loss of function in the damaged area.

REFERENCES

Grillner, S, & Wallen, P. (1985). Central program generators for locomotion, with special reference to vertebrates. *Annual Review of Neuroscience, 8,* 233–261.

Head, H. (192). *Studies in neurology* (Vol. 2). New York: Oxford University Press.

Houk, J, & Hennemou, E. (1967). Responses of Golgi tendon organs. *Journal of Neurophysiology, 30,* 466–489.

Kandel, ER, Schwartz, JH, & Jessel, TM. (1991). *Principles of neural science* (3rd ed.). Norwalk, CT: Appleton & Lange.

Moore, JC. (1974). The Golgi tendon organ and the muscle spindle. *American Journal of Occupational Therapy, 28,* 415–420.

Quillian, TA, & Ridley, A. (1971). The receptor community in the fingertip. *Journal of Physiology, 216,* 15–17.

Shepherd, RB. (1994, July 21–22). *Training motor control in individuals with movement dysfunction following brain lesions.* Conference at the Rehabilitation Institute of Chicago.

Scholz, J, & Campbell, S. (1981). Muscle spindles and the regulation of movement. *Physical Therapy, 60,* 1416–1424.

●●●●●●●●●●●●●●●●●●●●●●●●●●●●●●●●●●●●

SUGGESTED READINGS

Burt, AM. (1993). *Textbook of neuroanatomy*. Philadelphia: Saunders.

This comprehensive text of neuroanatomy is divided into seven sections, each of which deals with different anatomic topics. Some of the topics covered include the organization and development of the nervous system, neurocytology and neurotransmission, nervous system morphology, the sensory and motor systems, cranial nerves, and higher integrative centers.

Carpenter, MB. (1991). *Core text of neuroanatomy* (4th ed.). Baltimore: Williams & Wilkins.

This popular, readable, and thorough neuroanatomy text covers such neuroanatomic topics as gross morphology of the CNS, ascending and descending tracts, blood supply, and the meninges. It also separately considers the different sections of the CNS.

Cohen, H. (Ed.). (1993). *Neuroscience rehabilitation*. Philadelphia: Lippincott.

This neuroanatomy text writes to rehabilitation therapists as its audience. Its descriptions of neuroanatomy are complete, with an emphasis on clinical situations.

Guyton, AC. (1991). *Basic neuroscience–anatomy and physiology* (2nd ed.). Philadelphia: Saunders.

This basic but extensive neuroscience text is divided into seven sections that cover, among other topics, gross anatomy of the CNS and PNS, the cytoarchitecture of the nervous system, synapses, and neurotransmission. There are separate sections on general sensory, special sensory, and motor anatomy. The final six chapters discuss neural control of certain body functions (eg, contraction of skeletal muscle and control of heart functions).

Kandel, ER, Schwartz, JH, & Jessel, TM. (1995). *Essentials of neural science and behavior*. East Norwalk, CT: Appleton & Lange.

This is an extensive text that provides considerable information on the cellular mechanics of neuroscience, including neurotransmission. There is abundant material on such neural topics as cognition, perception, language, learning, and memory.

Littel, EH. (1990). *Basic neuroscience for the health professions*. Thorofare, NJ: Slack.

This thorough text of neuroscience is geared to those in the health professions. This text addresses all pertinent neuroanatomy topics covered in other fine neuroanatomy texts, but also includes review exercises at the end of each chapter that examine subjects covered in the chapter.

Analysis of Functional Mobility

LEARNING OBJECTIVES

After reading this chapter, you should be able to:

1. Describe the systems and task-oriented models and their relationship to the assessment model described in this chapter.
2. Understand the various movement strategies used by adults to complete the tasks of functional mobility.
3. Describe how impairments may result in abnormal movements, alter movement strategies, or both.
4. Discuss why functional mobility should be evaluated early in the assessment process.
5. Contrast the assessment model with traditional neurological assessment.
6. Discuss the recommended standardized scales that are to be used in conjunction with the assessment model.

One of the physical therapist's main assessment objectives in patients with neurological dysfunction is to determine if patients are experiencing limitations in functional mobility. The assessment then should include evaluation of the patient's ability to perform such basic movements as rolling from side to side in bed, moving from a supine position to standing, rising from sitting to standing, walking, and climbing stairs.

In the assessment model described in this chapter, the tasks of functional mobility are performed early in the examination process to enable the physical therapist to make a thorough assessment of the patient's abilities and disabilities. Assessing functional mobility first also affords the therapist more time to identify impairments that may contribute to disabilities. The sooner these problems are identified, the sooner the therapist can begin to implement helpful problem-solving strategies. Testing to identify specific impairments is performed after the assessment of functional mobility.

The physical therapist must also understand the functional anatomy of the nervous system, and be familiar with the patient's past and current medical history. Knowledge of the lesion's location can facilitate planning the assessment procedures and assist in the development of early treatment plans.

To help you understand the rationale behind the assessment procedure proposed in this text, we have provided preliminary information on the neurophysiologic theories of movement, and supplied an analysis of functional movements performed by individuals without disabilities. Following this important background material, the model for assessment is described. The assessment model recommended in this text is similar to a model proposed by Schenkman and Butler in 1989. Their model will be reviewed as it relates to the model on the assessment of disabilities and impairments presented in this chapter.

Before you move on to the next section, take a few minutes to read Display 3-1, which pre-

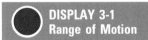

DISPLAY 3-1
Range of Motion

The range of motion (ROM) possible for a given joint is measured in degrees of a circle and encompasses maximum extension to maximum flexion, maximum abduction to maximum adduction, and maximum internal rotation to maximum external rotation. Range of motion can be assessed by having the patient perform, either alone (active ROM, AROM) or with the assistance of a therapist (passive ROM, or PROM), a series of exercises that involve the joints, muscles, and directional movements. The ROM for a given joint will depend on its type, but most can be tested using the following series of movements:

abduction: movement of a limb away from the body's axis
adduction: movement of a limb toward the body's axis
circumduction: circular movement of the limb that combines
                abduction, adduction, extension, and flexion
extension: movement that increases the angle between the two
                bones of a joint
flexion: movement that decreases the angle of adjoining bones
eversion: turning outward
inversion: turning inward
pronation: rotation that ends in the prone or face-down position
supination: rotation that ends in the supine or face-up position

sents and defines motion-related terms that will be referred to in the chapter.

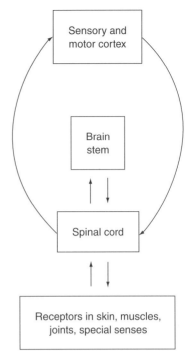

FIGURE 3-1. Reflex model of motor control.

NEUROPHYSIOLOGIC THEORIES OF MOVEMENT AND A MODEL OF NEUROLOGICAL REHABILITATION

Over the past 100 years, three models of movement have been described. These models have changed with our continually evolving knowledge of the physiology of the nervous system. The reflex model is based on research performed by Sir Charles Sherrington (1906) in the early 1900s. The hierarchical model was developed from the work of Hughlings Jackson in 1932 (Walsche, 1961), and the systems model is based on the 1932 work of the Russian neurologist Nicoli Bernstein (1962). In addition to these three traditional models, we have included a discussion of one of the models for neurological rehabilitation.

Reflex Model

Sherrington's research formed the foundation for the classic reflex theory of motor control (Shumway-Cook & Woollacott, 1995). The reflex model is peripherally based, in that stimuli applied to muscles or joints result in stereotypical responses that have been referred to as *reflex movement* (Horak, 1992). The premise of this model is that the sensory system must be intact for movement to occur. Once stimuli are provided, they create a chain of responses throughout the nervous system that ultimately results in movement.

Figure 3-1 is a diagram of the reflex model illustrating the chain effect of reflexes within the central nervous system (CNS) from the *initial stimulus* to the *periphery*.

Movement can be reflexive, volitional, or a combination of both. **Reflexive movement** is the purest example of the reflex stimulus model. A stimulus is provided and movement occurs, without the mediation of conscious thought. For example, stepping on a tack produces a reflexive movement of flexion away from the stimulus. You spend no time at all mulling over the need to make that particular move. **Volitional movement** results from a conscious or deliberate decision to move. Rising out of bed is a conscious decision. You decide that you would rather get up than stay in bed. In clinical practice, movement may be generated from a combination of reflexive and volitional activation, as described in the following example.

A clinical example of how the reflex model can create movement can be seen with a technique called **tapping.** In this technique, the therapist taps on weak muscles for the express purpose of forcing volitional contraction. Tapping on the muscle belly facilitates muscle activation by eliciting quick stretches of muscle spindles that contribute to the activation of the alpha motor neurons innervating **homonymous** and **synergistic** muscles (muscles that work together). This sensory information (ie, tapping), which activates a monosynaptic pathway; also ascends up the dorsal column–medial lemniscus system for integration into the sensory cortex. The physical therapist not only applies the stimulus of tapping, but provides verbal cues for the patient to actively contract the stimulated muscle.

Verbal cues may be perceived as an additional source of sensory stimulation (auditory stimulus), or they may encourage the patient to decide to engage in volitional movement. Tapping produces a stimulus response at the spinal cord level as well as the stimulus–response reflex in the brain stem and cortex via the ascending dorsal column–medial lemniscus system. The sensory stimulus activates a motor response at the spinal cord level or from higher cortical centers. The verbal cues provide a stimulus within the brain stem and cortex.

Another clinical example of a sensory-driven reflex movement is seen with the activation of the labyrinth, such as in righting, or equilibrium, reactions. Tilting the body to one side or another results in a head-righting response. An external perturbation that alters the center of gravity results in some type of extension or abduction of the extremities (or both) to maintain equilibrium. Both of these movements are reflexes generated in response to peripheral stimulation of the labyrinth.

A criticism of the reflex model is that volitional movement is not limited to responses from incoming peripheral stimuli. Reflex responses are seen with sensory stimuli such as labyrinth activation or in response to noxious stimuli (flexor withdrawal response); however, peripheral stimuli do not drive volitional movement. That is, a stimulus is not required for

activation of muscles resulting in movement. Taub (1976) and Polit and Bizzi (1979) have demonstrated that **deafferented** monkeys (those who have lost afferent nerve input) are able to complete normal movement patterns without somatosensory information. Volitional movement requires the integration of information from many systems (eg, muscles, joints, emotions, environment) and usually in the absence of external stimuli from the periphery. Movements, such as moving from sitting to standing or from sitting to walking, are not preceded by peripheral stimuli.

Hierarchical Model

Based on the work of the English physician Hughlings Jackson, the hierarchical model views the CNS as having higher, middle, and lower levels of control (Walsche, 1961). This model has been described as a "top-down" approach with each successive, anatomically higher level exerting control over the levels below.

The way in which the CNS matures from birth through early childhood supports the view that movement is controlled by successively more complex levels of the CNS (Gesell, 1954). At birth a child, no matter how advanced, is *apedal* (unable to walk) because the development of the brain stem and spinal cord do not support ambulation. Between 6 to 8 months of age, that child, supported by the development of the midbrain, begins to crawl. Another milestone occurs from 12 to 15 months, when the child begins to walk upright unsupported.

The highest level of motor control resides in the cortex, which is the most complex brain area and therefore the last to develop fully. Cortical control enables development of *bipedal* (two-legged) movement and equilibrium reactions (Fiorentino, 1981). The middle level, or midbrain, provides the *quadrupedal* (four-legged) mobility that is expressed in humans as crawling and righting reactions (Fiorentino,

1981). The brain stem and spinal cord occupy the lower levels, at which functional mobility is conspicuously absent.

Static (stationary) postures characterize the brain stem level, enabling one to maintain positions such as lying prone on the elbows or sitting. Brain stem level static postures include asymmetrical tonic neck, symmetrical tonic neck, tonic labyrinthine reflex, positive supporting reaction, and the negative supporting reaction. These static postures are described in Display 3-2.

Phasic reflexive movement characterizes the spinal level (Fiorentino, 1981) and results in nonpurposeful movement, which still contains primitive responses. In a description of reflexive development, Fiorentino (1981) stated that spinal level phasic movements include flexor withdrawal, extensor thrust, and crossed extension (see Display 3-2).

In a healthy, intact CNS, the cortical and midbrain levels control posture and movement. Individuals display equilibrium and righting reactions, are ambulatory, and make decisions about movement (ie, there is volitional activation of muscles). Reflexive movements associated with the spinal and brain stem levels are inhibited by higher CNS levels, which prevent static postures and phasic movements from occurring. Lesions that damage the cortex may prevent or limit bipedal mobility and equilibrium reactions. They may also release lower lev-

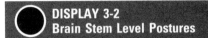

DISPLAY 3-2
Brain Stem Level Postures

A number of postures are associated with damage to or lesions of the mature brain stem.

Static

Asymmetrical tonic neck: A primitive reflex in which the head is turned to one side. The arm to which the face is turned extends, while the arm on the skull side is flexed.

Symmetrical tonic neck: A primitive reflex in which forward flexion of the head produces flexion of the arms and extension of the legs, and extension of the head produces extension of the arms and flexion of the legs.

Tonic labyrinthine reflex: The body assumes the extension tone when supine and the flexion tone when prone

Positive supporting reaction: The ability to bear weight on the legs when the feet are in contact with a hard surface

Negative supporting reaction: The inability to bear weight through the legs when the feet are in contact with a hard surface

Phasic

Flexor withdrawal syndrome: Flexion movement of one leg occurs in response to flexion of the opposite leg.

Extensor thrust: Extension of one leg occurs in response to flexion of the opposite leg.

Crossed extension: Adduction of one leg in occurs in response to a stimulus applied along the adductor muscles on the opposite leg.

els from cortical inhibition, thus producing the static postures mentioned above.

The hierarchical model has served as the basis for understanding the impairments displayed by patients with CNS lesions. One theory of spasticity is that it results from the release or loss of higher center control over lower subcortical levels. An example of this is the decorticate, or decerebrate, posture observed in patients who suffer bilateral damage at the midbrain region. The *decorticate posture* is caused by a bilateral lesion above the red nucleus, whereas the *decerebrate posture* is caused by a bilateral lesion below the red nucleus. Loss of cortical inhibition above or below the red nucleus results in flexion and extension or extension spasticity in the extremities.

In contrast to the reflex model, the hierarchical model is centrally based, with all activity for movement coming from within the CNS. Figure 3-2 illustrates the hierarchical anatomic levels that control muscle tone and equilibrium responses.

The hierarchical model has also been the basis for the development of treatment programs based on the intact levels of the CNS. If the brain stem was the highest intact system, then bipedal activities were not attempted. Similarly, the primitive reflexes and abnormal patterns of movement characteristic of the spinal and brain stem levels would be prevented or inhibited therapeutically to allow recovering higher centers of movement to return (Horak, 1992).

The hierarchical model's major shortcoming is that it focuses on one system, the CNS, as the primary source of movement. We now know that if other systems are involved, as indeed they are, then movement may be limited or abnormal. For example, a patient with a frozen shoulder provides evidence that the musculoskeletal system's involvement in movement is not to be discounted. Changes within the soft tissue of the joint limit normal movement of the humeral head within the glenoid fossa. To accomplish shoulder flexion, the patient must make the compensatory movements of shoulder elevation and retraction to raise the arm above the head.

Studies by Grillner and others showing that locomotion was possible in cats with spinal cord lesions suggest that other components for movement exist beyond hierarchical control (Grillner, 1981). The presence of *central program generators* (neurons located in various regions of the CNS that produce automatic movements), which could be activated without higher control, reinforced the concept that movement may occur without hierarchical domination (Horak, 1992). This information refutes the hierarchical model as the theoretical basis for movement.

Systems Model

The systems model was developed in 1932 by Bernstein, but the information was not read widely until it was translated into English in 1967. This model differs from the reflex and hierarchical models in that it is not focused on the nervous system, but on the interaction of the many systems that contribute to movement. Bernstein recognized that the forces needed to create movement may differ depending on two factors: (1) the environment in which the action occurs, and (2) the internal forces generated to accomplish the action (Bernstein, 1967). We use the simplified example of opening a door that you anticipate to be heavy to illustrate Bernstein's point.

Internal forces are generated in anticipation of overcoming the weight of the door. Because the door is, in actuality, very light, the force you have generated to open it becomes excessive. Should you decide to open the door a second time, you will adjust your actions to accommodate what you now know about the door's weight and the force needed to open it.

The diagram of the systems model is characterized by several circles looped together

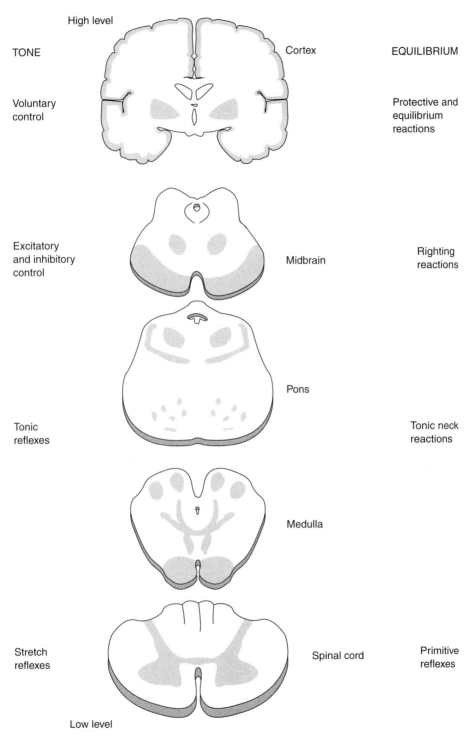

FIGURE 3-2. Hierarchical model of motor control.

High level

TONE   Cortex   EQUILIBRIUM

Voluntary control   Protective and equilibrium reactions

Excitatory and inhibitory control   Midbrain   Righting reactions

Pons

Tonic reflexes   Tonic neck reactions

Medulla

Stretch reflexes   Spinal cord   Primitive reflexes

Low level

(Fig. 3-3). Each circle represents a different system based on the task to be completed. In the previous example, the circles may represent the weight of the door, the angle of the line of pull of the arm, the internal forces created by the arm and body, the stability of the body as the weight of the object is pulled, and the activation of neural impulses to coordinate muscle activity to complete the action.

According to Horak (1992):

> A major assumption of the Systems Model is that the nervous system is organized to control the end points of motor behavior: the accomplishment of task goals. . . . normal movements are coordinated not because of muscle activation patterns prescribed by sensory pathways or by central programs, but because *strategies* of motion emerge from interaction of the systems. (p. 17)

The strategies of motion described by Horak are not restricted to the CNS but may include other systems as well (eg, muscles and joints). When moving from sitting positions to standing, the placement of the feet under the body (ie, the center of gravity) will have an impact on the movement. If the feet are placed too far in front of the center of gravity, the individual may not be able to stand. Successful completion of this task has as an integral component the alignment of joints to accommodate the shift in weight and adequate force generation from muscles. In the diagram of the systems model (see Fig. 3-3), joint alignment would be included as one of the circles.

In addition to proper joint alignment, movement also requires the interaction of the CNS and peripheral nervous system (PNS), the muscles, and the individual's motivation. Environmental characteristics could also factor in the successful performance of the task. For example, lifting the body up out of a low, cushioned seat requires the production of greater muscle force and weight shift than rising from a higher, firmer sitting surface. Individual desires or motivation can also affect the outcome of a task. For example, a basic need for food or drink could motivate someone to move out of the chair.

The systems approach to treatment in neurological rehabilitation is aimed primarily at task-oriented activities. The same task can be successfully accomplished with a wide variety of

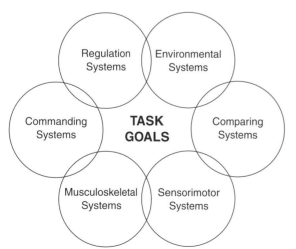

FIGURE 3-3.   The systems model of motor control.

movement patterns, based on internal and external factors. During the course of a day, people may use different movement strategies to rise from a chair. Internal factors here may include adequate strength in the arms and legs, range of motion (ROM) in the legs, and stable postures from which to move. External factors may include the surface of the environment (eg, whether the chair is soft or hard), the height of the chair, and the presence of arm rests. Variations of movement patterns displayed by individuals may include the use of arm supports, moving toward the edge of the seat, and aligning the feet under the body. Age can sometimes influence the way movement occurs. Young adults may stand up quickly without using their arms to push off the chair. An older adult may need to move to the edge of the chair, then push up with both arms to slowly lift the body out of the chair. In both examples, the task is accomplished, but by activating different systems of the body.

NEUROLOGICAL REHABILITATION MODELS

Horak (1992) describes three models of neurological rehabilitation:

1. Muscle re-education model of therapeutic exercise
2. Facilitation model of therapeutic rehabilitation
3. Task-oriented model of neurological rehabilitation

The muscle re-education model was advocated by Sister Kenny for the treatment of individuals with poliomyelitis. This model focused on the active contraction of individualized muscles. Developers of the facilitation model included the Bobaths; Kabat, Knott, and Voss; and Brunnstrom. This model was directed toward

affecting the CNS itself. Treatment did not target other systems such as the musculoskeletal system, which is frequently involved as a consequence of a lesion in the CNS. The task-oriented model described by Carr and Shepherd (1987), Gordon (1987), and Horak is the model emphasized in this text. It is also one of the theoretical perspectives on which the assessment model is based.

Task-Oriented Model

The task-oriented model can be viewed as a component of the systems model in that it "assumes that control of movement is organized around goal-directed, functional behaviors rather than on muscles or movement patterns" (Horak, 1992, p. 20). Similar to Bernstein's theory that the CNS seeks to control its own perceptions and actions for accomplishing tasks, the task-oriented model encourages the individual to actively participate in solving motor challenges.

Practice of a motor task requires the integration of systems and environmental factors integrated into the performance of the task. In rehabilitation, task-oriented activities should be functionally based. The activities of functional mobility should be practiced in a variety of contexts (Gordon, 1987) to enable the patient to develop and implement the strategies for performing tasks that will be continued after discharge from therapy.

Gordon's interpretation of Bernstein's systems model reinforces its relationship with the task-oriented model and emphasizes the need to practice task-oriented behaviors:

Bernstein proposed that all purposeful movement is organized to solve specific *motor problems* that arise from the interactions of our needs and desires with the environment. Thus, the specific form of a movement pattern is a means to an end: reaching the goal or solving the motor problem. The correctness of a movement pattern is not determined by whether it corresponds to some ideal form but by whether it is well adapted to the solution of a particular motor problem. The role of the therapist as teacher, therefore, should not simply be to stimulate or facilitate specific movement patterns but rather to select the tasks that are appropriate for the patient to begin to attempt to solve and to structure relevant conditions of the environment so that patients learn to solve these problems in a variety of contexts. (Gordon, 1987, p. 19)

DESCRIPTION OF FUNCTIONAL MOVEMENT

Examples of movement strategies used by healthy adults to perform the tasks of functional mobility are described below. Descriptions of normal movement strategies are provided to assist the reader in recognizing the compensatory strategies and abnormal movements that may result from impairments. Normal age-related changes in movement are also described. A patient who is 76 years old may have developed compensatory strategies related to the normal aging of the musculoskeletal system before suffering a stroke. The therapist must distinguish between normal compensatory changes that are a result of the aging process and those caused by the more recent neurological insult. The therapist should evaluate these tasks of functional mobility in the beginning of the assessment.

Movement Strategies in Healthy Adults

Rolling

Rolling may be performed to relieve pressure on the back, change position in bed, or as a component of moving from a supine position to sitting on the edge of the bed. Richter, VanSant, and Newton (1989) have concluded that there is more than one way to roll successfully. Some people may lift their arms above shoulder level and lead with their head and trunk, followed by unilateral lifting movements of the legs (Richter et al., 1989). Others may start with their legs in either a lifting pose or by placing their heels on the bed and pushing off. Given the variety of rolling patterns that may be used, it is recommended that the therapist determine which movement strategy the patient used before the disability developed.

Age-Related Movement Strategies. Age-related changes may contribute to slowed movement in this task. Patients may, in fact, be noted to abandon the strategy of segmental rolling, which is characteristic of adult movement, to revert to log rolling, a strategy seen in infants. In *segmental rolling*, the pelvis and shoulder move as two separate units, which may cause pain in a degenerative spine. There may be a noticeable limitation in ROM to enable segmental rolling to occur. In *log rolling*, the pelvis and shoulder move as a unit.

Supine to Sitting

Investigation into this specific movement strategy has not been reported. However, a great deal of variability was found in the strategies used to go from a supine position in bed to standing. Altogether, 89 patterns were found among 60 subjects tested in 10 trials (McCoy & VanSant, 1993; Sarnacki, 1985).

Before suffering a disability, patients' strategies for moving from a supine position to sitting may have included a combination of rolling as well as components of movements characteristic of the early phase of the supine-to-standing maneuver. Patients may roll to their sides and then push up, or initiate movements with sit-up maneuvers (as is also seen in supine-to-standing movements).

Age-Related Movement Strategies. In moving from a supine position to sitting, many older adults are unable to perform the sit-up maneuvers predominant in children and young adults. Instead, they may rely on their upper extremities to push their trunks up into sitting postures. These movements appear slow and deliberate because they are based on age-related weakness and joint changes.

Stable Sitting Posture

Assessment of stable sitting postures should include testing the patient's ability to sit unsupported while maintaining a symmetrical posture. Unsupported sitting consists of placing the feet on the floor and the hands on the thighs. To examine sitting posture symmetry, observe the patient's head position and the alignment of the shoulder and pelvis. Patients should be able to maintain this position for a functional period of time (eg, the time needed to don socks and shoes). They should also be able to maintain this position during the dynamic movements.

Age-Related Movement Strategies. Age-related changes may contribute to asymmetrical sitting postures due to postural deviations (eg, kyphosis, scoliosis), which may also alter the patient's center of gravity and balance in sitting. Older patients should be examined for any musculoskeletal limitations in the vertebral column and weakness in the muscles of back extension.

Sit-to-Stand Maneuver

The biomechanics of rising from sitting to standing have been documented in the literature (Millington, Myklebust, & Shambes, 1992; Schenkman, Berger, Riley, Mann, & Hodge, 1990). Moving to a standing position is a complex activity that incorporates the activation of several muscle groups, a change in the center of gravity, and the ability to balance on a bipedal base of support. There are four phases in the movement sequence of the sit-to-stand maneuver:

- Phase 1: flexion momentum
- Phase 2: momentum transfer
- Phase 3: extension
- Phase 4: stabilization (Millington et al., 1992)

The whole task is performed within 2 to 3 seconds. During phase 1, forward trunk flexion is needed to generate momentum. Early lift, or the momentum transfer phase, requires activation of the erector spinae, rectus femoris, vastus medialis, biceps femoris, gluteus maximus, and rectus abdominis (Millington et al., 1992). Initiating trunk flexion and the synergistic activation of multiple muscles can make the performance of this 2- to 3-second task difficult for patients who have muscle weakness and faulty timing and sequencing of muscle firing. The completion of the lift phase and the achievement of standing require strength, the proper timing and sequencing of muscle activation, and the patient's interaction with the environment in upright postures. When this task is successfully accomplished, the patient is able to move from a stable base of support in sitting to a bipedal posture with a narrower base of support.

Age-Related Movement Strategies. Arthritic joints in the weight-bearing extremities, weakness in the lower extremity or back extensor muscles, and the inability to rise to an upright posture due to joint changes in the vertebral column, hips, knees, or all three are just some of the age-related changes that can affect movement strategies.

Stable Standing Posture

The assessment of stable standing postures is similar to the assessment of stable sitting postures. Unsupported standing, body symmetry, and the ability to maintain the position should be evaluated. Unsupported standing is achieved when patients are able to maintain standing with symmetrical postures (eg, head position, shoulder and pelvis alignment) without hand support. Patients should be able to maintain this position long enough to complete a functional task, as well as during the dynamic movements required to accomplish the tasks of the activities of daily living.

Age-Related Movement Strategies. Forward flexed postures may be present in the aging population and are frequently indicative of forward flexed cervical spines and kyphotic changes in the thoracic spine. (*Kyphosis* refers to the excessive curvature of the spine with backward convexity.) This postural change alters the body's center of gravity by placing it anterior, and contributes to greater flexion in the hips and knees in an attempt to counterbalance the weight of the body.

To experience this, stand with your head projected forward, round your shoulders forward as far as possible, and flatten your lumbar lordosis. What you should feel is your center of gravity moving forward over the metatarsal heads of your feet. To compensate for this feeling of falling forward, flex your hips and knees. Forward flexed postures may contribute to restrictions in hip and knee extension, as a result of the compensation of hip and knee flexion. This posture may also appear to the examiner as a suspensory strategy. The *suspensory strategy* is the normal postural response of flexion of the hips and knees. Because this strategy lowers the body's center of gravity closer to the floor, it is used to assist in stabilizing balance. Older patients should be assessed for any musculoskeletal changes that may contribute to postural deviations and flexion of the hips and knees.

Transfers

Transferring from one sitting surface to another is not a functional movement that is incorporated into daily routines. It is rare to move from one sitting surface to another without walking between the two surfaces. It should come as no surprise, then, that some patients have difficulty comprehending the movement of stand, pivot, and sit. This movement sequence is not part of a daily movement repertoire and therefore may be difficult for neurologically impaired patients to comprehend.

The pivot transfer requires moving from a sitting posture to standing, followed by pivoting and sitting in a nearby chair. Normal movement strategies are unlikely to emerge because this task is unfamiliar. Therapists should be prepared to instruct patients on how to move, incorporating components of sit-to-stand maneuvers. Once these moves have been safely executed, therapists should instruct patients to pivot and then lower themselves onto the chair.

Age-Related Movement Strategies. The same age-related changes that applied for stable standing and moving from a sitting posture to standing also apply to this movement task.

Ambulation

Ambulation, like the sit-to-stand maneuver, is a complex activity. This movement strategy incorporates the activation of multiple muscle groups, shifting of the weight with change in the center of gravity in both the anterior/posterior and lateral planes, balancing on a single leg, and forward propulsion of the body. Environmental factors, such as rugs or outdoor terrain, contribute to the complexity of this task. Components of the gait cycle and muscle activity are described to enable readers to recognize abnormal movement and disability as a result of impairments from a neurological lesion.

Gait Cycle

Perry (1992) describes the *gait cycle,* or stride, as consisting of a stance period and a swing period. The *stance period* is divided into weight acceptance and single-limb support. The *swing period* is comprised of limb advancement. These periods are further divided into phases. Weight acceptance includes the *initial contact* phase, during which the leg that was swung forward touches down on the floor, and the *loading response,* during which that same leg accepts the weight of the body. Single-limb support encompasses the midstance, terminal stance, and preswing phases. The limb is advanced through space in a set of movements: the preswing, initial swing, mid-swing, and terminal swing (Fig. 3-4).

Muscle activation during the stance and swing periods is summarized in Figures 3-5 and 3-6. The extensor muscle sequence comprises muscle activation for the stance phase, and the flexor muscle sequence comprises muscle activation for swing phase.

Muscle Activation: Swing Period. In the swing sequence, the following muscles are active for the terminal stance: the soleus, gastrocnemius, flexor digitorum longus, flexor hallicus longus, and the adductor longus (Perry, 1992). Weak-

ness in any or all of these muscles may result in difficulty accelerating the body forward.

The *preswing phase* involves the activation of the anterior tibialis, extensor digitorum longus, extensor hallicus longus, and the rectus femoris in combination with the adductor longus (Perry, 1992). These muscles begin to draw the foot up off the ground to enable it to clear the walking surface during the swing phase.

Flexor muscles that are active during the preswing phase continue to fire during both the *initial swing* and *midswing phases.* In addition, the sartorius, gracilis, and iliacus advance the thigh forward, with the biceps femoris (short head) assisting knee flexion, allowing the foot to be lifted off the ground (Perry, 1992).

The *terminal swing* is accomplished with the activation of the hamstrings to decelerate hip flexion and knee extension, activation of the adductor magnus and gluteus maximus to continue hip deceleration without knee flexion, activation of the vastus muscle group to enable full knee extension at initial contact and to counteract the effects of the hamstrings, and the reactivation of the anterior tibialis to prepare the foot for the heel strike (Perry, 1992).

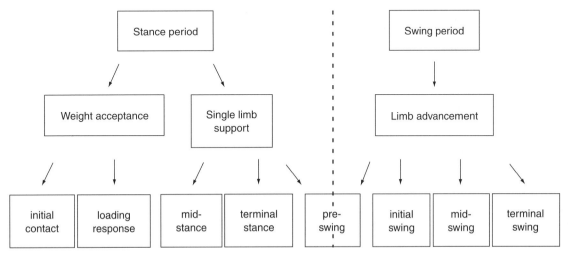

FIGURE 3-4. The stride of the gait cycle consists of the stance period and the swing period, which are further divided into their components.

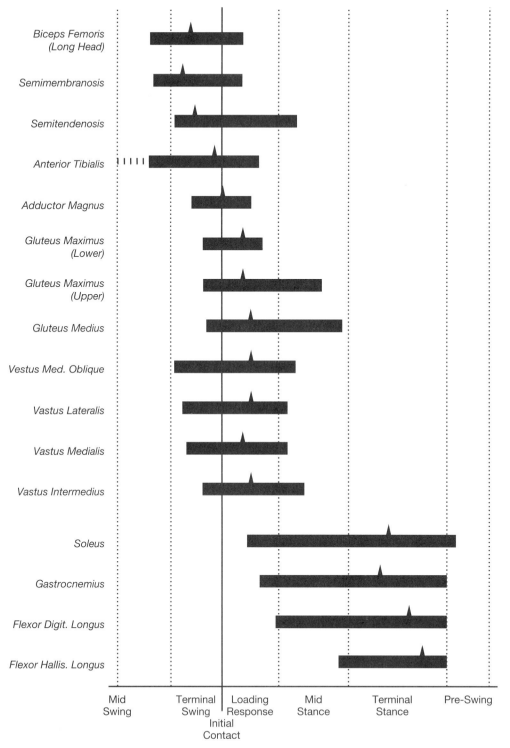

FIGURE 3-5. Extensor muscle sequence for stance.

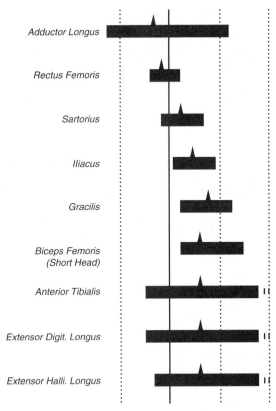

FIGURE 3-6. Flexor muscle sequence for swing.

Muscle Activation: Stance Period. Both the initial contact and the loading response rely on the extensor and flexor muscles working together to achieve stability in preparation for the stance phase. The adductor magnus and gluteus medius provide hip extension. The gluteus medius adds stability for the contralateral drop of the pelvis (Perry, 1992). The vastus muscles provide stable weight acceptance and control the knee flexion that occurs during initial loading and the body's forward momentum. The anterior tibialis decreases the rate of passive plantar flexion that occurs with initial loading.

The midstance and terminal stance are primarily controlled by the plantar flexors, the soleus and gastrocnemius. During the early phase of the midstance, the vastus muscles and the gluteus maximus and medius are active to accommodate knee extension and provide stability. However, "the primary responsibility for limb control is transferred to the ankle extensor muscles to provide graded progression over the supporting foot" (Perry, 1992, p. 161). Weakness in plantar flexors can result in decreased ankle ROM through the stance, decreased stance time, and limited forward acceleration of the body.

Age-Related Movement Strategies. The compensatory strategies used to accomplish this task (ie, the postural deviations of kyphosis, forward flexed posture) are similar to those seen in stable standing. They may also include movements to accommodate any weakness in the lower extremities that may alter the stance phase, the swing phase, or both. Weakness in the extensor muscles of the lower extremities, shortening of the flexor muscles, and painful weight-bearing joints (arthritis) may lead to an altered stance such as that seen in an *antalgic gait* (an alteration in movement undertaken for the relief of pain). The swing phase may be altered by a decrease in the length of the step and stride, as well as by shuffling of the feet.

Climbing Stairs

Climbing stairs incorporates the movement strategies used in ambulation and in rising from sitting to standing positions. Ascending stairs requires that the weight be shifted and that each leg be lifted in turn onto the stair through concentric muscle contractions. Once a step up has been achieved, the weight is shifted again, this time onto the elevated limb. This movement is followed by lifting or extending the body, as is done in the extension phase of the sit-to-stand maneuver. The trail leg follows the body up the stairs and may provide counterbalance.

Descending stairs is similar to ascending in that a shift in weight is involved, but now muscular contractions are predominantly *eccentric*. Lowering the body down steps may be analogous to moving from standing to sitting, except that descending stairs requires single-limb support.

Age-Related Movement Strategies. The musculoskeletal and sensory and perceptual changes that occur with normal aging may severely limit the older patient's ability to climb stairs. The majority of falls in public places are associated with descending stairs (Shumway-Cook & Woollacott, 1992). Individuals experiencing age-related changes in the musculoskeletal system may ascend stairs leading consistently with one foot instead of using the usual reciprocal pattern. This strategy may be used if there is diminished stance time on one extremity or an inability to flex one leg up onto a step. Descending stairs requires that the muscles possess enough eccentric strength to lower the body's weight, while the center of gravity moves forward down the step and forces generated in the patellofemoral joints increase. At the same time, perceptual processing of the environment may be altered resulting in fear of a misstep. The patient may clutch the handrail with two hands, use a nonreciprocal gait pattern, or proceed with slow, hesitant movements to avoid missteps.

Disabilities

Movement strategies that are inefficient, unsafe, and ineffectual can result in disabilities. A patient's inability to successfully and safely move within varied environments often develops from impairments associated with disease or injury to the CNS. Confusion, disorientation, lack of motivation, weakness, spasticity, soft tissue restrictions, joint limitations, balance disorders, incoordination, pain, and sensory or perceptual dysfunction are all examples of impairments that can contribute to disabilities. This text restricts its focus to four commonly occurring impairments, one of which is weakness.

In general, weakness may make it difficult to initiate, sustain, or complete a task. The presence of a balance dysfunction may eliminate the patient's ability to perform any type of movement from a static posture for fear of falling. If movement is possible, it may be slow and deliberate. Incoordination does not usually limit the patient's ability to perform tasks of functional mobility, unless it is accompanied by a balance dysfunction, but it may alter the quality of the movement strategies performed. For example, patients may be able to roll from side to side in bed. However, the movement of their lower extremities during this task may appear awkward or **ataxic** (characterized by a defect in muscular coordination during voluntary movements).

Sensory or perceptual dysfunction may limit tasks of functional mobility in a variety of ways. Diminished sensation may contribute to difficulty in the quality of a movement strategy. The movements may be excessive or awkward in appearance due to diminished sensory feedback. **Unilateral neglect** often results in a lack of awareness or recognition of the left side of the body, producing movements that incorporate only the right side of the body.

Detailed descriptions of how the tasks of functional mobility can be limited by the four major impairments of weakness, balance dysfunction, incoordination, and sensory and perceptual dysfunction are described in Section II of this text.

NEUROLOGICAL ASSESSMENT

Having reviewed the systems and task-oriented models, it should now be apparent to the reader that the assessment of tasks (ie, functional mobility) is an integral part of assessment. The systems model, which requires the integration of biopsychosocial and environmental factors, focuses on the accomplishment of tasks presented in the environment (Bernstein, 1967). As stated earlier by Horak (1992), "A major assumption of the Systems Model is that the nervous system is organized to control the end points of motor behavior: the accomplishment of task goals" (p. 17). The basis of the task-oriented model is the practice of motor tasks that require development or proficiency. An assessment of functional mobility is performed to determine which tasks require practice. The emphasis of the assessment model recommended in this text is on evaluating functional mobility as early in the process as possible. From this assesment the therapist can then identify any impairments that may contribute to the patient's disabilities.

The model for assessment of disabilities and impairments is given in Display 3-3. The first step in the assessment is patient observation, followed by evaluation of disabilities (functional mobility) and underlying impairments. Functional mobility is assessed early on to enable the therapist to identify limitations, as well as set patient goals and devise the best possible treatment plan to minimize or eliminate the disabilities. The therapists' problem-solving strategies are also tapped, as they try to identify the potential impairments that may be contributing to the disabilities exhibited. During the assessment of disabilities, patients are instructed to move or to assume positions that partially eliminate the disability and reduce the effect of impairment. Treatment is, in effect, initiated during the assessment procedure as the therapist begins to address limitations in functional mobility.

The next component of the assessment is patient reobservation, which is used to deter-

---

DISPLAY 3-3
Model for Assessment of Disabilities and Impairments

1. *Observation*
   Note the patient's level of awareness, cognition, body alignment and posture, position of extremities, ability to move, and use of any adaptive equipment or appliances.
2. *Assess for Disabilities*
   Have the patient perform the following movements and assess for any abnormalities indicative of disabilities: rolling side to side; supine-to-sit and back to supine; sit-to-stand and back to sit; transferring from bed to wheelchair and back (if wheelchair is used for mobility); ambulation; stair climbing; supine-to-stand from floor.
3. *Assess for Impairments*
   Examine the patient carefully, noting any weakness, tonal abnormalities or alignment problems, incoordination, balance dysfunction, and sensory or perceptual dysfunction.
4. *Reobservation*
   Observe the patient again after the evaluation.
5. *Community Mobility*
   Assess patients in environments that are similar to those in which they will function, work, shop, and engage in social and recreational activities.

mine the effectiveness of the evaluation and treatment. The goal of patient reobservation is to determine if any new motor behaviors were learned from the instruction provided during the assessment. Finally, patients are assessed for whether or not they are able to function within their total environments. The examination of the issues of community mobility focuses on activities such as going to work and shopping. The procedure for the assessment is described in greater detail later in this chapter.

Assessment Model—Rationale

The rationale for the design of this assessment model is supported by the clinical practice guidelines for rehabilitation after a stroke, established by the Agency for Health Care Policy and Research (AHCPR, 1985), which state that:

> . . . the first challenge facing a therapist is to determine which factors are contributing to movement or functional deficits. Assessment begins by observing a patient's attempts to accomplish functional tasks . . . . Thorough knowledge of the cause of impaired motor performance is needed to select appropriate exercises, treatment modalities, and activities. (p. 120)

The AHCPR (1985) also recommends that patients with stroke be encouraged to perform early mobilization as soon as medically feasible (within 24–48 hours of hospital admission). Assessment of mobility should include the:

> . . . patient's ability to turn from side to side and move up and sit in bed, and then progresses to examining the ability to sit on the edge of the bed . . . . Mobilization progresses to patient transfers to a chair, commode, sofa or wheelchair (and sitting on these); and finally coming to a standing position, bearing weight and walking. (p. 64)

Schenkman and Butler Model

The model for the assessment of disabilities and impairments is similar to a model proposed in 1989 by Schenkman and Butler, which was "intended to guide the clinician in identifying underlying causes of a patient's disability" (p. 538). The theoretical framework of the Schenkman and Butler model is based on the International Classification of Impairment, Disability, and Handicap (ICIDH), which was developed by the World Health Organization (see Chap. 1).

The primary difference between the two assessment models is where the assessment begins. The Schenkman and Butler model starts with the insult of the neurological occurrence (etiology) and progresses to neuroanatomic pathology, the direct effects of that pathology (impairments), and the resultant disability. The model in this text starts with the disability, progresses to the assessment of the underlying impairments that contribute to the disability, proceeds to a reassessment of functional mobility (disability), and ends with a discussion of the patient's community mobility (handicap). Figure 3-7 illustrates the difference in the direction of problem-solving proposed in the two models.

Schenkman and Butler also proposed starting with an assessment of the functional disability and progressing to an assessment of the impairment when the underlying pathology is not known. This particular variation on their model is more directly related to the model described in this chapter. The appeal of such an approach is that knowing the pathologic condition that the patient presents facilitates problem-solving and treatment planning. However, starting with the pathology and working through the impairments leads to the unnecessary testing of impairments that may not be related to the patient's particular disabilities. Evidence of unnecessary testing is described in the following section on traditional neurological assessment.

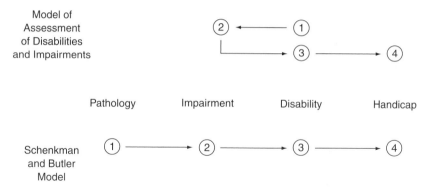

FIGURE 3-7. Comparison of Schenkman and Butler's model with the model of assessment of disabilities and impairments.

Schenkman and Butler also examined the direct effects of neuroanatomic pathology and the possible impairments that may result. Chapter 2 provides a similar discussion, emphasizing lesion locations along the movement pathway and the potential impairments that may result. The Schenkman and Butler table is reprinted here as Table 3-1 next to Table 3-2 to demonstrate the similarities in the impairments identified with lesions of the CNS.

Contrasting the Traditional Models for Neurological Assessment

The reader should recognize that the model for the assessment of disabilities and impairments described in this chapter is different from the traditional model for neurological assessment outlined in Display 3-4. Additional testing techniques beyond those listed in Display 3-4 may also be performed (eg, testing for the Babinski reflex, cranial nerve assessment). The traditional neurological assessment is a series of detailed tests designed to help the physical therapist identify the pathology or locate the lesion within the CNS. However, evaluation of functional mobility is left until the end of the clinical decision-making process (see Display 3-4). A traditional physical therapy assessment that includes *all* the components included in Display 3-4 is an inefficient use of the therapist's and the patient's time. Our model proposes a few modifications that maximize the efficiency of the therapist's assessment.

The assessment should not focus on measuring impairments that do not relate to patient disability (eg, Babinski reflex). If the therapist hypothesizes, through the observation of functional mobility, that the patient is impaired by muscle weakness, then a *detailed* sensory assessment may not be warranted. Specific testing to *rule in* the impairment of muscle weakness as a factor in the disability should be performed. The integrity of the sensory system can be determined by testing localized touch and proprioception. If localized touch and proprioception are not intact, then further sensory testing should be performed. If the postures or movements displayed by the patient suggest muscle weakness and sensory loss, then thorough assessments of both systems should be performed.

Not every traditional test to identify pathologies and impairments need be conducted for every patient; therapists can and should be selective in their assessment procedure. In this era of health care reform, therapists must be as efficient as possible in the assessment and treatment of patients.

TABLE 3-1. Schenkman and Butler Table of Neuroanatomic Pathology and Potential Impairments, With Table 2-4

Pathology	Impairment
Sensory	
Peripheral sensory neuropathy	Sensory loss
Parietal lesion	Perceptual loss, interpretive loss
Parietotemporal-occipital lesion	Attention loss
Motor	
Peripheral motor neuropathy	Motor loss
Anterior horn cell loss	Motor loss
Peripheral autonomic neuropathy	Loss of vasomotor tone
Integrative	
Basal ganglia	Diminished alerting mechanisms
	Loss of motor programming-planning
Prefrontal lobe lesion	Loss of ability to generate new motor plans
Cerebellar lesion	Loss of ability to correctly run motor programs

Schenkman, M., & Butler, R. B. (1989). A model for multisystem evaluation, interpretation, and treatment of individuals with neurologic dysfunction). *Physical Therapy*, *69*(7), 538–547.

TABLE 3-2. Lesion Sites and Impairments

Anatomic Region	Impairment
Primary motor cortex	Weakness or paralysis, change in tone
Sensory cortex	Loss of sensation, perception, proprioception, problems with motor control
Premotor region	Weakness from disuse, difficulty with planning motor tasks, apraxia
Supplemental motor region	Weakness from disuse, difficulty with complex motor tasks
Basal ganglia	Absence of movement, weakness from disuse, abnormal movements (chorea, tremor), or abnormal tone (rigidity)
Cerebellum	Incoordination, weakness from disuse, balance problems, changes in tone
Corticospinal tract	Weakness
Alpha motor neuron	Weakness or atrophy
Muscle	Weakness
Afferent sensory input	Loss of sensory awareness, uncoordinated movements, balance problems

ASSESSMENT PROCEDURES

The model for assessing disabilities and impairments is comprised of five steps:

1. Observe the patient and determine cognitive function.
2. Assess the patient's functional mobility; have the patient perform the various tasks that are used every day, to determine if disabilities exist.
3. Assess specific impairments that may contribute to limitations in functional mobility.
4. Observe the patient after the assessment or treatment, to determine responses to newly learned motor behaviors.

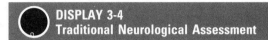

DISPLAY 3-4
Traditional Neurological Assessment

Demographic information
Medical history
Psychosocial history
Patient's chief complaint
Impact of disability on lifestyle
Mental status
Communication ability
Mobility

- Range of motion (ROM)
- Joint play
- Soft tissue
  - Skin condition
  - Compliance of muscle and connective tissue
  - Edema

Motor control

- Muscle tone
- Strength
- Abnormal reflexes
- Voluntary movement patterns
- Motor planning ability
- Coordination
- Balance—static/dynamic
- Developmental sequence
- Autonomic postural and equilibrium reactions

Vital functions
Autonomic nervous system
Sensation
Perceptual evaluation
Pain
Posture
Gait
Functional abilities
Equipment
Endurance/cardiorespiratory status

From Holden, M. (1985). Clinical decision making among neurologic patients: Stroke. In Wolf,
S. *Clinical decision making in physical therapy*. Philadelphia: Davis.

5. Assess the patient's potential difficulties with mobility within the community.

Step 1: Observation

The first step of the assessment should begin when the patient enters the clinic or when the therapist enters the patient's room. Therapists should look for:

- The patient's awareness of and response to the therapist's presence—the ability to communicate
- The patient's body alignment and posture and the position of the extremities
- The patient's ability to respond by moving when interacting with the therapist. Does the patient sit up straighter to attend to the discussion? Does the patient move the arms or legs appropriately to adjust position?
- The presence of adaptive equipment or appliances

The patient's awareness of the examiner's presence can be an indicator of cognitive status, the level of motivation to attend to the interaction at hand, or both. An impairment in cognition is indirectly related to a patient's functional mobility, so it must be assessed.

Determine the patient's orientation to person, place, and time and the ability to follow and interact with the therapist. Verbal interaction, including responses to questions, can reveal higher levels of cognitive processing and memory function. Deficits in cognition must also be distinguished from communication deficits, such as expressive, receptive, or global *aphasia,* commonly seen with patients who have had a stroke.

Patients who are oriented to person, place, and time may still have difficulty learning new motor tasks, relearning motor skills, and understanding treatment plans. In step 4 of this assessment model, observe the patient's ability to re-

tain motor activity sequences and to carry out simple motor tasks which have been demonstrated or for which verbal instruction was provided. It is necessary to use motor tasks that patients are physically capable of performing to assess motor learning. If patients are unable to repeat motor tasks because other behavioral or cognitive problems are displayed, refer them to appropriate health care providers for additional assessment.

Abnormal body alignment and extremity position may suggest the presence of weakness, as well as changes in muscle tone (Fig. 3-8).

During the patient–therapist interaction, any abnormal or depressed movements made by the patient may suggest muscle weakness, tonal changes, incoordination, or perceptual

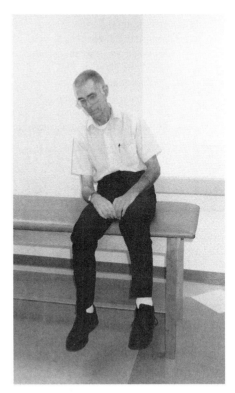

FIGURE 3-8.   The fact that the patient is listing to the right is indicative of poor alignment due to weakness.

deficits. The inability to correct slouching postures or to right the head could indicate weakness or balance dysfunction. The inability to
visually track to the left side of the body suggests
that the patient may have a perceptual problem
called *left-sided neglect.*

The presence of assistive devices, such as
ankle foot orthosis, cock-up splint, or a lap
board, suggests muscle weakness. Eyeglasses or
hearing aids suggest additional forms of sensory
impairment that must be considered. When observing an ambulatory patient entering the
clinic, be on the lookout for a quad cane. A
patient who uses this assistive device may have
weakness on one side of the body, a balance
problem, or an antalgic gait. All of these observations will facilitate testing by allowing the
therapist to narrow the focus to the most likely
impairments and disabilities.

Step 2: Testing for Disabilities

Functional mobility, observed in step 2, consists
of the following tasks, which are traditionally
tested in the given sequence:

- Rolling from side to side in bed
- Moving from the supine position to sit-
  ting at the edge of the bed
- Maintaining a stable sitting posture
- Transferring from one support surface to
  another
- Maintaining standing postures
- Walking
- Ascending and descending stairs

The assessment of adult functional mobility
should be inclusive but not necessarily in a systematic sequence. For example, a patient who
arrives in the physical therapy department in a
wheelchair and displays a symmetrical sitting
posture could be assessed for standing and ambulation before rolling activities. The symmetrical sitting posture of this patient suggests that

there is adequate trunk strength to maintain
sitting, and potentially adequate trunk strength
for standing and ambulation with or without
assistance. The therapist may choose to start
with an assessment of a higher level functional
skill, but should not exclude lower level skills.
This same patient, who can maintain a symmetrical sitting posture and is able to stand,
may be unable to roll to the noninvolved
side.

Conversely, a patient sitting with an asymmetrical posture and poor positioning of the extremities (eg, right arm off the arm rest, and
right leg externally rotated and off the foot
rest), may have weakness, sensory loss, or balance dysfunction. Unilateral neglect can usually
be ruled out since the lesion did not occur
in the right cerebral hemisphere. However, a
detailed sensory assessment should be performed to remove any doubt.

Identifying the impairment(s) contributing
to this disability in sitting should follow the assessment of functional mobility. The assessment
of functional mobility should start with placing
the patient in a stable sitting posture. Depending on the response to this position, the patient
can progress directly to standing and transfer
activities or be instructed to perform the less
strenuous rolling and supine-to-sitting maneuvers.

Keep in mind that the patient who is unable
to maintain a stable sitting posture will most
likely be unsuccessful in standing. All patients
should be assessed for their ability to stand and
ambulate within the first few days of treatment,
regardless of how they respond to the demands
of stable sitting. This enables the therapist to
determine a baseline of functional mobility
from which the goals and treatment plan are
to be established. Patients in a coma, or those
with other medical complications that prevent
standing or ambulation, are exceptions to
this rule.

The functional movements that should be
assessed to determine the presence of disabili-

ties are listed in Display 3-5. There are other tasks of functional mobility beyond those listed in this table that may be assessed based on the patient's needs and abilities at the time of assessment.

Determining Movement Strategies

The therapist would do well to remember a few things about the nature of movement strategies. First, adults may use more than one movement pattern to execute the functional movements in their repertoire (Green & Williams, 1992; McCoy & VanSant, 1993; Sarnacki, 1985; VanSant, 1988). Second, the presence of impairments may alter the movement strategy before the disability becomes apparent. During the assessment of functional mobility, the therapist must recognize the movement strategies that are unique to each patient and consider the unique challenges posed by the patient's environment.

Impairments.   Movement strategies altered by impairments can be assessed through observation of the task and knowledge of normal movement strategies. Take, for example, the task of moving from a supine position to sitting on the edge of the bed. Ask the patient to sit up from the supine position. Observe closely for the strategies used to accomplish this movement. Does the patient attempt to sit up directly from the supine posture? Does the patient roll over completely onto one side and push up to sit? Or does the patient sit up halfway and begin to roll to the side? Take note of the movement strategies attempted by the patient so that you can incorporate them into the treatment program to retrain previously intact motor programs (Schmidt, 1991).

When asked to move toward their involved side, patients with **hemiplegia** (one-sided paralysis) may demonstrate the movement strategies that they used before the onset of weakness. Close observation of the movement of the non-involved extremities is required to identify past strategies. Does the head turn first? Does the patient reach forward with a protracted shoulder with the noninvolved arm? Does the non-involved leg flex at the hip and knee to assist with pushing the body over? These selected movement strategies should be incorporated into the therapist's instruction to the patient to roll toward the noninvolved side with the involved extremities.

Patients with complete *paraplegia* (paralysis of the lower body and legs) or *quadriplegia* (paralysis of the arms, legs, and torso) probably

DISPLAY 3-5
Functional Movements to Assess Disability

1. Rolling from side to side in bed.
2. Moving from a supine position to sitting at the edge of the bed
3. Maintaining a stable sitting posture
4. Moving back to a supine position from sitting
5. Moving from a sitting position to standing
6. Maintaining a stable standing posture
7. Moving back to a sitting position from standing
8. Transferring from the bed to wheelchair and back (if wheelchair is used for mobility)
9. Walking
10. Ascending and descending stairs

will be unable to incorporate previously learned motor programs into relearning mobility tasks. The lack of ascending and descending tracts within the spinal cord renders the involved extremities nonfunctional. Individuals with paraplegia or quadriplegia require intensive training to compensate for movement and sensory loss in their upper extremities, trunk, and lower extremities. Without this training, they cannot accomplish functional movement. (For additional information on training patients with spinal cord lesions, see the suggested readings at the end of this chapter.)

Environments. Different environments may alter movement strategies to complete the same task. For example, the sequence of motions differs depending on the properties of a chair. Is a chair a hard kitchen chair or a soft, low, overstuffed chair? Rolling from side to side in a hospital bed can be accomplished using bed rails. This alternate strategy may be impossible to achieve in a regular bed, which is not outfitted with rails. Bed rails may enhance patient performance for another reason: They provide a measure of safety against falling, which may allay patients' fears of rolling off the bed. This knowledge may encourage patients to test movement strategies that might be dangerous under less secure conditions. Rising from the supine position to sitting at the edge of the bed is easier to accomplish in a hospital bed, especially if the head of the bed is elevated. Patients who move independently in a hospital bed (with the above-mentioned assistive devices) are often not independent in this task at home.

The assessment of functional mobility, either initially or during the treatment phase, must include evaluation of the functional task in the environment wherein the patient will ultimately reside. Functional movements should be practiced in varied environments. This has the two-fold benefit of assisting the patient to develop reliable problem-solving skills to devise and execute various movement strategies. Treatment should also include an opportunity to practice tasks in an environment similar to the discharge environment. This will facilitate transfer of the learned motor behavior to the new environment (Winstein, 1991), enhance home and community interaction, and limit potentially handicapping conditions.

Other Tasks. Two additional tasks that may be assessed later during treatment are (1) standing up from a supine position on the floor, and (2) opening a closed door and walking through the doorway. These movements, particularly the latter, will also test the patient's perceptual abilities.

As always, test the patient's abilities as soon as possible so that you can develop the most effective treatment plans possible. Tasks of functional mobility that patients are unable to perform safely and efficiently should be incorporated in treatment planning and practiced.

For example, the patient in Figure 3-9 has difficulty ascending stairs with his involved leg. To address this problem, have the patient step up and down one set of steps of varying heights repeatedly with the involved extremity. After repeating this activity several times, the patient should practice climbing up the four stairs using a reciprocal pattern.

Step 3: Testing for the Presence of Impairments

Patients who have difficulty initiating, sustaining, or completing functional movements may have weakness. The absence of stabilizing postures may be the result of balance dysfunctions or weakness. The absence of or any reduction in movement quality may indicate coordination problems or abnormalities of tone. Disregard for movement of half of the body may be an indication of perceptual neglect. A limited

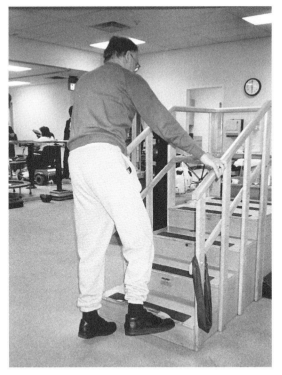

FIGURE 3-9. Patient has difficulty ascending the stairs with his involved leg.

ROM or abnormal movement patterns suggest abnormal muscle tone or weakness.

Once the therapist has carefully observed the patient in motion, the assessment can progress to the identification of the impairments that are contributing to the disability. The major impairments that limit functional mobility are:

- Muscle weakness
- Muscle tone abnormalities and alignment problems
- Incoordination
- Balance dysfunction
- Sensory or perceptual dysfunction

It is not unusual to test for the presence of two or three impairments, although the thera-

pist should be selective in the choice of tests used to identify these impairments. There is no reason to perform a detailed assessment for every impairment, unless the preliminary tests suggest that such comprehensive testing is warranted.

For example, if the patient is sitting asymmetrically in a wheelchair and leaning excessively to the right, test for weakness. If, however, sensory tests of localized touch or proprioception are abnormal, then further sensory assessment should be performed in addition to testing for weakness. The test for localized touch and proprioception confirms the integrity of sensory reception in the PNS and CNS and the integration of sensory information at the cortex.

Weakness

Weakness is an impairment in the quantity of active ROM or in the strength available to perform tasks. Weakness may result from lesions within the CNS, PNS, or the musculoskeletal system. Determining the origin of muscle weakness is a necessary first step toward achieving the most effective treatment outcome. Assessing *deep tendon reflexes* (*DTRs*), a muscular contraction elicited by a sharp tap, can assist in determining if the PNS is involved. If the reflex arcs are intact, then strength can be increased by using treatment aimed at the cortically activated movements that will transmit impulses to muscle via the alpha motor neurons. The absence of reflex arcs may suggest more palliative treatment (eg, passive ROM, positioning, electric stimulation with monophasic current).

Chapter 5 describes in detail the standardized assessment procedures used to measure strength, as well as the treatment approaches used to increase strength. Weakness is an impairment in the quantity of active ROM or in the strength available to perform tasks.

Muscle Abnormalities and Abnormal Alignment

The physiologic basis for tone abnormalities is the subject of much debate. Recent investigations have suggested that peripheral input is a factor in the generation of hypertonicity in muscles (Carey & Brughardt, 1993; Craik, 1994; Hufschmidt & Mauritz, 1985). Hypertonicity has been defined by Shepherd (1994) as resistance to passive ROM that could be the result of muscle shortening. Spasticity has been defined as the state of *hyperreflexia* (hyperactive deep tendon reflex) (Shepherd, 1994). Hypertonicity, when present, can create joint or extremity malalignment, which may contribute to postural changes, and therefore affect patient movement. Treatment of tone is discussed in Chapter 5.

Incoordination

Coordination deficits result in a deterioration of the quality of movement. In tests of coordination, patients should exhibit adequate strength and ROM to perform the desired movements. The quality of movement is determined by the timing and sequencing of muscle activity. The speed of movement should be increased to assess the motor unit's ability to rapidly turn on and off. Additionally, the range of movement for the task should be increased to further test the ability of the muscles to move within a sequenced pattern at a lengthened range. Chapter 7 describes the available testing procedures to measure coordination and the appropriate treatment strategies for enhancing movement quality.

Balance Dysfunction

Balance dysfunction may result from lesions within the cerebellum and the vestibular and somatosensory systems. It may also result from lack of muscle strength or be the byproduct of compensatory strategies used to maintain stable postures.

In assessing balance, pay particular attention to determining the specific causes of the observed balance dysfunction. The origin of the impairment (location of the lesion) will suggest the type of treatment program to be implemented. Chapter 8 describes in detail the various etiologies of balance dysfunctions, as well as assessment procedures and appropriate treatments based on the origin of the problem.

Sensory or Perceptual Deficits

Sensory or perceptual deficits that commonly impair the successful completion of movement tasks include visual impairments, left-sided neglect, and lack of proprioception, body awareness, and spatial orientation. The inability to receive or process sensory information that contributes to movement can result in disability. Chapter 6 describes assessment procedures to identify impairments in sensory integration or perceptual processing and provides recommendations for treatment techniques.

Table 3-3 is a general overview of testing techniques that may be performed to determine which impairments are present. Testing techniques for each of the four major types of impairments are discussed in greater detail in Chapters 5 to 8 of this text.

Step 4: Observation After Assessment

Assessment is most often a combination of treatment and evaluation. During the assessment, treatment interventions are often performed. The therapist may, for example, instruct patients to move in ways to reduce their disabilities, or to change their postures to reduce impairments or disabilities. At the end of the evaluation and treatment session, therapists

TABLE 3-3. General Overview of Testing Techniques*	
Impairment	**Testing Technique**
Weakness	Active range of motion, (AROM), passive range of motion (PROM), and strength testing
Tonal abnormalities	Observe a movement pattern, patient's ability to actively correct his or her own alignment or hold alignment statically once you have placed the extremity in alignment and PROM
Incoordination	Coordination tests including changes in range of movement and speed
Balance dysfunction	Ability to statically hold postures in sitting and standing; ability to move out of these static postures into dynamic functional movements
Sensory/perceptual dysfunction	Assess visual field, proprioception, kinesthesia, body awareness, and spatial awareness

* The reader is referred to chapters 5 through 8 for a detailed description of assessment procedures and treatment applications for each of the impairments listed.

should again observe patients to determine if they have retained any recently learned strategies for improving posture alignment or movement.

For example, if patients were instructed during the positioning of the extremity to maintain joint alignment and support, observe if this new positioning has been incorporated at the completion of the treatment session. If patients were instructed in ambulation, note whether or not they made any attempt to incorporate the suggestions into their gait patterns as they left the department. Observing patients after the assessment may provide insight into their motivation to change, the ability to retain new motor tasks, and their motor ability to begin to incorporate the task into their motor repertoire.

Figure 3-10 shows a patient's sitting posture after conclusion of the assessment. (Compare it with Fig. 3-8.)

Step 5: Community Mobility

The external environment must also be considered when assessing a patient's functional abilities. When patients are assessed and trained in ambulation on hard-floored, uncluttered physical therapy departments, their performance may not reflect how they will function in their home or community environments, where various support surfaces abound. Make every effort to vary the therapeutic environment so that patients encounter and learn to negotiate the real-world variables that can interfere with their mobility:

- Introduce soft and hard surfaces and chairs or beds of varying heights.
- Have the patient practice ambulation on carpeting or outdoors. Also have them walk in busy or cluttered environments.

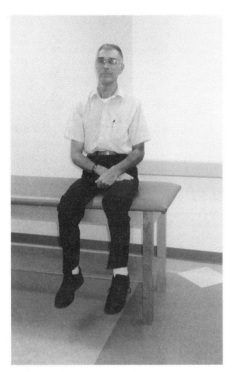

FIGURE 3-10. Patient exhibits improved posture after instruction in strategies to improve alignment.

- Instruct them to ascend and descend curbs.

Not only will these exercises enable you to better assess your patients' abilities, but they will help you to plan appropriate treatment interventions to promote your patients' functional independence at home and within their communities.

STANDARDIZED SCALES FOR FUNCTIONAL ASSESSMENT

Standardized scales that measure disability are recommended for use in combination with the assessment model. Together, these tools assist in quantifying the patient's initial status and changes over time. They also facilitate the documentation of assessment procedures and enhance communication among various rehabilitation disciplines.

The Functional Independence Measure (FIM), the Barthel Index, and the Rivermead Mobility Index are the standardized scales that we recommend for use in conjunction with this assessment model. Scales that are specific to a diagnosis, such as the National Institutes of Health Stroke Scale, the Kurtzke Scale (multiple sclerosis), and the Rappaport Scale (head injury), are used only with patients who have the specific problems the tests are designed to assess. A similar limitation is found with the Fugl–Meyer, the Motor Assessment Scale, and the Motricity Index, all of which measure weakness, and the Berg Balance Scale, which specifically detects balance dysfunction (AHCPR, 1985).

The FIM, the Barthel Index, and the Rivermead Mobility Index, presented in Appendix A, are valid and reliable. The AHCPR recommends the use of the FIM and Barthel to measure disability in the basic activities of daily living, and the Rivermead Mobility Index to measure mobility. These scales have two serious shortcomings: (1) they are not sensitive to change in patients in whom the disability is not severe, and (2) they do not contribute to the identification of impairments that contribute to disabilities (AHCPR, 1985). Use of these scales in conjunction with the assessment model addresses the second of these limitations.

SUMMARY

- The systems and task-oriented models are the basis of the assessment model described in this chapter.

- Knowledge of the various movement strategies used to complete the tasks of functional mobility in adults assists the therapist in recognizing abnormal movements, movement strategies that are unsuccessful in patients, or both.
- Functional mobility should be evaluated early in the assessment process to give the therapist guidance in problem-solving to identify impairments that contribute to disabilities.
- An understanding of how impairments may alter functional mobility is necessary in identifying factors that contribute to disabilities.
- The focus of the model for the assessment of disabilities and impairments is supported by the recommendations of the AHCPR.
- The standardized scales recommended for use in conjunction with the assessment model are the FIM, the Barthel Index, and the Rivermead Mobility Index.

REFERENCES

Agency for Health Care Policy and Research. (1985). *Clinical practice guidelines, post-stroke rehabilitation.* Washington, DC: U.S. Department of Health and Human Services.

Bernstein, N. (1967). *The coordination and regulation of movement.* London: Pergamon Press.

Carey, JR, & Burghardt, TP. (1993). Movement dysfunction following central nervous system lesions: A problem of neurologic or muscular impairment. *Physical Therapy, 73*(8), 538–547.

Carr, JH, & Shepherd, RB. (Eds.). (1987). *Movement science, foundations for physical therapy rehabilitation.* Rockville, MD: Aspen.

Craik, RL. (1994). *Mechanisms and spasticity.* Presented at APTA Combined Sections Meeting, San Antonio, TX.

Fiorentino, MR. (1981). *Reflex testing methods for evaluating CNS development* (2nd ed.). Springfield, IL: Thomas.

Gesell, A. (1954). Behavior patterns of fetal-infant and child. *Genetics. Proceedings of the Association for Research in Nervous and Mental Disease, 33,* 114.

Gordon, J. (1987). Assumptions underlying physical therapy intervention: Theoretical and historical perspectives. In JH Carr & RB Shepherd (Eds.). *Movement science, foundations for physical therapy rehabilitation.* Rockville, MD: Aspen.

Green, LN, & Williams, K. (1992). Differences in developmental movement patterns used by active versus sedentary middle-aged adults coming from a supine position to erect stance. *Physical Therapy, 72*(8), 560–568.

Grillner, S. (1981). Control of locomotion in bipeds, tetrapods and fish. In SR Geiger (Ed.). *Handbook of physiology* (Vol. 2, pp. 1179–1236). Bethesda, MD: American Psychological Society.

Horak, F. (1992). Assumptions underlying motor control for neurologic rehabilitation. In *Contemporary management of motor control problems.* Proceedings of the II-Step Conference, Foundation for Physical Therapy, Alexandria, VA.

Hufschmidt, A, & Mauritz, K-H. (1985). Chronic transformation of muscle in spasticity: A peripheral contribution to increased tone. *Journal of Neurology, Neurosurgery, and Psychiatry, 48,* 676–685.

McCoy, AO, & VanSant, AF. (1993). Movement patterns of adolescents rising from a bed. *Physical Therapy, 73,* 182–193.

Millington, PJ, Myklebust, BM, & Shambes, GM. (1992). Biomechanical analysis of the sit-to-stand motion in elderly persons. *Archives of Physical Medicine and Rehabilitation, 73,* 609–617.

Perry, J. (1992). *Gait analysis: Normal and pathological function.* Thorofare, NJ: Slack.

Polit, A, & Bizzi, E. (1979). Characteristics of motor programs underlying arm movements in monkeys. *Journal of Neurophysiology, 42,* 183–194.

Richter, RR, VanSant, AF, & Newton. RA. (1989). Description of adult rolling movements and hypothesis of developmental sequences. *Physical Therapy, 69*(1), 63–71.

Sarnacki, SJ. (1985). Rising from supine on a bed: A description of adult movement and hypothesis of developmental sequences. Unpublished master's thesis, Virginia Commonwealth University, Richmond.

Schenkman, M, Berger, RA, Riley, P, Mann, RW, & Hodge, WA. (1990). Whole-body movements during rising to standing from sitting. *Physical Therapy, 70*(10), 638–648.

Schenkman, M, & Butler, RB. (1989). A model for multisystem evaluation, interpretation, and treatment of individuals with neurologic dysfunction. *Physical Therapy, 69*(7), 538–547.

Schmidt, RA. (1991). Motor learning principles for physical therapy. In *Contemporary management of motor control problems.* Proceedings of the II Step Conference, Foundation for Physical Therapy, Alexandria, VA.

Shepherd, RB. (1994, July 21–22). *Training motor control in individuals with movement dysfunction following brain lesions.* Conference at Rehabilitation Institute of Chicago.

Sherrington, CS. (1906). *The integrative action of the nervous system* (p. 7). New Haven, CT: Yale University Press.

Shumway-Cook, A, & Woollacott, M. (1995). *Motor control, theory and practical applications.* Philadelphia: Williams & Wilkins.

Taub, E. (1976). Motor behavior following deafferentation in the developing and motorically mature monkey. *Advances in Behavioral Biology, 18,* 675–705.

VanSant, AF. (1988). Rising from a supine position to erect stance. *Physical Therapy, 68*(2), 185–192.

Walsche, FMP. (1961). Contribution of John Hughlings Jackson to neurology. *Archives of Neurology, 5,* 99–133.

Winstein, CJ. (1991). Designing practice for motor learning: Clinical implications. In *Contemporary management of motor control problems.* Proceedings of the II Step Conference, Foundation for Physical Therapy, Alexandria, VA.

SUGGESTED READINGS

Agency for Health Care Policy and Research. (1995). *Post-stroke rehabilitation, clinical practice guidelines.* Washington, DC: U.S. Department of Health and Human Services.

Convened by the AHCPR, a panel of experts representing medical and rehabilitation specialists in stroke rehabilitation produced the clinical guidelines. The guidelines are comprehensive and include the epidemiology and natural history of stroke, assessment methods, rehabilitation during acute care, screening for rehabilitation settings, managing rehabilitation, and transition to the community.

Fiorentino, MR. (1981). *Reflex testing methods for evaluating CNS development* (2nd ed.). Springfield, IL: Thomas.

This 53-page text has been used for understanding reflexive development from the spinal cord to the cortex. In addition to detailed descriptions on reflexes associated with the spinal, brain stem, midbrain, and cortical levels, descriptions are also provided of automatic movement reactions. Charts on reflex testing and motor development are also provided.

O'Sullivan, SB, & Schmidt, TJ. (1994). *Physical rehabilitation: Assessment and treatment* (3rd ed.). Philadelphia: Davis.

Early chapters focus on clinical decision-making and the assessment of specific systems. Additional chapters describe the assessment of commonly occurring diagnoses requiring rehabilitation (eg, stroke, arthritis, burns, spinal cord injury). Each of these chapters provides an overview of anatomy, pathophysiology, and medical and rehabilitative management.

Palmer, ML, & Toms, JE. (1992). *Manual for functional training* (3rd ed.). Philadelphia: Davis.

This text presents issues related to the mobility of patients who have suffered spinal cord injury, head trauma, and amputations. Chapters describe wheelchair mobility, home modifications, orthotics and prosthetics, functional activities for the patient populations addressed, and guarding issues.

Perry, J. (1992). *Gait analysis, normal and pathological function.* Thorofare, NJ: Slack.

This is a comprehensive text of normal and pathologic gait. The text is divided into four sections that describe the fundamentals of gait, including normal gait, pathologic gait, and gait analysis systems. Normal and pathologic gait are described in detail in terms of the forces acting on the joints, joint ROM, and muscular activity.

Wade, DT. (1992). *Measurement in neurological rehabilitation.* New York: Oxford University Press.

This is an in-depth review of the measurement tools associated with neurological rehabilitation. The four sections of the text include background on the choice and use of instrument, measurement at different levels (eg, motor and sensory, cognitive and emotional, handicap and quality of life), measurement in practice (ie, measurement issues specific to disease or diagnosis), and measures for neurological disability (impairment based, disabilities, and diagnosis specific).

Whiting, HTA. (1985). Human motor actions, Bernstein reassessed. *Advances in Psychology, 17.*

This text contains the English translations of six of the original writings of Nicoli Bernstein. In addition, there are two original writings by scientists who attended an international conference where each of Bernstein's six chapters were discussed. The six chapters written by Bernstein cover the techniques of the study of movement, the problem of the interrelation of coordination and localization, the biodynamics of locomotion, some emergent problems of the regulation of motor acts, trends and problems in the study of physiology of activity, and trends in physiology and their relation to cybernetics.

Theoretical Approach to Treatment

LEARNING OBJECTIVES

After reading this chapter, you should be able to:

1. Discuss the traditional theories of treatment in the rehabilitation of patients with neurological dysfunction.
2. Contrast the task-oriented theory of treatment with the traditional theories.
3. Recognize the appropriate use of selected techniques of facilitation in the treatment of low-functioning patients.
4. Understand how the systems and motor control theories are related to the task-oriented model.
5. Describe how motor learning should be incorporated into the task-oriented model.
6. Describe an integrated approach to treatment with the task-oriented model.

Theoretical approaches that serve as the basis of treatment for patients with lesions affecting the nervous system have been based on our continually evolving understanding of neurophysiology. Traditional theoretical approaches such as neurodevelopmental treatment (NDT), proprioceptive neuromuscular facilitation (PNF), and the strategies devised by Brunnstrom and Rood, were based on both the reflex–stimulus model and the hierarchical model (described in Chap. 3). Recent advances in the understanding of how the central nervous system (CNS) functions has led to the incorporation of the contemporary task-oriented model for treatment into the systems model, which holds that the CNS is just one of a network of systems responsible for movement.

Many traditional theories incorporated abnormal movement patterns, manual techniques, or both to *inhibit* (to hold back or keep from some action) or *facilitate* (to make easy or easier) movement. The effectiveness of these traditional therapies has recently been questioned because little evidence shows that gains made with this treatment approach carry over to improved function in daily life (Gordon, 1987). The contemporary task-oriented model is functionally based and incorporates multiple systems working together to complete a task.

This chapter describes the various theoretical treatments that have been used in the past and the task-oriented model for treatment that is recommended in this text. Our present understanding of neurophysiology supports functional, task-oriented treatment approaches. The traditional theories are presented for several reasons:

- To assist the reader in understanding the evolution of rehabilitation therapies for patients with neurological dysfunction
- To acknowledge the contributions of the theorists
- To recognize that traditional treatment techniques of facilitation may be appropriate to use in task-related activities in low-functioning patients

Low-functioning patients require manual assistance to perform functional movement. They may benefit from the application of selected facilitation techniques to promote motor activity in a posture or during a functional movement. **High-functioning patients** are capable of performing the tasks, but their movement strategies may be inefficient, unsafe, or both.

TRADITIONAL THEORISTS AND THEIR APPROACHES

The traditional theoretical approaches described are based on the work of Margaret Rood; Berta and Karl Bobath (NDT); Signe

Brunnstrom; and Herman Kabat, Margaret Knott, and Dorothy Voss (PNF).

Rood

Margaret Rood's contribution to the treatment of neurologically impaired patients covered two major areas: (1) motor development, or *designs of movement*, and (2) sensory stimulation techniques (Flanagan, 1966). According to Rood, the sequence of motor development encompasses these four concepts: mobility, stability, controlled mobility, and skill.

Rood grouped sensory stimuli that she used as either **phasic** (pertaining to the phases of movement) or **tonic** (holding contraction, stationary), and closely linked them to the type of motor pattern (mobility or stability) that was sought in treatment (Stockmeyer, 1966). To achieve a holding contraction, such as is attained with arm support in sitting, tonic stimuli such as **approximation** (a physical therapy technique in which the bones of a joint are brought together) or **joint compression** (the application of pressure to a joint) would be used. Phasic stimuli such as quick stretches are used for any activity requiring movement, such as reaching forward with the arm.

Stockmeyer (1966) defined Rood's four stages of motor development as follows:

Mobility: free, flexible movement that encompasses qualities of range and speed
Stability: motor function that fixes the body to enable weight-bearing and later in the motor progression enables dynamic holding during movement
Controlled mobility (initially termed ''mobility superimposed on stability'' by Rood): fixation of the distal segment of an extremity with movement of the proximal segment. An example of this is rocking forward and backward in the quadruped position. The hands and knees are fixed

in weight-bearing positions while the shoulder, pelvis, and trunk move.

Skill: a coordinated movement that enables the distal segment of an extremity to manipulate an object while in a stabilized posture. In the quadruped position, skill is demonstrated by reaching up with one upper extremity to explore the environment as the opposite upper extremity provides stability.

Rood advocated the use of sensory stimuli to facilitate or inhibit responses. The sensory stimuli she used are categorized according to whether they facilitate or inhibit movement (Display 4-1). Brief descriptions of how each stimulus is applied are provided in Chapter 5.

These sensory stimuli may facilitate a muscle response or inhibit unwanted postural or muscle tone. The physiologic response to the sensory techniques is most often based on the activation of **muscle spindles** (receptors sensitive to length of muscle), Golgi tendon organs, or **cutaneous receptors** (receptors sensitive to touch). The carotid sinus is an exception because it activates **baroreceptors** (receptors sensitive to changes in blood pressure). The premise of Rood's techniques is based on the work of Sherrington and the reflex stimulus model.

Once the desired response is obtained (ie, muscle activation or inhibition), the sensory stimulus should be withdrawn. Repeated application of the stimulus should be occasional, not

 DISPLAY 4-1
Sensory Stimuli

Rehabilitation therapists use a variety of sensory stimuli to elicit responses from their patients. These stimuli can either facilitate or inhibit a desired response.

Facilitation

Approximation: drawing the bones of a joint together (the application of pressure to a joint)

Ice applications (3–5 seconds): quick stroking of an ice cube on the skin

Joint compression: the application of pressure to a joint

Light touch: the application of a gentle touch, such as with a cotton swab

Quick stretch: a quick elongation of a muscle at its lengthened state or during a contraction

Resistance: a strengthening exercise done by applying an outside force to a muscle to force it to develop greater tension. Resistance may be applied manually by the therapist, or mechanically, through the application of weights.

Tapping: the tapping of the muscle belly of weak muscles to produce volitional contraction

Traction: drawing or pulling of the joints of spine or extremities

Inhibition

Prolonged stretch or deep pressure
Warm or neutral temperature
Prolonged cold (15–20 minutes)
Slow stroking down posterior rami
Carotid reflex

consistent, to avoid having the patient make a conditioned response to the stimulus. The treatment goal is muscle activation, or performance of the task, which should occur independently of the therapist's application of a sensory stimulus.

In this text, we advocate the application of selected facilitation techniques during a functional task. For example, a patient who is having difficulty maintaining weight on an involved lower extremity should practice weight-shifting while standing. This is a functional task that incorporates joint approximation in the hip and knee, an exercise that facilitates contraction of the muscles of extension around the joint.

Similarly, to promote extension of the triceps, support the patient's arm on a table with the elbow flexed. Have the patient achieve extension by reaching out for a cup. If motor activation is not occurring, tap on the muscle belly with your hand. Theoretically, tapping activates muscle spindles in much the same way that a quick muscle stretch does. When muscle spindles are activated, a signal that a muscle is being stretched is sent, exciting alpha motor neurons within the spinal cord. This, in turn, causes the muscle to contract. Tapping is performed while the patient is reaching for an object to provide an added stimulus for the muscle to fire. Facilitation techniques may be beneficial in assisting muscle activation during a functional task.

Karl and Berta Bobath: Neurodevelopmental Treatment (NDT)

Neurodevelopmental treatment is also referred to as the Bobath approach after its founding theorists, Dr. Karl Bobath and Berta Bobath. Karl Bobath, a physician, and Berta Bobath, a physical therapist, spent much of their professional careers treating children with cerebral palsy (CP) and adults with hemiplegia. In both populations, the Bobaths observed that abnormal tone and coordination problems (or muscular imbalances) were due to the release of *abnormal postural reflexes* (primitive reflexes seen at brain stem or spinal cord levels; see Display 3-2) that inhibited righting reactions, equilibrium reactions, and automatic movements. Abnormal patterns of posture and movement resulted from the loss of CNS control as a consequence of disease or injury (Semans, 1966).

Loss of righting reactions, equilibrium reactions, and automatic responses limit normal development, which is the primary model used in NDT. Neurodevelopmental treatment is based on the hierarchical model of neurophysiologic function. Montgomery (1991) states that "NDT identifies the problem as release of abnormal and widespread reflex patterns of posture and movement from inhibition, specifically brainstem, cerebellum, midbrain, basal ganglia, and cortex" (p.135).

According to Montgomery, the general goal of NDT is to "achieve a balance between muscle groups and to decrease the effects of abnormal tonal influence on automatic responses and movement patterns" (p. 135).

The developmental sequence (Fig. 4-1) served as the basis of treatment of the NDT approach for many years. Treatment emphasized normalizing muscle tone, inhibiting primitive reflexes, and facilitating normal postural reactions through the developmental sequence (Montgomery & Connolly, 1991). This was accomplished by handling. During **handling,** the therapists put their hands on the patient in specific regions (**key points of control**) to facilitate targeted movements and inhibit other, unwanted movements.

The treatment principles for NDT are:

- To change abnormal patterns of movement with **dynamic reflex inhibiting patterns** (**RIPs**) (a specific handling technique to produce inhibition of excessive tone)

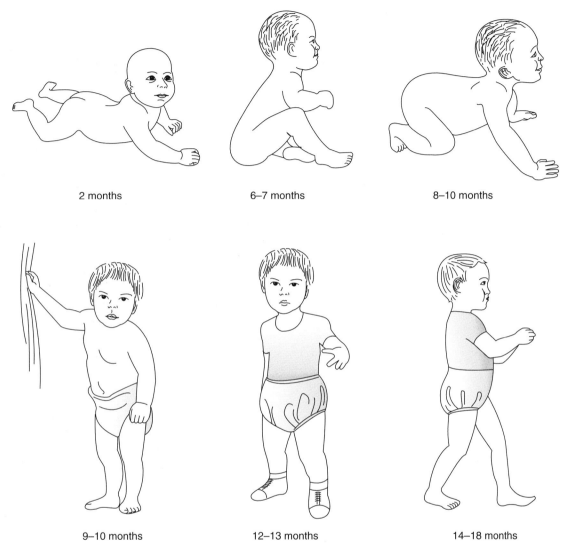

2 months   6–7 months   8–10 months

9–10 months   12–13 months   14–18 months

FIGURE 4-1. Developmental sequence: Motor skills emerge as the child develops postural control.

- To use key points of control (neck and spine, shoulders, pelvis, toes and ankles, and fingers and wrists) as manual contacts
- To replace abnormal tone or patterns of movement immediately with normal movement patterns (Ostrosky, 1990)

The RIPs are used to move the extremities out of the abnormal positions that developed from abnormal tone and into antagonistic patterns. For example, an arm that is flexed and internally rotated is extended and externally rotated. The RIP decreases abnormal tone in flexor components, while dynamically positioning the extremity for the activation of extensor muscles.

The RIP can be considered a handling technique because it allows the therapist to manually assist the patient to achieve alignment, righting, or equilibrium reactions using principles similar to those involving the key points of control. Patients who assume slouched sitting postures with lower extremity extension may require manual assistance from the therapist in moving the pelvis anteriorly before placing the feet under the chair so that they can attempt to stand. Abnormal tone may or may not be present in the lower extremity, but manually assisting the patient at a key point of control assists in the biomechanical performance of the task.

Other components of NDT include:

- Varying the activity level according to the level of difficulty the patient can handle
- Varying the context in which the activity occurs
- Adhering to the developmental sequence is used, although not necessarily in series (Ostrosky, 1990)

Varying the difficulty of activities and the environment in which they are performed are principles that NDT shares with the motor control theory. Just as in weight lifting, where the goal of increasing muscle strength can be achieved only if the amount of weight lifted is continually increased, tasks are made increasingly difficult so that individuals can progress beyond their current level. Changing environments may also increase the difficulty of the task, but it should enable the patient to transfer the task to other environments.

Neurodevelopmental treatment has evolved over the past several years to incorporate activities that encourage functional carryover. Most activities used in NDT are functional activities that patients performed before onset of their disability.

Brunnstrom

Signe Brunnstrom identified seven stages of recovery, based on observing her patients after a stroke (Display 4-2). Brunnstrom's theory was based on the hierarchical model developed by Hughlings Jackson. Brunnstrom believed that movement *synergies* (patterns of muscle activity) occurred at a spinal cord level as a result of the hierarchical organization of the CNS (VanSant, 1992). This concept of synergistic movement at the spinal cord level is still popular today, although synergies now go by the name of *functional movement patterns* (Brooks, 1986).

The seven recovery stages described by Brunnstrom are used extensively to document motor recovery seen in patients with stroke. Knowledge of these stages is universal among physicians and nurses, as well as occupational, speech, and physical therapists. Recovery starts with a period of flaccidity (stage 1) and may progress through full recovery (stage 7), with the return of normal motor function.

Brunnstrom believed that introducing sensory input from the periphery was beneficial to developing the desired motor responses. In this regard, she was incorporating the reflex stimulus model. She advocated the use of cutaneous and muscle sensations and maximally resisting voluntary movement of normally innervated muscles to create overflow to recruit the involved musculature (Sigwarth, 1990). For example, tapping over the biceps brachii muscle belly was used to activate cutaneous receptors and muscle spindles to increase the contractile response from the muscle. Resisting the contraction of synergistic muscles (such as wrist flexors) was also used to activate the involved biceps muscle via the **overflow phenomenon,** the process by which activity is detected in an unexercised muscle during excitation of a muscle in another part of the body.

During the early recovery stages, Brunnstrom encouraged control of limb synergy pat-

DISPLAY 4-2
Brunnstrom's Seven Stages of Recovery

Stage 1. Immediately following the acute episode, flaccidity of the involved limbs is present, and no movement, on either a reflex or a voluntary basis, can be initiated.

Stage 2. As recovery begins, the basic limb synergies or some of their components may appear as associated reactions, or minimal voluntary movement responses may be present. Spasticity begins to develop and may be particularly evident in muscle groups that dominate synergy movement (eg, elbow flexors, knee extensors).

Stage 3. The patient gains voluntary control of the movement synergies, although full range of all synergy components does not necessarily develop. Spasticity, which may become severe in some cases, reaches its peak. This stage in the recovery process may be thought of as semivoluntary in that the patient is able to initiate movement in the involved limbs on a volitional basis but is unable to control the form of the resulting movement, which will be the basic limb synergies.

Stage 4. Some movement combinations that do not follow the paths of the basic limb synergies are mastered, first with difficulty, then with increasing ease. Spasticity begins to decline, but the influence of spasticity on nonsynergistic movements is still readily observable.

Stage 5. If recovery continues, more difficult movement combinations are mastered as the basic limb synergies lose their dominance over motor acts. Spasticity continues to decline.

Stage 6. Individual joint movements become possible, and coordination approaches normalcy. As spasticity disappears, the patient becomes capable of a full spectrum of movement patterns.

Stage 7. As the last recovery stage, normal motor function is restored.

terns, with the use of afferent stimuli of proprioceptive and exteroreceptive (pertaining to organs that receive stimuli from outside the body) origin. Selected primitive postural reflexes (eg, asymmetrical tonic neck, associated reactions) were used to elicit voluntary movement. This treatment approach was contrary to what was proposed by other traditional theorists because it had the *unintended* result of emphasizing abnormal movement patterns.

Brunnstrom's contributions to understanding motor recovery from stroke were monumental. However, her emphasis on reinforcing abnormal movement patterns is rarely used now because, once learned, the abnormal movement patterns become difficult, if not impossible, to break.

Kabat, Knott, and Voss: Proprioceptive Neuromuscular Facilitation (PNF)

Proprioceptive neuromuscular facilitation was originally developed in the early 1950s by Dr. Herman Kabat, a neurophysiologist and physician, and Maggie Knott, a physical therapist. The goal of this therapeutic technique was to strengthen muscles in the movement patterns in which they were designed to function. Later Dorothy Voss, a physical therapist, added to the development of clinical techniques used today.

The patterns of motion used in PNF are **mass movement patterns,** which are characteristic of normal motor activity. These patterns are *spiral* and *diagonal,* in keeping with the spiral and rotary characteristics of skeletal muscle, and closely resemble the movements used in sports and work activities. The diagonal patterns were designed to address specific problems, such as weakness through partial ranges, lack of stability, and weakness in eccentric contractions.

The total patterns of movement in PNF are based on the developmental sequence and the sequential mastery of those motor milestones (Duesterhaus, 1991). The hierarchical model is the framework for the theoretical development of PNF. The original theoretical goal of PNF was to lay down **gross motor patterns** within the CNS; "to 'engram' movement patterns as close to normal as possible into the central nervous system" (Duesterhaus, 1991, p. 139). This could be a limiting aspect of PNF because there are many varieties of movement patterns; it would be useless to lay down only one or two patterns of movement for any given task.

In PNF, two diagonals of motion exist for each major part of the body, and each diagonal is made up of two patterns that are antagonistic to each other. This is done to address muscle imbalances (Voss, Ionta, & Myers, 1985). Each pattern has a major component of flexion or extension (D1 flexion, D1 extension, D2 flexion, D2 extension). In addition, each diagonal involves movement toward and across the midline or movement across and away from the midline. Each diagonal also includes rotation with the flexion or extension pattern.

Treatment techniques are added to the diagonals to increase muscle activation or range of motion. Some of these techniques include:

- Slow reversal and slow reversal hold
- Repeated contractions with quick stretch
- Agonistic reversal
- Rhythmic initiation
- Hold relax active movement
- Hold relax or contract relax
- Rhythmic stabilization

These techniques, which are explained in Chapter 5, are examples of the use of sensory information to facilitate a movement pattern. Manual contacts used in PNF facilitate underlying muscles and are used to apply resistance in the movement pattern to activate muscle spindles or Golgi tendon organs.

Summary of Traditional Theorists' Contributions

The contributions of the traditional theorists mentioned are numerous. Their theories provided the framework for which treatment programs were developed. They also added to our current understanding of the CNS and abnormal movement observed when damage occurs to the system. Some of the treatment techniques advocated by Rood (eg, techniques of facilitation) and the Bobaths are continually practiced, and are beneficial to function when incorporated into task-oriented behavior.

CONTEMPORARY TASK-ORIENTED MODEL

The systems model described by Bernstein (1967) is the general theoretical basis for the task-oriented model. As described in Chapter 3, the systems approach to treatment is geared primarily to task-oriented activities inclusive of the interaction of multiple physiologic systems (ie, muscles, joints, CNS), the environment, and the individual's motivation to complete the task.

In the systems model, no one system dominates another (as is characteristic of the hierarchical model). The model is rather egalitarian in its integration of all the factors that have as a common goal the accomplishment of a specific task. Thus, rehabilitation of patients with neurological dysfunction who may have a variety of problems (eg, muscle weakness, ataxia, soft tissue restrictions) should be best served by a task-oriented approach. The focus of the task-oriented model in this text is on the practice of those tasks in functional mobility that are inefficient, unsafe, or cannot be performed. It is not uncommon for a patient to present with a combination of these problems.

We avoid using the term "motor control" in our discussion of the task-oriented model because there is currently no singular definition of this theoretical approach. However, the reader should recognize that the task-oriented model is embedded in motor control theory, which is itself an integral part of the systems theory (Fig. 4-2). It is also our belief that the

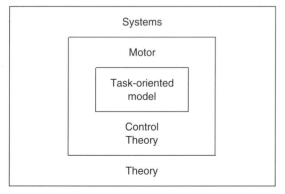

FIGURE 4-2. Integration of task-oriented model within motor control and systems theories.

task-oriented model is a comprehensive term that includes theories of motor learning as well as those of motor control. The theories of motor control and motor learning are described later in this chapter.

Researchers who have contributed to our understanding of the task-oriented model are Carr and Shepherd, Gordon, and Horak, each of whom is discussed below.

Carr and Shepherd

Janet Carr and Roberta Shepherd (1987) were the first to refer to physical therapists as "applied movement scientists," a term which we enthusiastically endorse. The analysis and practice of task- specific activities are emphasized in the Carr and Shepherd Motor Relearning Program (Display 4-3). Therapists are able to identify those factors that limit successful completion of the requested activity by analyzing the tasks to be performed and comparing them to normal biomechanical movement. A similar model for assessment is described in Chapter 3, which emphasizes observing the tasks of functional mobility to determine which impairments contribute to disability.

Carr and Shepherd believe that the role of movement scientists in treatment is to create an environment in which patients practice goal-directed behavior that will enable them to relearn the task. Practice sessions may include breaking the task into discrete components, followed by practice of the whole task. Verbal and visual feedback should be provided to facilitate relearning of the task. Manual guidance is provided as needed, but emphasis is placed on using the patient's own **internal biofeedback** systems for learning (ie, somatosensory and visual systems) (Carr & Shepherd, 1987).

Carr and Shepherd, like many other rehabilitation therapists, stress having the patient practice the task in a variety of environments. They also encourage therapists to work with the pa-

---

DISPLAY 4-3
Carr and Shepherd's Motor Relearning Program

Step 1: Analysis of Task
        Observation
        Comparison
        Analysis
Step 2: Practice of Missing Components
        Explanation—identification of goal
        Instruction
        Practice plus verbal and visual feedback plus manual guidance
Step 3: Practice of Task
        Explanation—identification of goal
        Instruction
        Practice plus verbal and visual feedback plus manual guidance
        Reevaluation
        Encourage flexibility
Step 4: Transference of Training
        Opportunity to practice in context
        Consistency of practice
        Organization of self-monitored practice
        Structured learning environment
        Involvement of relatives and staff

---

tient on achieving flexibility of movement patterns.

Gordon

Understanding the problems faced by the CNS in controlling movement is a key assumption of the task-oriented model according to James Gordon (1987). The problems may include changes within the musculoskeletal system, previously learned movement strategies stored in the brain, and the challenges of the environment.

For example, imagine that you have decided to take up a new sport–curling. Your bowling skills are fairly good, so you anticipate that curling should be easy to master. Your CNS may, however, have more of an adjustment to make than you might think. Examine a few of the problems that the CNS has to solve in completing this new task:

- It has to recall the previously learned movement strategies you used to roll a bowling ball.
- Then it has to adapt those movement patterns to an environment that now consists of ice.
- It must concentrate on maintaining your equilibrium so that you can balance on the ice surface.
- The CNS must determine how the musculoskeletal system will respond to the new environment, how the previously

learned movement strategies need to be altered, and how to produce a movement pattern to accomplish this task.

Multiple systems are integrated by the CNS in this whole process. How the CNS coordinates all of these problems was first formulated by Bernstein (1967) in the systems model. Once you understand the complexity of curling from the CNS's perspective, it is easy to understand that you will need time to learn this new motor task. It will require multiple repetitions, in varying environments (Gordon, 1987). This is analogous to the rehabilitation tasks facing the disabled patient.

Horak

Fay Horak also views the task-oriented model as a component of motor control and the larger systems theory:

> From the systems model of motor control, the task-oriented model assumes that control of movement is organized around goal-directed, functional behaviors rather than on muscles or movement patterns. (Horak, 1992, p. 20)

Horak also emphasizes that different people can perform the same task differently. As a result, she insists on the therapist's training the patient in more than one movement pattern. This will allow the patient to use alternative movement strategies to accomplish the **functional tasks** efficiently.

Horak also recognized a few limitations of the task-oriented model. First and foremost, it is difficult to quantify the effectiveness and efficiency of movement patterns used to accomplish the task at hand. The model de-emphasizes hands-on treatment by the therapist and instead emphasizes how the patient uses cognitive information to explore the best strategies for movement. Although this approach has

its merits, patients who have severe neurological impairments may have difficulty with the hands-off approach. The techniques of facilitation may be of use in treating these severely impaired patients.

Summary of the Task-Oriented Model

The task-oriented model is based on systems theory, which itself is an integral part of both the motor control and motor learning theories. Carr and Shepherd provide insight into how the model can be used to identify limitations of movement (impairments). They also advocate the use of part-task activities to assist in developing successful whole-task movement.

Gordon, Carr and Shepherd, and Horak all emphasize the role of motor learning in the model and focus on tasks that are functionally goal directed.

THEORIES OF MOTOR CONTROL AND MOTOR LEARNING

There are several definitions, or theories, of motor control. Shumway-Cook and Woollacott (1995) define *motor control* "as the study of the nature and cause of movement" (p. 3). Their theories of motor control include:

- All of the neurophysiologic theories described in Chapter 3 (reflex, hierarchical, systems)
- Task-oriented theory
- Motor programming theories
- Dynamical action theory
- Parallel distributed processing theory
- Ecological theories

Horak (1992) includes the reflex, hierarchical, and systems theories as models of motor control, but describes the task-oriented model as a component of a larger neurological rehabilitation model. Burtner and Woollacott (1996) describe the reflex, hierarchical, and systems theories as theories of motor control, and also include a modular theory and dynamical systems theory.

One would conclude from these three references that theories of motor control are numerous and not definitive. It may be safe to summarize the many theories by saying that motor control is a discipline that "pursues an understanding of how motor activities are planned, initiated, and carried efficiently and accurately to completion" (Fredericks & Saladin, 1996, p. 107).

Motor learning has been defined as the acquisition of skill (Schmidt, 1991). In the case of patients with neurological disabilities, motor relearning is focused on the reacquisition of previously learned skills with a CNS that has been damaged. If motor control is the study of the nature and cause of movement, then motor learning is the acquisition of the movement.

Numerous textbooks and articles have been written on motor learning, particularly in healthy individuals. Schmidt (1991) and Winstein (1991) have explored the relationship between motor learning and the practice of skill acquisition in physical therapy.

Schmidt (1991) makes a distinction between the performance of motor tasks and learning, which is an important factor to be included in the task-oriented model. Proper performance of a task in a physical therapy clinic has no bearing on whether the patient has learned that task and can transfer its motor component to other environments. Performance implies only that the motor behavior can be repeated with practice in that specific environment under certain conditions. Learning requires that the skill in question be retained and transferred to other environments.

Performance is seen when the patient is able to stand up from a seated position on a low mat table in the physical therapy clinic. With practice, the patient performs the task in the physical therapy clinic moving from a specific surface. The patient who has learned the motor task will be able to transfer these sitting-to-standing skills to different environments. The inability to transfer the task to other environments implies that the patient never learned the movement pattern in the first place, but was simply capable of performing the task in a restricted setting.

Two principles of practice, blocked and random, are used in motor learning (Schmidt, 1991). **Blocked practice** occurs when the learner practices one task or activity before moving on to the next activity. **Random practice** occurs when tasks or activities to be learned are practiced together. For example, when teaching the sit-to-stand maneuver and ambulation in blocked practice, the patient would be required to repeat the first maneuver several times before practicing ambulation. However, in random practice the two movement patterns would be practiced together repeatedly. Research has demonstrated that random practice results in greater retention of motor skills (Shea & Morgan, 1975).

Feedback to facilitate the acquisition of motor skills has been provided in a variety of forms, most often verbal. In the 1980s, it was believed that more frequent and more immediate feedback was beneficial for motor learning (Schmidt, 1991). This type of feedback was effective in promoting the performance of the activity but ineffective in facilitating retention of the motor skill (Schmidt, 1991).

Learning a motor skill is enhanced by providing feedback or information about how a task was performed. This is known as communicating the **knowledge of results.** This information is useful when provided after the skill has been completed; it is not particularly helpful when communicated during the activity. Winstein

(1991) reported that randomly offered knowledge of results was superior to blocked or scheduled knowledge of results. Blocked knowledge of results may be considered part of the conditioning model described by Pavlov.

Certainly, cuing patients during every aspect of the motor activity is a conditioned response. How often have you overheard a therapist during gait training repeatedly give the cues "cane, right foot, left foot, cane. . ."? This type of feedback conditions patients to move when they hear verbal stimuli; it does not facilitate learning motor skills. What would happen if cuing were suddenly not provided? In most cases, patients would experience difficulty completing the motor task without the conditioned verbal stimulus.

Internal feedback, such as proprioception, should be used in addition to verbal feedback to facilitate learning of activities. Instruct patients to think about placement of their extremities or how their bodies move during an activity. They may need to visually watch their extremities or the movement to increase proprioceptive awareness. This can be enhanced with the use of a mirror or by videotaping them during the task and replaying the tape to provide knowledge of results. Ask patients to analyze their movement during the replay of the tape to increase their awareness of how they move.

Provide manual assistance to enable patients to "feel" how the movement is to be performed when neither verbal nor visual feedback is sufficient. Manual assistance may be provided to achieve a correct posture (as in moving the pelvis anterior during sitting) or to assist in a dynamic movement (such as during the swing phase of the involved extremity).

Another factor to be considered in learning a motor skill is breaking the task down into its parts. Carr and Shepherd (1987) advocated using part-task movements as a means of achieving whole-task movement. Although some complex whole tasks can be broken into subunits and practiced piecemeal, this strategy is not appropriate for all motor tasks. Whole tasks must have natural subunits that can be practiced in isolation.

Winstein and colleagues (1989) reported that weight-shifting in standing did not transfer to weight-shifting during gait. She hypothesized that the weight-shifting phase of gait (*loading response*) may not be a natural subunit of gait. This may be due to the continuous dynamic nature of gait, which is different from the intermittent weight-shifting done in standing. Determining which part-task activities are appropriate may be a challenge because identification of part-task activities for whole tasks has not been consistently reported in the literature. Winstein (1991) does, however, suggest that forward trunk flexion in preparation for the whole sit-to-stand movement is a natural subunit of the whole task. It can thus be used as a part-task activity for sit-to-stand.

Naylor and Briggs (1963) suggest that whole tasks that involve continuous movements and last less than 200 msec may not be appropriate for part-task practice. Movements that are *serial*, or step-by step in their pattern, are more likely candidates for this type of practice.

We recommend that the performance of whole tasks be incorporated into the task-oriented model as the primary focus of retraining motor skills. Part-task activities should be incorporated when the whole task is difficult to perform and it lends itself to being broken down into discrete subunits. When using part-task activities, always incorporate whole-task activities within the same treatment sessions (Carr & Shepherd, 1987). The part-task activities that we recommend in Section 2 have not been reported to be natural subunits, and therefore may or may not be successful in retraining whole tasks. The part-task activities suggested in this text were chosen because biomechanical analysis of the whole task proved them to be likely candidates for part-task practice.

Key factors for motor control and motor learning include:

- Varying the practice setting and environment to facilitate learning of the motor skill
- Having the patient practice the tasks randomly
- Providing feedback on the desired outcome of the task after the patient has completed the task and incorporating patient biofeedback as often as possible to improve or reinforce learning the task
- Having the patient practice the whole task and incorporate part-task activities as needed

In the varied environments in which our patients will need to move, the most efficient treatment approach to enable safe, proficient mobility must be provided by therapists.

INTEGRATED TREATMENT IN THE TASK-ORIENTED MODEL

Research supports the use of task-oriented treatment as effective in relearning functional activities. Patients who are low functioning (eg, those who need maximal assistance with bed mobility and accomplishing the supine-to-sit maneuver) should be treated with a task-oriented model; however, it may be appropriate to include specific traditional treatments to facilitate motor activity.

For example, when practicing supported sitting with a patient who is low functioning, placing the involved upper extremity out to the side of the body on the mat or bed may encourage weight-bearing through the extremity. This placement of the involved extremity and weight-bearing through the arm uses the technique of joint approximation. Tapping the triceps brachii muscle belly in this position is an-

other adjunctive treatment to activating a muscle response in a functional position.

A similar type of patient who has difficulty with weight-bearing in an involved lower extremity should be placed in standing position, which produces manual compression of the hip and knee joint. Tapping of the involved quadriceps muscle, while standing and weight-bearing, may encourage additional muscle activity in this functional position.

As stated by Carr and Shepherd (1987), physical therapists are movement scientists. As such, they should examine patient movement patterns before intervening with instruction on a "standard" way to move. Before the disability, each patient relied on movement strategies that had been learned while taking age, musculoskeletal structure, and other comorbidities (eg, arthritis) into consideration. Keep this in mind as you observe the movement strategies used by your patients. Intervene as needed to maintain a safe environment and to assist with completion of the task. New movement strategies may be developed based on the physical abilities of the patient. Provide opportunities for patients to solve the problem of their own movement difficulties. This will encourage them to develop new movements and reinforce learning of the motor skills needed to accomplish the task being taught.

SUMMARY

- The traditional theoretical approaches attributed to Rood; Karl and Berta Bobath (NDT); Brunnstrom; and Kabat, Knott, and Voss (PNF) are based on the reflex–stimulus model and the hierarchical model. Many of the traditional techniques developed by these theorists are incorporated in retraining the patient in task-oriented behavior.

- Selected traditional treatment approaches may still be appropriate with low-functioning patients when performed in functional postures or during functional movement.
- The systems and motor control theories serve as the foundations for the task-oriented model. The systems theory holds that functional movement relies on the successful integration of input from many systems. Motor control theories are set forth to understand movement in terms of how it is planned, initiated, and executed.
- Motor learning should be incorporated into the task-oriented model.
- Creating varied environments for practice of motor skills and incorporating patients' internal biofeedback will aid patients as they relearn specific movement patterns.

REFERENCES

Bernstein, N. (1967). *The coordination and regulation of movement.* London: Pergamon Press.

Brooks, VB. (1986). *The neural basis of motor control.* New York: Oxford University Press.

Burtner, PA, & Woollacott, MH. (1996). Theories of motor control. In CM Fredericks & LK Saladin (Eds.). *Pathophysiology of the motor systems: Principles and clinical presentations.* Philadelphia: Davis.

Carr, JH, & Shepherd, RB. (1987). *Movement science, foundations for physical therapy rehabilitation.* Rockville, MD: Aspen.

Duesterhaus, MA. (1991). Proprioceptive neuromuscular facilitation and the approach of Rood. In *Contemporary management of motor control problems.* Proceedings of the II Step Conference. Foundation for Physical Therapy, Alexandria, VA.

Flanagan, EM. (1966). Methods for facilitation and inhibition of motor activity. *American Journal of Physical Medicine, 46*(1), 1006–1011.

Fredericks, CM, & Saladin, LK. (Eds.). (1996) *Pathophysiology of the motor systems: Principles and clinical presentations.* Philadelphia: Davis.

Gordon, J. (1987). Assumptions underlying physical therapy intervention: Theoretical and historical perspectives. In *Movement science, foundations for physical therapy rehabilitation.* Rockville, MD: Aspen.

Horak, F. (1991). Assumptions underlying motor control for neurologic rehabilitation. In *Contemporary management of motor control problems.* Proceedings of the II Step Conference. Foundation for Physical Therapy, Alexandria, VA.

Montgomery, PC. (1991). Neurodevelopmental treatment and sensory integrative theory. In *Contemporary management of motor control problems.* Proceedings of the II Step Conference. Foundation for Physical Therapy, Alexandria, VA.

Montgomery, PC, & Connolly, BH. (1991). *Motor control and physical therapy: Theoretical framework and practical applications.* Hixson, TN: Chattanooga Group.

Naylor, J, & Briggs, G. (1963). Effects of task complexity and task organization on the relative efficiency of part and whole training methods. *Journal of Experimental Psychology, 65,* 217.

Ostrosky, KM. (1990, May/June). Facilitation vs motor control. *Clinical Management, 10,* 34–40.

Schmidt, RA. (1991). Motor learning principles for physical therapy. In *Contemporary management of motor control problems.* Proceedings of the II Step Conference. Foundation for Physical Therapy, Alexandria, VA.

Semans, S. (1966). The Bobath concept in treatment of neurological disorders. *American Journal of Physical Medicine, 46*(1), 732–785.

Shea, JB, & Morgan, RL. (1975). Contextual interference effects on the acquisition, retention, and transfer of a motor skill. *Journal Experimental Psychology [Human Learning Memory]. 5,* 179–187.

Shumway-Cook, A, & Woollacott, M. (1995). *Motor control, theory and practical applications.* Baltimore: Williams & Wilkins.

Sigwarth, DM. (1990). Therapeutic exercise programs for neurologic patients: A survey of entry-level physical therapy programs. *Neurology Report, 14*(4), 8–13.

Stockmeyer, SA. (1966). An interpretation of the approach of Rood to the Treatment of neuromuscular dysfunction. *American Journal of Physical Medicine, 46*(1), 900–946.

VanSant, A. (1992). Brunnstrom's treatment approach in the light of contemporary motor-control concepts. In Sawner, K, & LaVigne, J. (Eds.). *Brunnstrom's movement therapy in hemiplegia, a neurophysiological approach* (2nd ed.). Philadelphia: Lippincott.

Voss, DE, Ionta, MK, & Myers, BJ. (1985). *Propriocep-tive neuromuscular facilitation, patterns and techniques* (3rd ed.). Philadelphia: Harper & Row.

Winstein, C. (1991). Designing practice for motor learning. In *Contemporary management of motor control problems.* Proceedings of the II Step Conference. Foundation for Physical Therapy, Alexandria, VA.

Winstein, CJ, Gardner, ER, McNeal, DR, Barto, PS, Nicholson, DE. (1989). Standing balance training: Effect on balance and locomotion in hemiparetic adults. *Archives Physical Medicine and Rehabilitation, 70,* 755–762.

●●

SUGGESTED READINGS

Carr, JH, & Shepherd, RB. (1987). *Movement science, foundations for physical therapy rehabilitation.* Rockville, MD: Aspen.

The text begins with the role of the physical therapist as a movement scientist and reviews the various traditional theoretical perspectives that have guided treatment, the advent of the systems theory as a basis for motor control, and the task-oriented model. The motor relearning program developed by Carr and Shepherd is described in detail. Contributor Ann Gentile discusses skill acquisition for action, movement, and neuromotor processes; Jean Held discusses recovery of function after brain damage and its theoretical implications.

Fredericks, CM, & Saladin. LK. (1996). *Pathophysiology of the motor systems: Principles and clinical presentations.* Philadelphia: Davis.

This text is comprehensive in its presentation of the pathophysiology of the motor system and the description, by disease, of changes occurring within the system. The six sections of this text include: basic components of the motor systems from a cellular and tissue perspective, control of motor activity including systems that regulate and coordinate movement (described at each anatomic level), clinical manifestations of motor dysfunction, disorders of the motor unit including neuromuscular diseases, disorders of central motor control (described by disease), and the consequences of immobilization.

Sawner, K, & LaVigne, J. (1992). *Brunnstrom's movement therapy in hemiplegia, a neurophysiological approach* (2nd ed.). Philadelphia: Lippincott.

Sawner and LaVigne provide an update of the Brunnstrom approach to treatment with emphasis on the motor behavior of adults with hemiplegia, recovery stages and evaluation procedures, training procedures for the trunk and upper extremity, gait patterns in hemiplegia, walking preparation, and gait training. Brunnstrom's approach is also considered in light of the new motor control theories. The chapter on recovery stages is of particular interest.

Shumway-Cook, A, & Woollacott, M. (1995). *Motor control, theory and practical applications.* Baltimore: Williams & Wilkins.

The text is presented in four sections: theoretical framework, posture and balance, mobility functions, and upper extremity control. Numerous case studies are interspersed throughout the text to assist the reader in applying the material to clinical situations. Life span changes are discussed as they relate to posture, balance, and mobility functions.

Voss, DE, Ionta, MK, & Myers, BJ. (1985). *Proprioceptive neuromuscular facilitation* (3rd ed.). Philadelphia: Harper & Row.

A brief history of the development and evolution of PNF is presented in this edition, along with chapters on the patterns of motion for all extremities and the trunk, techniques for facilitation, stimulation of vital and related functions, PNF and joint mobilization, evaluation and treatment programs, and a discussion of practice and motor learning. Of particular interest are the chapters on patterns of movement and techniques of facilitation.

Weakness

Learning Objectives

After reading this chapter, you should be able to:

1. Define weakness and describe how it develops with lesions of the nervous system.
2. Analyze how weakness limits a patient's ability to perform tasks of functional mobility.
3. Describe the tests available to determine if weakness is a contributor to disability.
4. Describe the effects of spasticity or synergy on movement or the ability of the muscle to contract.
5. Identify and discuss treatments to strengthen patients with flaccidity.
6. Identify and discuss treatments to strengthen patients with weakness.
7. Discuss the significance of the systems and task-oriented models as they relate to the treatment of weakness.

Muscle weakness can occur with a variety of musculoskeletal and neuromuscular problems. In fact, it is often the primary cause of disability. Lack of muscle strength can be seen in a variety of patients, such as those who have traumatic brain injury (TBI), stroke, spinal cord injury, multiple sclerosis (MS), Parkinson's disease, Guillain Barré syndrome, or myasthenia gravis. These injuries or disease processes can result in flaccid paralysis, paresis, bradykinesia, or the inability to perform repeated muscle contractions. Muscle weakness also occurs with **deconditioning,** a process by which the body loses strength and cardiovascular endurance as a result of long-term disuse associated with illness, hospitalization, or chronic neurological conditions. In this context, endurance may be a problem associated with muscle weakness, and the treatment approach must address that factor as well.

This chapter describes the evaluation techniques used to measure strength and treatment applications for patients who demonstrate weakness. The section on treatment is divided into two parts: the first concentrates on strengthening the muscles of patients with flaccidity, and the second focuses on rehabilitating patients with weakness.

Flaccidity is characterized by the absence of muscle tone and the inability to generate any form of muscle contraction. If patients progress out of flaccidity, some muscle tone becomes evident; however, they are unable to generate normal levels of muscle force and henceforth have weakness. A variety of treatment applications are presented, with an emphasis on task-oriented activities to increase strength and reduce or eliminate disabilities.

IMPAIRMENT— MUSCLE WEAKNESS

Strength

Strength is a concept that is expressed or operationalized in different ways. In this text, **strength** is expressed as a measure of the force output

of a contracting muscle, and is directly related to the amount of tension produced in that muscle (Kisner & Colby, 1990). Muscle tension reflects both the number of motor units and the rate at which they fire. This tension can be increased by recruiting additional motor units based on the size principle (ie, small motor units are recruited first, followed by larger motor units); increasing firing rates in those motor units already firing; or both (Craik, 1991).

Muscle tension, or muscle force, is generated as a result of muscle contraction and varies depending on the type of contraction. **Eccentric contractions** (those that involve an active lengthening of muscle) provide the greatest muscle tension, followed by isometric and then isotonic contractions. **Isometric contractions** produce high levels of tension in the absence of limb movement; **isotonic contractions** produce equal levels of tension throughout the range of limb movement.

Muscle length at the time of contraction contributes to the amount of tension produced. The normal resting length of muscle produces the greatest tension in a contraction. Longer resting lengths cause higher resting muscle tension, and result in less muscle force development (Fig. 5-1) (Guyton & Hall, 1996).

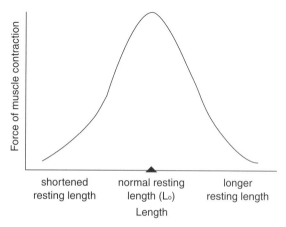

FIGURE 5-1.   Relation of different resting lengths of force production during muscle contraction.

Muscle Weakness

Weakness may be defined as the inability to generate normal levels of muscle force. Weakness is related to a low rate of motor unit firing or the inability of the motor units to fire. Lack of motor unit activity may result from any of the following conditions:

- Cortical lesions with inadequate cortico-spinal activation
- Disruption of the impulses sent by alpha motor neurons to muscle fibers
- Synaptic dysfunction (eg, neuromuscular junction)
- Damage within muscle tissue

In upper motor neuron lesions, reduced firing rates of motor units have been reported (Rosenfalck & Andreassen, 1980). Research has demonstrated that individuals with stroke display "atrophy" in muscle units on the paretic side. Remaining motor units require more time to contract, and they fatigue more rapidly. It has been suggested that altered recruitment and decreased motor unit firing account for this weakness, but evidence is still conflicting (Craik, 1991). These same recruitment problems may be evident in lesions of the peripheral nervous system (PNS) or muscle tissue.

Changes in muscle tissue resulting from an upper motor neuron lesion suggest that muscle may not be as "strong" due to changes in viscoelasticity (a property that allows muscle to resist movement and return to resting lengths after being lengthened) and the presence of denervated muscle fibers (those that lack normal innervation) (Craik, 1991). Research (Lenman, 1959; Light, 1996; McCartney, Moroz, Garner, & McComas, 1988; Peach, 1990; Rose, Giuliani, & Light, 1992; Vignos, 1983) has illustrated the benefits of strength training in neurologically involved individuals as a possible means of preventing or slowing down the viscoelastic changes and denervation of muscle fibers.

Abnormal Tone

As patients progress out of the stage of flaccidity, muscle tone begins to return. In the early phases of recovery of muscle function, the tone in affected muscles is below normal. If recovery continues, muscle tone will increase, at times exceeding the level of normal tone. When muscle tone exceeds normal levels, it is referred to as spastic and can be felt as resistance to passive elongation of the affected muscle. The presence of spasticity can interfere with active movement, especially in muscles that are antagonistic to spastic muscles.

Hufschmidt and Mauritz (1985) and McComas (1991), suggest that spasticity may originate in the periphery, within the biomechanical properties of muscle. Previous research supported the hypothesis that spasticity was the result of loss of cortical inhibition on subcortical and spinal neurons. This hypothesis was based on the controversial theory of hierarchical organization of the nervous system (see Chap. 3). It is now believed that spasticity may result from an imbalance in the mechanisms that regulate reflex motor activities at the spinal cord level (Lewis & Mueller, 1993).

Craik (1991) suggests that the complexity of the neural mechanisms in the spinal cord, including input from **flexor reflex afferents** (**FRAs**) and the processing of afferent information in the spinal cord, may contribute to the development of hyperactive reflexes. Changes in the viscoelastic properties of muscle, as well as in associated connective tissue, tendons, ligaments, joint structure, and alignment, may also be factors in the development of spasticity (Craik, 1991). Correctly aligning a spastic extremity that is in a flexion or extension pattern immediately reduces the resistance felt with passive movement and usually results in improved active movement.

Haley and Inacio (1990) state that the clinical evaluation of spasticity is complex due to

. . . the difficulty of reproducing consistent levels of spasticity at rest and during volitional movements, and the influence of emotional, behavioral and systematic factors on the clinical manifestations of spasticity. (p.71)

Clinically, it is known that changes in body position result in changes in resistance to movement that can be assessed passively. Is this change in resistance to movement the result of the orientation of the **labyrinth,** as originally thought; a change in joint alignment; or a change in muscle, tendon, and ligament length? If resistance to passive movement fluctuates with changes in position, movement, and emotional and systemic factors, then can the measures of spasticity be valid and reliable?

Bohannon and Smith (1987a) attempted to determine the reliability of the Modified Ashworth Scale, which has been used to assess resistance felt by the examiner during passive movement. However, there are potential problems with that study (Bohannon & Smith, 1987a). The study included the assessment of only one muscle (biceps brachii) and one testing position (supine), and the raters of the test were the investigators of the study.

Testing the tone of one muscle that is easy to manipulate passively through a **range of motion** (ROM) is not reflective of consistent measures of tone in other muscles. To establish the reliability of the Modified Ashworth Scale, the therapist should test several muscles that have different functions and are more difficult to passively guide through ROM. This might be achieved by testing muscles such as the flexor carpi radialis and ulnaris, the adductor magnus, the quadriceps, and the gastrocnemius.

Performance of the Modified Ashworth Scale in one position does not ensure that the measures would be consistent if the same patient were assessed in a different position. For example, the simple act of sitting changes joint alignment in the shoulder, elbow, wrist, and hand. These changes may alter the presence of spasticity. Sitting also alters the position of the head

and the labyrinth, which may change the degree of spasticity resulting from the primitive tonic labyrinthine reflex. When this reflex is present, there is an increase in muscle tone in the extensors when the patient is lying supine.

Results of the study by Bohannon and Smith (1987a) may have been biased because these investigators also were raters of the Modified Ashworth Scale. Ideally, raters should be individuals who are unaware of the intent of the study and therefore do not present with any bias toward the outcome of the study.

The reader should surmise that a variety of factors limit the reliability of measuring spasticity. The problem of measuring spasticity with a patient lying supine was described earlier. The influence of a primitive tonic labyrinthine reflex (see Chap. 3, Display 3-2) is removed as soon as the patient is put in a side-lying, prone, or sitting position. The alignment of joints in the lower extremities is also altered in standing because the ankle, which is in a weight-bearing posture, is put in a neutral or in dorsiflexed position, both of which diminish abnormal muscle tone in the lower extremity.

Another factor that limits reliability in passive movement is the rate of movement applied by the therapist. The rate of passive movement has been correlated with the amount of resistance palpated during passive movements. The greater the speed of the passive movement, the greater the muscle's resistance to movement. This may prove to be especially problematic when more than one therapist assesses spasticity in a single patient using variable rates of passive movement.

The majority of tests that have been developed to measure spasticity are performed with passive movements. This is because active voluntary movement of the antagonist muscle(s) does not yield objective values of spasticity. For example, if spasticity were present in the biceps brachii muscle, the patient might or might not be able to activate the triceps brachii muscle sufficiently to extend the elbow. Muscle activity in the biceps brachii may physiologically inhibit muscle activity in the triceps brachii muscle. Therefore, in this example, assessment of active movement of the triceps brachii muscle reveals nothing about the presence of spasticity in the biceps brachii.

Resistance to passive movement is not related to any difficulty patients may experience with active movement. For example, from the above scenario, one cannot infer good active movement in the triceps brachii muscle from observed mild spasticity in the biceps brachii muscle. Similarly, moderate spasticity in the biceps brachii does not imply poor active movement in the triceps brachii muscle. Resistance to passive movement in agonist muscles has no relationship to the amount of active, or functional, movement in antagonist muscles.

It is our opinion that current measurement techniques fail to provide valid and objective measures of spasticity that are related to functional mobility. Therefore, we do not advocate the assessment of spasticity. We have chosen instead to focus on achieving muscle balance by strengthening weak agonist and antagonist muscles. Treatments to facilitate motor unit recruitment in muscles with low tone, or to strengthen muscles around joints placed in normal alignment, can do as much, if not more, to alleviate impairments caused by spasticity than treatments to inhibit tone.

In treatment of abnormal tone, traditional techniques such as prolonged stretch, deep pressure, or the prolonged application of ice have preceded strengthening exercises for antagonist muscles. A more efficient treatment would be to have the patient perform strengthening activities with the extremity in normal alignment. These activities would emphasize contraction of the agonist and antagonist muscles surrounding the joint(s). Strengthening programs that benefit spastic muscles as well as weak antagonists will facilitate the functional cooperation of the muscles surrounding the affected joints. These strengthening programs should be performed in functional positions, such as standing in a weight-bearing posture, stepping up onto a stair, and reaching out with the involved upper extremity during standing or sitting.

ANATOMY OVERVIEW

Volitional muscle contractions result from activity within the central nervous system (CNS) and PNS, as well as within muscle fibers. Descending upper motor neurons (eg, the lateral and anterior corticospinal tracts, vestibulospinal tract, rubrospinal tract, reticulospinal tract) terminate directly or indirectly on the spinal cord motor neurons in ventral gray matter.

When action potentials transmitted along alpha motor neurons reach neuromuscular junctions, synaptic vesicles within presynaptic motor endplates release the neurotransmitter acetylcholine. This neurochemical messenger crosses the synaptic cleft to reach the postsynaptic muscle fiber. This activates chemical reactions within the muscle fiber. **Actin,** a muscle protein found on the I band of the sarcomere, and **myosin,** a muscle protein found on the A band of the sarcomere, engage. The energy liberated from their engagement causes these filaments to ''slide'' across one another to produce muscle contraction (Fig. 5-2). These chemical reactions produce muscle contractions that, along with other components such as oxygen from capillary beds, help maintain muscle viability (Hasson, 1994).

Axons of alpha motor neurons branch into several collaterals, each innervating a single muscle fiber at neuromuscular junctions. All muscle fibers innervated by a single motor neuron are activated when that motor neuron is stimulated. The frequency of motor neuron activation influences the force of contractions. As a result, twitch contractions have forces approximately 33% that of tetanic contractions.

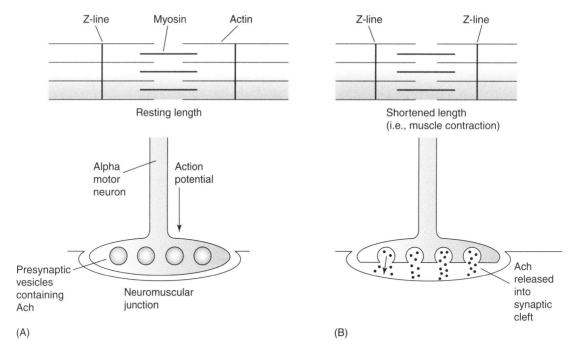

FIGURE 5-2.   Events that produce an active muscle contraction. (*A*) An action potential arrives at the neuromuscular junction. (*B*) Acetylcholine (Ach) is released from vesicles into the synaptic cleft, causing actin and myosin to "slide" across each other.

(**Twitch contractions** are simple, spasmodic contractions that occur independent of stimulation, whereas **tetanic contractions** are sustained and generally induced by stimulation.) Simply increasing the frequency of motor neuron activation can augment the development of muscle force (Hasson, 1994).

Another means of increasing muscle force output is to activate greater numbers of muscle fibers by recruiting more alpha motor neurons. Recruitment is based on the "size" of the alpha motor neuron. That is, the threshold for the recruitment of small motor neurons is low, whereas that for large motor neurons is higher.

When smaller muscle forces are needed, low-threshold, or small motor neurons, are activated. As required forces increase, larger, high-threshold motor neurons are sequentially recruited. This suggests that low-intensity activi-

ties use predominantly small motor neurons, and high-intensity activities require additional larger motor neurons (Hasson, 1994). As muscle force requirements decrease, motor neurons are "derecruited" in reverse order. Large motor neurons are deactivated first and small motor neurons last (Hasson, 1994).

Lesions

Lesions within the CNS, PNS, or muscular system can produce weakness or flaccid paralysis. Lesions in the CNS most often result in other impairments in addition to weakness, such as muscle tone abnormalities, balance dysfunction, lack of coordination, or sensory dysfunction. Weakness patterns or paralysis seen with CNS lesions is most often hemiparetic, paraplegic, or quadriplegic. The pattern of muscle weakness or paralysis that occurs with these lesion sites can result in severe disabilities or lead to additional impairments.

Within 2 months of the insult, patients with hemiparesis resulting from stroke show significant reductions (ie, up to 50%) in motor units on affected sides (McComas, 1991). Possible reasons for this include transsynaptic dysfunction, resulting in loss of the *trophic,* or nutritional, influences of muscle on spinal motor neurons (McComas, 1991).

Interestingly, when the muscle is at rest, neither normal nor spastic muscle shows any **electromyographic activity.** This is also true of normal and spastic muscle during slow passive movements. Tone associated with normal and spastic muscle is due to intrinsic muscular properties and not to continuous motor neuron activity (Hufschmidt & Mauritz, 1985). In spastic muscle, an increased plastic resistance has been found, but this resistance is not due to tonic innervation of the muscle (Hufschmidt & Mauritz, 1985).

Lesions within the PNS can be isolated to one group of muscles, or they can be diffused throughout the entire body, as in the case of Guillain-Barré syndrome. Peripheral nerve lesions often result in muscle atrophy as a result of denervation. Damage to peripheral nerves can include motor and sensory losses, so an additional impairment of sensory dysfunction could be present (Umphred, 1995). Muscle weakness can also produce incoordination, but in this case lack of coordination is the result of a deficiency in movement rather than a control problem (Umphred, 1995).

Based on clinical observation, the majority of patients with PNS lesions do not usually present with disabilities that are as severe as those of patients with CNS lesions. One exception occurs when the PNS lesion is diffused throughout the entire system, as occurs in Guillain-Barré syndrome. Various neurological disorders are associated with changes in the number of functioning motor units (Dantes & McComas, 1991;

Hufschmidt & Mauritz, 1985; McComas, 1991). Significant decreases in the number of motor units have been reported in the muscles of patients with amyotrophic lateral sclerosis (ALS), even in muscles that have not been shown clinically to have weakened (Dantes & McComas, 1991; McComas, 1991). This reduction in the number of motor units has been reported to equal 50% every 6 months once the denervating process begins. Neuronal recovery has been documented in some instances (Dantes & McComas, 1991; McComas, 1991).

Persons with postpolio syndrome have decreased numbers of motor units, along with enlargement of those surviving motor units (McComas, 1991). Various peripheral neuropathies have been associated with different degrees of motor unit loss. Diabetic neuropathies appear to produce axonal dysfunctions associated with demyelination along with associated collateral **reinnervation,** the process of reintroducing nervous innervation after a period of denervation. Patients with acute idiopathic polyneuritis (eg, those with Guillain-Barré syndrome) show a decrease in the number of motor units during the active disease process. Numbers increase with recovery. In fact, those with the best recovery are those who have demonstrated motor unit numbers that are within normal ranges (McComas, 1991).

Patients diagnosed with toxic neuropathies show remodeling of motor units. Collateral sprouting to neighboring muscle fibers occurs during the active disease process. However, as recovery occurs, the "original" motor neurons are recaptured by the original muscle fiber (McComas, 1991).

Disease processes affecting the muscular system can produce muscle weakness that progresses to muscle atrophy. In these cases, denervation will occur as muscle fibers degenerate. In addition to muscle weakness, patients may present with decreased muscle tone, which may result in joint abnormalities or malalignments. Degeneration of muscle fibers is generally restricted to muscular dystrophies (ie, Duchenne's, limb-girdle, and facioscapulohumeral), but may also result from malnutrition, metabolic disorders, systemic infections, or some combination of these factors. Muscular dystrophies, especially Duchenne's, can result in severe disability for patients because the degeneration of muscle fibers occurs throughout the body.

Muscle tissue can also undergo structural changes and weakness as a result of immobility or disuse. Weakness and changes in tissue structure are two of the underlying problems in motor unit recruitment with lesions of the CNS or PNS. Immobility of the joint or extremity, or disuse of the muscle as a result of a nervous system lesion, results in disuse atrophy and changes within the tissue and cellular state of the muscle.

ASSESSING DISABILITIES RESULTING FROM MUSCLE WEAKNESS

The first two steps in a neurological assessment are the observation and assessment of functional mobility. Initial observation enables the examiner to gather general information regarding a patient's state of awareness and to make preliminary observations of the patient's movement dysfunctions.

Assessment of functional mobility allows examiners to determine which activities are difficult or impossible for patients to perform because of underlying impairments. To determine disabilities, you must assess the patient's ability to perform various **functional tasks.** Difficulty initiating, sustaining, or completing movements may result from muscle weakness. The range of disabilities presented by patients with muscle weakness is related to

the variety of lesions that produce the impairment.

Functional mobility, previously described in Chapter 3, is repeated here to illustrate how weakness could limit or interfere with the patient's ability to move. Alternative movement strategies are those outside the range of normative movements described in the literature. For example, moving from supine to sitting by using the involved leg to hook the noninvolved leg is considered an alternative means by which the patient can move both the lower extremities and the pelvis over the edge of the bed.

Rolling

This movement may be limited in patients with diffuse weakness or hemiplegia. Patients who have generalized weakness throughout their bodies may be unable to accomplish any or a combination of the following movements:

- Lifting the arms forward
- Rotating the head and trunk
- Unilaterally lifting the legs
- Pushing off from the bed with the heels

Patients with hemiplegia may be able to roll to the involved side with the noninvolved upper extremity pulling the body over to a side-lying position. Rolling to the noninvolved side may be difficult if the patient is unable to protract the involved shoulder and reach across the body. Patients with paraplegia will frequently use the upper body to push up onto their elbows from a supine position to roll over onto their sides.

Supine-to-Sitting Maneuver

A patient with weakness may exhibit limited movement or alternative movement strategies when rising from the supine position to sit at the edge of the bed. Patients with generalized weakness may attempt to prop themselves up on their forearms (if adequate upper extremity strength is present), and then press up into a long sitting posture. Alternatively, they may push themselves over into a side-lying posture (Fig. 5-3). From the side-lying position, patients can use their upper extremities to bring their legs over to the edge of the bed and press up into sitting with their upper extremities. If upper extremity strength is graded less than fair, patients may be unable to accomplish this task without the therapist's assistance.

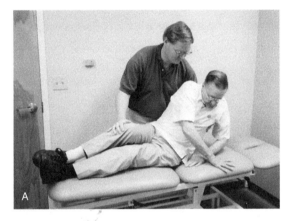

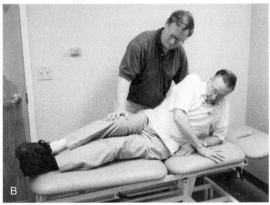

FIGURE 5-3. (*A,B*) The patient moves from a supine to an upright posture.

Weakness on one side of the body may interfere with the patient's ability to move from supine to sitting on the edge of the bed. If a sit-up maneuver was previously used, the weakness-induced inability to lift the head and shoulders may prevent the patient from accomplishing this task. The patient may use alternative movement strategies to accomplish this task. Rolling into side-lying on the involved side and pushing with the noninvolved upper extremity may be the patient's strategy of choice.

Rolling to a side-lying position and then moving to sitting may have been the movement strategy used before a stroke. In this case, the difficulty may be in rolling to the noninvolved side as described in the section on rolling. The patient may roll onto the involved side by pushing up into sitting with the noninvolved upper extremity.

Stable Sitting Posture

When assessing stable sitting postures, look for the patient's ability to sit, unsupported, in a symmetrical posture for a period of time. Patients with generalized weakness may be unable to maintain a sitting posture without the therapist's support. The posture of this patient is generally slumped forward, and a posterior pelvic tilt is evident. The patient with hemiplegia may have an asymmetrical sitting posture in which the involved shoulder is depressed and a posterior pelvic tilt is evident. Although the patient may be able to maintain this position, prolonged sitting in this position contributes to postural abnormalities and muscle imbalances. Moving from this position to standing is impossible without moving the pelvis anteriorly (Berta Bobath, 1982). Elevation of the depressed shoulder to a more "correct" position will also assist in raising the upper trunk. This postural adjustment assists with the early lift phase of the sitting-to-standing maneuver. Symmetrical sitting should be emphasized often to develop muscle strength and alignment.

Sit-to-Stand Maneuver

The biomechanics of moving from a sitting to a standing position have been documented (Millington, Myklebust, & Shambes, 1992; Schenkman, Berger, Riley, Mann, & Hodge, 1990). There are four phases in this sequence: (1) flexion momentum, (2) early lift, (3) extension, and (4) stabilization (Schenkman et al., 1991). Patients with generalized weakness or hemiplegia may have difficulty during each phase due to inadequate strength. Early momentum may be difficult, especially if the patient sits with a posterior pelvic tilt (Berta Bobath, 1982). Trunk forward flexion is needed to generate momentum. Early lift requires activation of the erector spinae, rectus femoris, vastus medialis, biceps femoris, gluteus maximus, and rectus abdominis (Millington et al., 1992).

Completing a 2- to 3-second sit-to-stand maneuver is difficult when weakness is present. Patients who have faulty timing and inappropriate sequencing of muscle firing have difficulty with this movement. Patients with generalized weakness or hemiplegia may rely excessively on their upper extremities to flex their trunk forward, to initiate early lift. They may continue to push with their upper extremities during the extension phase. On standing, upper extremity support on an assistance device may be needed if weakness in the lower extremities prevents adequate stability for weight bearing. Patients with hemiplegia may also incorporate use of an asymmetrical movement pattern to accomplish the task (Fig. 5-4). Shifting the center of gravity toward the noninvolved side during the sit-to-stand maneuver allows for the completion of the task without the use of the involved extremities. However, asymmetrical movement will be exaggerated.

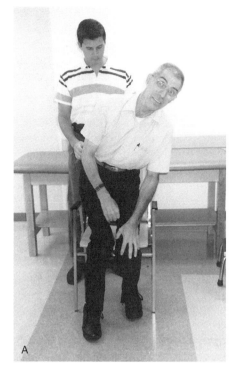

FIGURE 5-4. (*A*) The patient displays asymmetry when moving from sitting to standing.

Stable Standing Posture

The assessment of stable standing postures should include an evaluation of the patient's ability to maintain an unsupported standing posture that incorporates body symmetry. Patients with generalized weakness in a lower extremity and sufficient upper extremity strength will rely excessively on a walker or parallel bars to maintain standing. Weakness throughout the body will most likely prevent the patient from standing without assistance from the therapist. Patients with hemiplegia often stand asymmetrically with the involved shoulder depressed, while the noninvolved upper extremity is supported by parallel bars or another assistive device.

Asymmetrical weight-bearing through the noninvolved lower extremity contributes to **pelvic obliquity,** an inclination or slanting of the

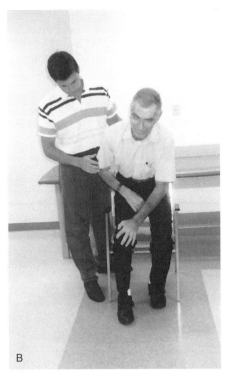

B

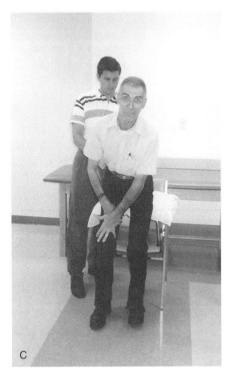

C

FIGURE 5-4. (*B*) With the therapist's assistance, the patient achieves an increase in symmetry of movement as he maintains his center of gravity over the body's midline.

FIGURE 5-4. (*C*) The patient completes the maneuver.

pelvis. Use of the noninvolved upper extremity in weight-bearing contributes to a shift in the center of gravity toward the noninvolved side. Standing may be maintained by the assumption of an asymmetrical posture that incorporates upper extremity support. However, prolonged standing in this position contributes to the development of postural abnormalities and muscle imbalances.

Transfers

The majority of transfers performed use a stand-pivot or lateral slide board. Pivot transfers require that muscles be activated as described for sit-to-stand transfers, followed by pivoting and

lowering of the body into a chair. Difficulties described in sit-to-stand transfers may be evident in this movement task. Traditionally, patients are instructed to pivot toward their stronger side; in hemiplegia, they are asked to pivot toward the noninvolved side. This movement reinforces the shift in weight onto the stronger or noninvolved side, and diminishes the ability to bear weight through the involved lower extremity.

During the pivot, patients often display a "hopping step" with their noninvolved lower extremity. "Hopping steps" are used as an alternative movement strategy to compensate for diminished weight-bearing through the involved lower extremity.

Lowering the body into a chair from a standing posture is difficult for patients whose weakness derives from a deficiency in the eccentric activity of the muscles used to lift the body out of the chair. With weakness, lowering activities often result in a quick descent, or "plop" into the chair. This movement should be assessed by patients slowly lowering themselves into the chair. Upper extremity support during a transfer is often evident with patients who display weakness. Support may involve weight-bearing through their arms to achieve stability during standing and pivot. The upper extremities may be used to assist in generating momentum forward and through the lift phase during the sit-to-stand maneuver.

Lateral transfers, with or without a sliding board, are another means of moving from one surface to another. Lateral transfers are indicated for those who may be unable to bear weight on their lower extremities, although they have good function and strength in their upper extremities. A patient with MS with bilateral lower extremity weakness or paralysis is a good example of someone who fits this description. To perform a lateral transfer, the patient must have dynamic sitting balance and upper extremity strength. Otherwise, it will be impossible to slide the buttocks across the board or lift the body up and onto the new surface. Patients who have difficulty maintaining sitting balance, or inadequate upper extremity strength, will require that the therapist assist them in completing this transfer.

Ambulation

The stance and swing phase of gait can be affected by weakness and may result in atypical mobility patterns. When weakness is present in both lower extremities, the patient's ability to function is greatly reduced (Perry, 1992).

Stance Phase: Muscle Activation

Initial contact and the loading response result from extensor and flexor muscles working together to achieve stability in preparation for the stance phase. The adductor magnus and the gluteus medius assist in hip extension; the gluteus medius also provides the stability needed for the contralateral drop of the pelvis. The vastus lateralis, medialis, and intermedius provide stable weight acceptance and control the knee flexion that occurs with initial loading and forward momentum of the body. The anterior tibialis decreases the rate of passive plantar flexion that occurs with initial loading. The heel may fail to strike the floor during initial contact as a result of anterior tibialis weakness, which produces a characteristic "foot slap." Weakness in extensor sequence muscles can result in buckling of the weight-bearing extremity on initial contact or during the loading response.

The midstance and terminal stance are primarily controlled by the plantar flexors, the soleus and gastrocnemius. During the early phase of midstance, the vastus muscles, along with the gluteus maximus and medius, are active to assist knee extension and stability. However, "the primary responsibility for limb control is transferred to the ankle extensor muscles to provide graded progression over the supporting foot" (Perry, 1992, p. 161). Weakness in the plantar flexors can result in decreased ankle ROM through stance, decreased stance time, and limited acceleration of the body forward.

Isolated weakness in a single muscle or groups of muscles may result in alternative gait patterns. For example, the compensation for quadriceps weakness may be a stiff, or extended, knee throughout the stance period, whereas weak dorsiflexors may be compensated for by excessive hip flexion, or a hiking up of the hip, to clear the foot off the ground. Paresis or paralysis on one side of the body or in one extremity affects the flexor and extensor muscle sequence of gait. Therefore, patients may display difficulty with weight shift, stance, and swing periods. Because initiating gait from a static standing posture requires that the weight be shifted, assess the patient's ability to shift the weight laterally and move through each phase.

Also determine the amount of time spent in each phase. Table 5-1 summarizes the problems that can occur in the stance phase of gait and the muscles associated with these abnormalities. A scissored gait is frequently seen when the adductor muscles are spastic, resulting in the leg crossing over midline of the body, or with weakness of the gluteus medius. Toe-off refers to the last stage of terminal stance just before the foot (toes) leaves the floor for swing phase.

Swing Phase: Muscle Activation

The preswing phase involves activation of the anterior tibialis, extensor digitorum longus, extensor hallicus longus, and the rectus femoris in combination with the adductor longus. These muscles begin to draw the leg up off the ground to allow for foot clearance during the swing phase. Those flexor muscles active during preswing continue to fire during the initial swing and midswing periods. In addition, the sartorius, gracilis, and iliacus advance the thigh forward with the biceps femoris (short head) aiding knee flexion for lifting the foot off the ground.

The final component of the swing phase (ie, terminal swing) is accomplished in a series of steps:

1. The hamstrings are activated to decelerate hip flexion and knee extension.
2. The adductor magnus and gluteus maximus are activated to continue hip deceleration without knee flexion.
3. The vastus muscle group is activated to enable full knee extension at initial contact and to counteract the effect of the hamstrings.
4. The anterior tibialis is reactivated to prepare the foot for the heel strike.

Weakness of flexor sequence muscles will limit clearance of the foot during the swing phase, which may result in dragging or "catching" the foot on the ground and stumbling.

The alternative movement strategies of hip hiking and circumduction may also be seen with weakness of flexor muscles. Table 5-2 summarizes the problems that can occur during the swing phase and the muscles associated with these abnormalities.

Clinical Examples of Gait Abnormalities. Patients with Parkinson's disease may have trouble initiating gait because of the inherent difficulty of moving their centers of gravity in preparation for the lateral shift in weight. Their gait displays the characteristic shuffling pattern, in which there is no clear delineation between the stance and swing phases. Gait components, beginning with the weight shift, must be introduced and practiced repeatedly.

Therapists should be aware that the majority of patients with hemiplegia first develop motor recovery in the lower extremity in the extensor muscle sequence. This will enable them to practice weight-bearing and weight-shifting early in the rehabilitation program. Slow recovery of the flexor muscle sequence can impede relearning of the phases of the swing period. Because of excessive weakness in flexor muscles, these patients develop compensatory or alternative movement strategies to advance the involved extremity forward.

The most common gait abnormality seen with hemiplegic patients is circumduction. When hemiplegic patients attempt to move out of the stance phase and into the swing phase, they may find that they are unable to initiate or complete the swing due to a failure of activation in the flexor muscles. The result is a circumducted gait, one in which the hip is elevated and the limb swings into abduction. Therapists must be aware of alternative strategies. They must also know when to provide patients with visual or verbal cues and manual assistance as they move through correct patterns.

Climbing Stairs. Ascending stairs requires that the weight be shifted onto one stable lower

TABLE 5-1. Gait Cycle Abnormalities Due to Weakness: Stance Phase

Components of Stance Phase	Weakness Muscles Involved						Muscle Imbalance* Muscles Involved	
	Anterior Tibialis	Quadriceps	Gastroc–Soleus	Iliopsoas	Gluteus Medius	Hamstrings	Gastroc–Soleus	Hamstrings
Foot contact loading	X (foot flat, or foot slap)						X	X (inadequate knee extension)
Mid-stance								
recurvatum		X					X	
persistent knee flexion			X					
forward trunk lean		X (compensatory movement)						
backward trunk lean				X (compensatory movement)				
lateral lean					X			
drop in pelvis					X (contralateral)			
scissored gait					X	X		
Terminal stance								
inadequate toe-off			X					

* These muscles are stronger than their antagonists.

	Weakness **Muscles Involved**		**Muscle Imbalance*** **Muscles Involved/Synergy**		
Components of Swing Phase	Iliopsoas	Hamstrings	Adductors	Hamstrings	Flexor Synergy
Inadequate hip flexion	X				
Mid-swing					
Inadequate knee flexion		X			
Excessive adduction			X		
Terminal Swing					
Inadequate knee extension				X	X

TABLE 5-2. Gait Cycle Abnormalities Due to Weakness: Swing Phase

* The muscles identified are stronger than their antagonists.

extremity while the opposite extremity is lifted and placed onto a higher step. Weight shift onto the stable limb requires adequate strength in the extensor and abductor muscles to maintain support while the other limb advances up the stair. The ascending limb must have adequate hip, knee, and ankle flexion to lift the extremity up onto the step and adequate extension to lift the body up onto the step. Climbing stairs is usually performed in a reciprocal pattern, with each limb alternating movements of weight-bearing and elevation.

Bilateral weakness in the lower extremities may make climbing stairs impossible, especially if the patient is unable to advance one leg up onto the stair. In patients with hemiplegia, involved limbs may be advanced onto the step with hip elevation and circumduction or lateral trunk flexion. The pattern in hemiplegia is usually nonreciprocal, with the involved leg trailing when ascending stairs and leading when descending stairs. Reliance on handrails for support is another strategy used to compensate for instability during this maneuver.

Descending stairs is similar to ascending them, in that a shift in weight is involved. Lowering the body onto steps may be analogous to

moving from standing to sitting, in that eccentric contractions are required. The one exception is that descending steps requires single-limb support. Patients with hemiplegia may lower themselves with their noninvolved limbs and may display **genu recurvatum,** or buckling of the involved limbs, as the weight is shifted onto the involved descending limbs. Hand support may be used to compensate for the instability of involved limbs during the weight-bearing phase.

Case Study

Admission

Mr. Jones was admitted to the hospital with sudden onset of weakness in his right arm and leg, and a facial droop. Computed tomography (CT) revealed infarction of the left precentral gyrus, (primary motor cortex). Physical therapy evaluation was performed at bedside 48 hours after admission. The patient was supine with an intravenous line in his left forearm and an indwelling catheter.

Assessment of the Disability

Ask the patient to roll toward his right side and observe what strategies are used. Does he display any preexisting movement strategies? Does he turn his head and protract his left shoulder to reach across his body in rolling to the right side? Does his left hip and knee flex to bring the pelvis forward, or does he push off the bed with the noninvolved extremity? Is the patient able to accomplish the task independently or does he need assistance?

Now ask the patient to roll to his left side. Does his right arm move? If it does move, is its pattern similar to that used by the left arm? Is the patient able to move the right lower extremity in the same way he moves his left to assist with rolling? Can he accomplish the task without assistance?

The patient's failure to initiate movement on the right side of the body suggests weakness. As you assist the patient in rolling toward the left side, consider the weight of the right extremities: Are they heavy with diminished muscle tone? Is there resistance as the muscle is lengthened during the movement pattern? Assistance provided in rolling or movement of the right extremities aids in determining the extent of muscle weakness or the presence of excessive tone that limits normal movement.

Progress this patient to sitting from side-lying on the involved side. What happens to the pelvis during the movement from side-lying to sitting? Can the patient push up into sitting with the involved right upper extremity? Can he support himself on his right upper extremity? Can the patient move both lower extremities forward off the edge of the bed? Is the involved leg assisted in movement by the left leg? The inability to push off with the right arm and the inability to support the upper body on the right suggest muscle weak-

ness. Use of the left leg to advance the right leg forward and off the bed is another sign of potential weakness.

When sitting, is the patient able to maintain an upright, stable symmetrical sitting posture? Inability to maintain an upright sitting posture may be due to weakness, balance dysfunction, or sensory impairment. Patients who display difficulty in rolling and supine-to-sit transfers, and those who are unable to maintain upright sitting postures may have weakness.

Attempt to stand this patient to determine a baseline for standing posture and potential ambulation. How much assistance is required to move the patient from sitting to standing? Does the patient move in a symmetrical pattern? Is weight borne through both lower extremities? Is he able to achieve a stable standing posture? Is the standing posture symmetrical? Does the patient need hand support to maintain an upright stance or can he stand without hand support? Are both lower extremities providing support of the body in weight bearing?

Results of Assessment of Functional Mobility

- Rolling to right—independent.
- Rolling to left—moderate assistance to protract shoulder and advance right hip forward.
- Supine-to-sit—moderate assistance, unable to use right arm to push up, and unable to bear weight on the right arm. Left leg is used to push right leg off the side of the bed.
- Stable sitting—requires minimal assistance to maintain sitting, which is asymmetrical. Patient also supports himself with left upper extremity.

- Sit-to-stand and standing—requires maximal assistance. He does not appear to bear weight on the involved lower extremity and leans excessively toward the involved side.
- Ambulation is not attempted due to the difficulty of coming to a standing posture.

ASSESSING THE IMPAIRMENT— MUSCLE WEAKNESS

Muscle strength is evaluated to determine the presence of weakness that may have an impact on the patient's ability to perform the tasks required for functional mobility. The following measures have been documented in the literature as appropriate measures to assess muscle strength.

- Active range of motion (AROM)
- Manual muscle test
- Hand-held dynamometer
- Isokinetic dynamometer
- Electromyography (EMG)

Active Range of Motion

Assess AROM first. If patients are unable to actively move through the full range, then perform passive ROM (PROM) to determine the presence of joint restrictions or spasticity. When patients present with limited joint ROM, an objective measure of strength is limited because the muscle cannot move through its full length. Limitations in AROM may have an impact on the patient's ability to successfully perform functional tasks. The elimination or reduction of joint restrictions should be addressed in treatment plans, to enable normal muscle strength to develop within the full range.

When patients present with spasticity, determine if normal muscle length and joint ROM are achievable, or if secondary soft tissue changes now limit the ROM. The presence of soft tissue restrictions would indicate a need to increase the elasticity of the tissue to enable increased ROM.

Patients who have full PROM but who are unable to move through the AROM probably have weakness. The recruitment of synergistic muscles to perform a movement is also an indicator of weakness. For example, any attempt at shoulder flexion that is accompanied by the synergistic movements of shoulder elevation and scapular retraction is evidence of weakness. The synergistic movements seen in recovery from stroke have been documented by Signe Brunnstrom (Display 5-1).

Active ROM of weak muscles against a force such as gravity may reinforce synergistic movements with **biomechanical substitution** as a means to accomplish motor tasks. This can lead to muscle imbalance and the inability to develop normal movement patterns.

Manual Muscle Test

Manual muscle tests are performed to assess the strength of muscles during isolated movements (Danneskiold-Samsoe et al., 1984; Demeurisse, Demol, & Robaye, 1980; Kleyweg, Frans, Meche, & Schmitz, 1991; Milner-Brown & Miller, 1989). Specific testing techniques have been reported by Kendall, McCreary, and Provance (1993) and by Daniels and Worthingham (1986). Muscles are graded from zero (no response of muscle) to five (normal strength).

Kendall's concept of "break" test is used to determine the difference between good and normal strength. The break test is frequently performed at midrange, with the therapist attempting to break the isometric contraction maintained by the patient. Daniels and Wor-

DISPLAY 5-1
Brunnstrom Synergies of Motor Recovery

Stage 1. Immediately following the acute episode, flaccidity of the involved limbs is present, and no movement, on either a reflex or voluntary basis, can be initiated.

Stage 2. As recovery begins, the basic limb synergies, or some of their components, may appear as associated reactions, or minimal voluntary movement responses may be present. Spasticity begins to develop and may be particularly evident in muscle groups that dominate synergy movement (eg, elbow flexors, knee extensors).

Stage 3. The patient gains voluntary control of the movement synergies, although full range of all synergy components does not necessarily develop. Spasticity, which may become severe in some cases, reaches its peak. This stage in the recovery process may be thought of as semivoluntary in that the patient is able to initiate movement in the involved limbs on a volitional basis but is unable to control the form of the resulting movement, which will be the basic limb synergies.

Stage 4. Some movement combinations that do not follow the paths of basic limb synergy are mastered, first with difficulty, then with increasing ease. Spasticity begins to decline, but the influence of spasticity on nonsynergistic movements is still readily observable.

Stage 5. If recovery continues, more difficult movement combinations are mastered as the basic limb synergies lose their dominance over motor acts. Spasticity continues to decline.

Stage 6. Individual joint movements become possible and coordination approaches normalcy. As spasticity disappears, the patient becomes capable of a full spectrum of movement patterns.

Stage 7. As the last recovery stage, normal function is restored.

From Sawner, K, & LaVigne, J. (Eds.). *Brunnstrom's Movement Therapy in Hemiplegia: A Neurophysiological Approach* (2nd ed.). Philadelphia: Lippincott.

thingham use full ROM with resistance applied throughout to differentiate between good and normal strength. Because it provides information about the strength of the muscle at any length, we recommend the consistent use of resistance throughout ROM as the preferred technique for manual muscle testing.

Manual muscle testing has been reported to be reliable within one-half muscle grade. However, interrater reliability for grades ''good'' and ''normal'' have been questioned because of the variability of resistance applied by different examiners. Figure 5-5 demonstrates the technique of manual muscle testing as applied to the left hip flexors.

Hand-Held Dynamometer

Hand-held dynamometers have gained some acceptance because they are easy to apply and test a variety of muscles. Several muscles have been

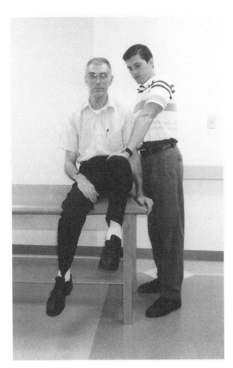

FIGURE 5-5. Manual muscle testing of the left hip.

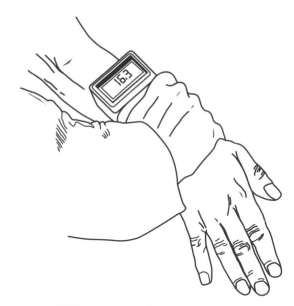

FIGURE 5-6. A hand-held dynamometer.

evaluated with hand-held dynamometers, but testing is limited to static contractions (Bohannon & Smith, 1987b). Introducing dynamic movements with hand-held dynamometers distorts the speed of the movement generated by the patient and the resistance applied by the examiner.

To apply a hand-held dynamometer, place it on the desired body part and apply sufficient force to overcome the patient's isometric contractions (Fig. 5-6). At the point where the examiner overcomes patient strength, readings on the dynamometer are recorded. Reliability of this type of testing has not been reported. Hand-grip dynamometers have been used to objectively measure grip strength (Hamrin et al., 1982; Heller et al., 1987; Grimby et al., 1992; Rosenfalck & Andreassen, 1980; Sunderland, Tinson, Bradley, & Hewer, 1989) and to predict

recovery of upper extremity function (Sunderland et al., 1989) (Fig. 5-7).

Isokinetic Dynamometer

Isokinetic dynamometers are the most widely used devices for objectively measuring muscle strength (Cress, Johnson, & Agre, 1991; Falkel, 1978; Fisher et al., 1993; Graves et al., 1990; Hasue, Fujiwara, & Kikuchi, 1980; Larsson, Brimby, & Karlsson, 1979; Lord, Aitkens, McCrory, & Bernauer, 1992; Milner-Brown, Mellenthin, & Miller, 1986; Newton & Waddell, 1993; Nicholas, Robinson, Logan, & Robertson, 1989; Pedersen & Oberg, 1993; Perry, Mulroy, & Renwick, 1993; Pitetti, 1990; Ringsberg, 1993; Rosenfalck & Andreassen, 1980; Rothstein, Lamb, & Mayhew, 1987; Suomi, Surburg, & Lecius, 1993). Isokinetic dynamometers enable patients to move through an ROM of varying resistances while the amount of force generated

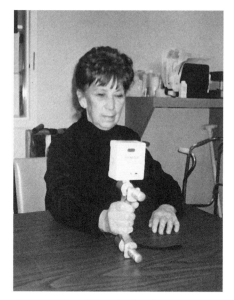

FIGURE 5-7.   A hand-grip dynamometer.

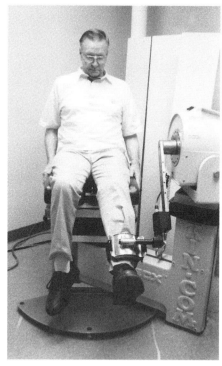

FIGURE 5-8.   Isokinetic knee extension in sitting, an open chain activity.

in the involved muscles is recorded. The speed of movement can be varied to alter the tension required by contracting muscles. Adaptive pieces can be added to the machine to allow for measuring most major muscle groups, including back extensors and abdominal muscles.

A limitation to strength measurement with isokinetic dynamometers is the limited use of **closed chain activities,** which are performed with the distal part of an extremity in a weight-bearing position. In most testing setups, the lower extremities are not in weight-bearing positions (Fig. 5-8), which limits the functional application of the findings.

Electromyography

Indwelling EMG recordings provide information about the relative numbers of motor units firing and the types of muscle fibers that are contracting. EMG is most often used in diagnostic tests to confirm or rule out peripheral lesions

of the CNS and has been used in research to measure the changes in muscle strength that result from treatment intervention (Glendinning & Enoka, 1994; Leonard, 1993; Milner-Brown et al., 1986; Pedersen & Oberg, 1993). Rarely is it used clinically to routinely measure strength changes because the test is time-consuming to conduct.

ASSESSING STRENGTH IN PATIENTS WITH SYNERGY

Assessing strength in patients with upper motor neuron lesions (eg, stroke) remains a controversial topic. Given Jules Rothstein's commentary on

Bohannon's (1989) article on strength testing muscles in synergy, it is evident that more research is needed. At this time it is not known if strength measurements in individuals with nervous system dysfunctions are valid. Further research may make it apparent that patients who display synergistic movement should not be tested with the strength assessment tools outlined above.

True measures of isolated muscle contractions may be difficult to obtain in upper motor neuron lesions where synergy is present. In synergistic movements, several muscles fire to assist the activation of weak muscles, as seen in Figure 5-9, where the patient is attempting active hip flexion. As evidenced by Figure 5-9, isolated hip flexion cannot be determined because of the additional activity of synergistic muscles.

Synergy is seen not only in neurologically involved patients but in nonneurologically in-

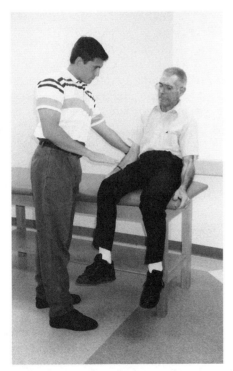

FIGURE 5-9. The patient exhibits hip flexion with synergy during AROM.

volved persons as well. Synergy may be evident in patients who have musculoskeletal conditions involving muscle weakness. For example, patients with humeral fractures use shoulder elevation to perform shoulder flexion. Synergistic firing may result from **recruitment overflow** in neighboring alpha motor neurons in the spinal cord, or it may be the result of biomechanical substitution. Recruitment of neighboring alpha motor neurons from higher centers may exceed what is needed to accomplish tasks, or it may be related to inappropriate timing and sequencing problems in the recruitment of motor units (Gentile, 1987).

Biomechanical substitution may occur as patients attempt to complete desired movements, using other muscles to assist in the movement patterns. A good example of this occurs with elbow flexion and the associated elevation of the shoulder. To attempt to contract a weak biceps brachii muscle, a patient will have to elevate the shoulder to mechanically assist in flexing the elbow. You can perform this same mechanical recruitment on yourself. Maximally resist elbow flexion and you will feel tension develop in your anterior deltoids and upper trapezius. You do not display the typical flexion synergy patterns that are seen with stroke patients, but activation of synergistic muscles does occur.

Percent of Isolated Active Range of Motion

Many clinicians have begun to classify the motor recovery seen with synergy by describing the percent of active range of motion present when a muscle functions in isolation. To use this technique the therapist must examine functional ranges of motion in primary joints such as:

Shoulder—flexion/extension, abduction/
 adduction
Elbow—flexion/extension
Wrist—flexion/extension
Hand—flexion/extension

Hip—flexion/extension, abduction/adduction

Knee—flexion/extension

Ankle—dorsiflexion/plantar flexion, inversion/eversion

In addition, if the patient is unable to activate a muscle in isolation (without other synergistic muscles firing) in a gravity plane, the therapist may need to describe the isolated movements present in both gravity *and* gravity eliminated planes. For example:

> The patient has 25% AROM of isolated shoulder flexion against gravity, and 75% AROM of isolated shoulder flexion in antigravity. This tells you that in sitting the patient can move the shoulder through 25% AROM before synergy starts to occur. The presence of synergy would be indicated by shoulder elevation or retraction, or elbow flexion. When the effects of gravity are eliminated, the isolated AROM increases to 75% AROM. Hence, the patient unconsciously recruits synergistic muscles in a gravity-dependent plane due to weakness in the muscle being tested.

Brunnstrom's Stages of Motor Recovery

Developed by Signe Brunnstrom, the stages of motor recovery were based on her observations of patterns of movements exhibited by stroke patients. Brunnstrom's stages (see Display 5-1) are commonly used to describe synergistic movement patterns displayed by patients with stroke. They do not, however, measure strength. Repetition of the Brunnstrom stages to document the recovery of motor function may impede the development of normal isolated movements, and the repetition of synergistic movement appears to reinforce biomechanical substitution and synergistic overflow.

Figure 5-10 depicts a patient performing AROM of both upper extremities. Synergy displayed on the right extremity is apparent and is described as indicative of Brunnstrom's stage 4.

ASSESSING STRENGTH IN PATIENTS WITH SPASTICITY

Assessing strength in spastic muscle is not believed to be a valid means of measuring the numbers of motor units recruited to accomplish muscle contractions. Motor units may be recruited inappropriately in spastic muscles because of the heightened synaptic activity at the alpha and gamma motor neurons. This produces abnormal tone, which is particularly evident during movement.

Abnormal tone is also present in spastic muscle at rest, as evidenced by the presence of hyperactive deep tendon reflexes (DTRs). Eliciting DTRs reveals information concerning the sensitivity of muscle spindles brought about by either supraspinal or spinal center influences. During volitional activation, the motor units in spastic muscle are inappropriately recruited, or are recruited with delays in timing and sequencing that may affect the production of muscle force.

Case Study

Assessment of the Impairment

Mr. Jones experienced difficulty in rolling to the left side and moving from supine to a sitting posture. Sitting required minimal assistance and the support of his noninvolved left arm on the bed. Moving from sitting to standing, and standing alone, both required the therapist's maximal assistance. The difficulties experienced with functional mobility are indicators of muscle

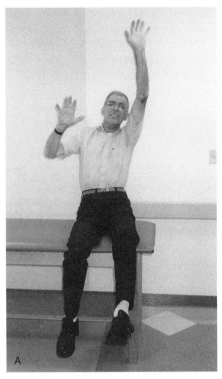
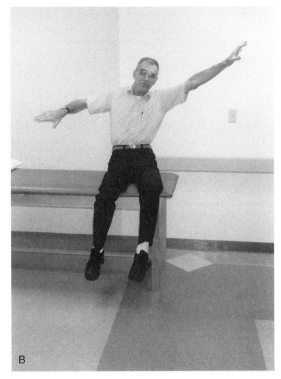

FIGURE 5-10 (*A,B*) The patient displays marked right-side synergy during active range of motion (AROM) exercises of the upper extremities.

weakness, sensory dysfunction, or balance dysfunction. To confirm the suspicion of weakness, assess the AROM of the involved extremities. In assessing AROM, look for quantity of movement.

Full AROM should be present for Mr. Jones to have a manual muscle test grade of "fair." Less than full AROM suggests weakness, soft tissue restrictions, abnormal tone, painful joints, or bony blocks. To determine what is preventing full AROM, assess PROM. Full PROM and limited AROM confirm weakness as the underlying impairment. Limited PROM, if present, may be due to soft tissue adhesions, abnormal tone, or bony blocks. To assess tone, passively range the joint to assess resistance to passive movement. Evidence of resistance to passive movement suggests the presence of abnormal tone. Place all joints of the involved extremity in normal alignment and then repeat PROM. Full PROM with normal joint alignment confirms that abnormal tone is the cause of limited PROM.

To rule out sensory dysfunction as an impairment, assess localization to touch and proprioception. If these two modalities are intact, diminished sensation is not contributing to the disabilities.

Balance dysfunction may be difficult to assess at this point because of the patient's low functional level. Ask the patient if nausea and vertigo were experienced with rolling to either side or moving to a sitting posture. Examine the patient for nystagmus immediately after he rolls or sits upright. The absence of vertigo, nystagmus, or nausea and the integrity of the sensory system would appear to rule out a balance dysfunction caused by anything other than weakness.

Results of Impairment Testing

- AROM—limited in right upper and lower extremities, with appearance of synergistic movement as the patient attempts isolated movement.
- PROM—within normal limits and no resistance to PROM felt.
- Sensory—localization and proprioception intact.
- Balance assessment—negative for vertigo, nausea, or nystagmus with positional changes.

TREATMENT OF MUSCLE WEAKNESS

In the past, based on the teachings of traditional theorists such as Bobath and Brunnstrom, therapists did not strength train muscles weakened by neurological disease or injury (see Chap. 4). Therapists attempted to inhibit or facilitate muscle to normalize muscle tone. Today, research indicates that strength training muscles weakened by neurological disease or injury is appropriate when the joints are in normal alignment (Lenman, 1959; Light, 1996; McCartney et al., 1988; Peach, 1990; Rose et al., 1992; Vignos, 1983).

This section is divided into two parts: (1) strengthening patients with flaccidity, and (2) strengthening patients with weakness. Treatment interventions that have been cited in the literature and are appropriate for patients with neurological disability are discussed. Current rehabilitation practice focuses on task-oriented activities. However, some exercises referenced in this chapter are based on the traditional theoretical approach incorporated in a functional task.

Treating the impairment of weakness with exercise alone may increase muscle strength, but it will not necessarily reduce disabilities. Treatment should be designed to minimize or eliminate disabilities and impairments through the practice of functional tasks. Treatment should also aim to assist patients in learning new motor strategies to reduce their disabilities.

Treatment for patients with neurological weakness or paralysis should be modified based on the level of motor unit activation displayed. Patients with stroke who have flaccid extremities must have their muscle tone developed and their joints stabilized by strengthening the surrounding muscle. They may require treatment with static functional positioning (ie, static positions that provide joint stability) and facilitation activities.

As motor unit activation becomes evident by visible muscle contraction, treatment programs should progress from static positioning and facilitation techniques to task-oriented activities that require movement. Have patients practice previously performed activities to retrain motor unit activation and develop adequate strength to accomplish common functional tasks. Development of skill and control are discussed in Chapter 7.

STRENGTHENING PATIENTS WITH FLACCIDITY

The emphasis of treatment for patients with flaccidity should be on the establishment of stability in a functional position (Flanagan,

1966). Functional positioning may include side-lying, sitting, or standing. You may assist patients into these positions as needed.

Task-Oriented Activities

Treatment emphasis should be on initiating stable postures and assisting the patient in functional movements that will be repeated as motor recovery occurs. For patients with flaccidity, rolling side-to-side and moving from a supine position to sitting will be difficult and may require the therapist's assistance. However, these are important functional tasks that must be initiated early on in the rehabilitative process to enable the patient to relieve pressure on bony prominences and obtain an upright sitting posture needed for pulmonary hygiene. Repetitive practice of these tasks requires activation of intact muscles and manual assistance by the therapist for PROM and weight bearing on the involved extremities.

Other functional tasks that should be practiced are transfers from bed to chair and sit-to-stand activities. In these tasks, as with those required for bed mobility, the therapist must manually assist the patient in passive movement and stabilization of the involved extremities. The physiologic stimulation produced in completion of these functional tasks will generate tremendous sensory stimulation and will increase cardiovascular and pulmonary function.

Selected Techniques of Facilitation to Enhance Functional Postures or Movement

To increase motor unit firing in flaccid muscles to maintain stable postures, therapists may choose to incorporate facilitation techniques that are based on the reflex model described in Chapter 3. When these techniques are used, they stimulate the spinal cord, which may result in a reflex motor response. For example, tapping on a muscle activates, among other things, muscle spindles. The Ia afferent neurons from the spindles travel to the spinal cord to excite alpha motor neurons that cause muscle contraction.

We recommend that facilitation techniques be incorporated during functional positioning or functional mobility. This will ensure that the muscle contraction becomes part of a functional task. The facilitation techniques of traditional neurorehabilitation theorists, such as Rood, that may be used to enhance functional positioning or movement include:

- Approximation
- Quick stretch
- Tapping
- Visual input

Performing facilitation techniques alone provides little effect if these techniques are not combined with stable and dynamic postures or functional movement. Inclusion of stable and dynamic postures and functional movements are based on the systems and task-oriented models.

Approximation

To apply this technique, place patients in weight-bearing positions that produce joint approximation. For the upper extremities, this can be accomplished by having patients sit in a weight-bearing position with the involved upper extremity extended to the side on a mat. Provide manual assistance as needed to stabilize the elbow. As the patient leans toward the involved side, weight-bearing through the upper extremity produces joint approximation (Fig. 5-11). The patient may also stand with the involved hand placed on a tabletop and the elbow extended to bear weight through the extremity. Recent evidence supports the effectiveness of upper extremity weight-bearing in normalizing and activating corticospinal facilitation of motor units in the muscles of hemiparetic patients (Brouwer & Ambury, 1994).

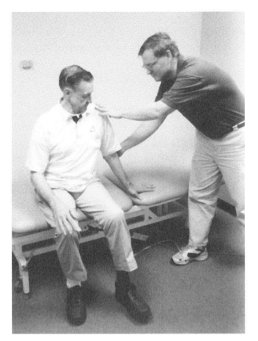

FIGURE 5-11.   The patient leans on the involved arm for joint approximation.

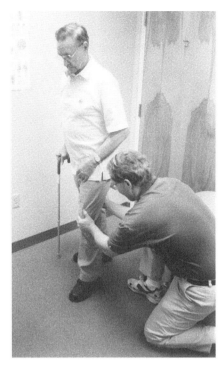

FIGURE 5-12.   The therapist assists the patient in weight-bearing through the involved knee by stabilizing that joint.

Joint approximation in the lower extremities is most easily accomplished by having the patient stand and shift weight onto the involved limbs. Again, manual assistance or use of an *airsplint* (an inflatable cylinder that prevents the extremity inside the splint from moving) may be needed to prevent the knee from buckling (Fig. 5-12).

If patients are unable to stand, weight-bearing (and, therefore, joint approximation) can be accomplished in the **hook-lying position.** In this position, the patient lies supine with the knees flexed so that both feet can be positioned flat on the surface on which the person is lying. Once in the hook-lying position, the patient may use **bridging,** fully extending the hips, thereby lifting the trunk off the surface, to attain approximation (Fig. 5-13).

Approximation techniques can be applied to several joints using a variety of positions (eg,

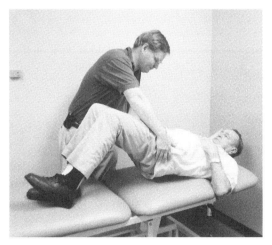

FIGURE 5-13.   Weight-bearing with bridging.

sitting, prone on elbows, quadruped, kneeling, standing) to challenge the patient. Tilt tables are effective for positioning patients upright and for enabling them to bear weight through the lower extremities. Upright postures that can be obtained on a tilt table produce joint approximation in the lower extremities, as well as vestibular activation when the head is upright. Standing with the support of a tilt table is not a functional position. However, the physiologic benefits of positioning a flaccid patient upright may outweigh the lack of functional carryover.

Quick Stretch

This technique is used with PROM or AROM. With the muscle in a lengthened position, quick stretch is applied to activate muscle spindles to produce excitatory impulses along the afferent pathways to alpha motor neurons. Quick stretch incorporates the monosynaptic reflex arc to activate motor units. This technique should be used in conjunction with the therapist verbally cuing the patient to contract the targeted muscle to perform a functional movement. An example of this is a quick stretch to the triceps muscle while the arm is supported on a table. This technique can be used to initiate elbow extension to reach for a glass placed in front of the patient.

Tapping

Tapping is similar to quick stretch in that it also incorporates the activation of muscle spindles. To perform this technique, tap the flaccid muscle belly while instructing the patient to contract the targeted muscle. A series of taps on the muscle is similar to repetitively eliciting a tendon tap with a reflex hammer. Figure 5-14 shows a therapist tapping the triceps muscle as the patient attempts to contract the muscle to maintain elbow extension in a weight-bearing posture. In this position, joint approximation may also contribute to activation of the triceps.

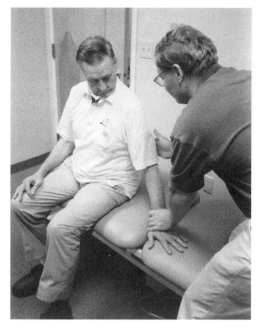

FIGURE 5-14. The therapist taps the patient's triceps muscle as the patient tries to contract it to maintain extension.

Visual Input

Visual input uses the patient's vision to view muscles contracting. This, in essence, serves as a form of movement-related biofeedback. Patients may be directed by the therapist to look at their arm or leg to provide feedback about stability or movement, or they may use a mirror to provide the visual feedback.

It is important to note that all of these techniques should be used only occasionally during treatment sessions. For example, when tapping the triceps muscle, provide stimuli for the first few contractions in functional positions, then, while withholding stimuli, ask the patient to contract the muscle without tapping. The goal is to activate muscles to assist patients in relearning how to move functionally. If facilitation techniques are applied consistently, patients may become conditioned to contract muscles or move only when stimuli are applied.

Other Treatment for Flaccidity

Therapists may choose to use electric stimulation to activate flaccid muscles. Low-frequency electric stimulation has been used to generate movement in paralyzed limbs and to increase strength in weak muscles. Electric stimulation can be applied to flaccid muscles to promote activation of the muscle fibers that are not receiving impulses from higher centers. Although the impulse from higher centers is absent, patients should be cued to attempt volitional contraction of the muscle as the electric impulse is received. Electric stimulation without the patient's volitional activation of contraction does not assist in developing strength. Whenever possible, the electric stimulation should be used in functional positions or movements. Examples of situations in which electric stimulation might be used successfully include:

- On the triceps when sitting and weight-bearing on the arm
- On the quadriceps during the stance phase
- On the anterior tibialis during swing phase

The benefits of electric stimulation include increased strength and endurance and prevention of disuse atrophy in partially denervated muscles (Gordon & Mao, 1994). Training methods with electric stimulation vary across rehabilitation centers, so comparisons of the efficacy of different training protocols have not been established.

Progression of Treatment for Patients With Flaccidity

As patients begin to contract muscles in stable postures or move without facilitation, increase the emphasis on volitional contraction and cease to use facilitation techniques. Patients are now no longer classified as suffering from flaccidity but rather from muscle weakness. As muscle activation occurs, provide additional task-oriented activities that focus on movement. This will allow the patient to capitalize on motor unit activity.

A simple progression is illustrated with the task of reaching for a cup. In the flaccid patient, we may start with weight-bearing in sitting to emphasize stability and then perform PROM with facilitation to start a movement of reaching for the cup. From here, we progress to **active assistive exercise** (**AAE**) in functional, **gravity-eliminated** planes. Having the patient support the exercised arm on a tabletop is one way of eliminating the force of gravity. Progress the patient through AROM with gravity eliminated to AROM *against* gravity.

Adding movement to weight-bearing activities will allow the patient to shift into and out of stable postures. For example, as patients sit and bear weight through their involved upper extremities, have them gently bend and then straighten their elbows (Fig. 5-15). This incorporates joint approximation and active movement in the upper extremity with resistance of the body weight through the limb. In the lower extremity, hook-lying positions can be used to initiate weight-bearing. Patients can be verbally cued to engage in active movement by suggesting that they lift the buttocks off the mat into a bridged position (ie, joint approximation with active movement), then slowly lower the buttocks back to the mat. Patients can perform this activity repeatedly, or, while in bridged positions, they can move their knees into abduction and adduction (Fig. 5-16).

Another dynamic activity in bridged positions is extending one leg while bearing weight on the opposite leg. Alternating legs will increase the stability of the weight-bearing leg and introduce dynamic activities in the opposite extremity. Practice of these activities in the hook-lying position may not carry over to

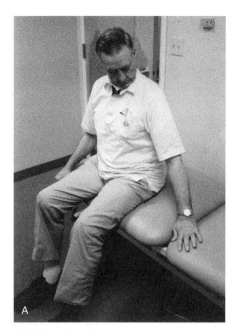
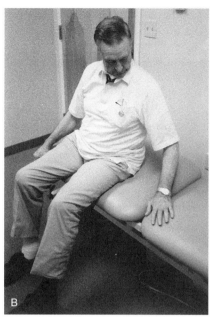

FIGURE 5-15. Add movement to weight-bearing activities in the involved limb to enable the patient to shift into and out of stable postures. (*A*) The patient extends and then (*B*) flexes the elbow.

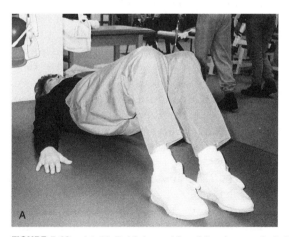
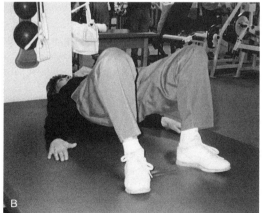

FIGURE 5-16 (*A,B*) Bridging with adduction and abduction of the legs.

improved functional mobility. However, re-educating the gluteus and quadriceps to contract while in the hook-lying position may be of some value when the patient attempts to contract the muscle in a more functional position (eg, while standing or moving from sitting to standing).

A more functional activity for the patient would be standing and repeatedly stepping forward and back with one foot. The lower extremity that provides support remains fixed distally while the proximal joints are in motion. The patient alternates between the legs to accommodate the stance and swing phases of the gait cycle.

Moving into and out of positions that comprise the tasks of functional mobility is another form of introducing dynamic activities and increasing stability. Patients may start in any position and progress to the reclining or upright position, depending on the functional mobility that needs to be developed. For example, if the patient starts in a sitting position, introduce weight-shifting from side to side and anteriorly and posteriorly. Then have the patient stand or assume a side-lying posture. Shifting the weight from side to side prepares the patient for moving into a side-lying position. Weight-shifting to the side is needed to achieve the recumbent position. Shifting the weight anteriorly and posteriorly (with emphasis on anterior weight shift) is part of the sit-to-stand activity.

One major problem that patients with stroke develop is the inability to shift their weight anteriorly while trying to stand. Functional mobility should be incorporated into static and dynamic activities for the patient progressing out of flaccidity. Manual assistance may be needed with these activities depending on the extent of weakness.

Patients should be allowed to progress into more advanced activities as soon as possible. (See the next section on strengthening for the patient with weakness.) Remember, patient strength will increase only if resistance in-

creases. Patients should not be set up for failure and frustration; be prepared to provide manual assistance as needed to enable them to accomplish the task. For example, if the patient is unable to move from a low-seated position to standing, provide manual assistance to initiate momentum or assist with the lifting phase of the movement. To repeat the task, modify the surface to a chair with a higher seat and gradually reintroduce the lower seat at a later time.

●●●●●●●●●●●●●●●●●●●●●●●●●●●●●●●●●●

STRENGTHENING PATIENTS WITH WEAKNESS

Strengthening programs for neurological patients with muscle weakness can progress from isometric to eccentric to concentric contractions (Berta Bobath, 1982), all of which are needed to complete functional tasks. (**Concentric contractions** are those that produce limb movement.) The purpose of this progression is to prevent the development of synergies, which usually occur as patients attempt to concentrically contract weakened muscles through full ROM (Berta Bobath, 1982).

Isometric contractions should be performed at midrange to produce the greatest tension in muscle, which promotes the greatest success in contracting. For example, if the task is to reach into the cabinet for a cup, start with an isometric contraction at the level of shoulder flexion needed to reach the cabinet. Eccentric contractions enable continued tension to develop in muscle as it lengthens. Once the patient has maintained the isometric contraction, have the patient slowly lower the arm from the initial position to produce a lengthening contraction. Concentric contractions should be developed as well because they are used to bring the hand to the mouth, to step forward in gait, and to climb stairs. However, if concentric contractions result in synergistic movement, continue to build strength in the isometric and eccentric modes, or position the extremity in a gravity-eliminated plane to work concentric contractions. Reintroduce gravity as the concentric movement is performed without synergistic overflow.

Therapeutically, concentric and eccentric contractions are produced during AAE, AROM, and **active resistive exercises (ARE),** those performed with resistance provided by a therapist or by other resistive equipment, such as free weights. Once the patient is able to perform AROM successfully, add resistance. Having the patient perform ARE allows for the recruitment of additional motor units and the strengthening of muscle. Repeated muscle contraction without resistance will not increase a patient's strength.

Task-Oriented Activities

The task-oriented activities to use for strength training should be based on the assessment of the patient's functional mobility (or identification of disabilities). Tasks that patients have difficulty performing should become the major emphasis of the strengthening program and should be practiced as whole-task activities whenever possible. By repeating functional tasks several times, patients learn the movement sequence and exercise the muscles needed to perform the tasks.

The environment should be modified to enable patients to accomplish the tasks, then gradually changed to make the tasks harder. For example, when transferring from a sitting position to standing, patients should begin the task

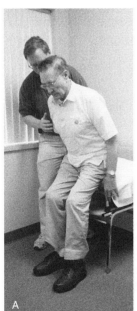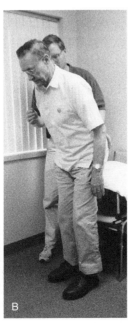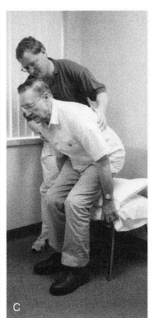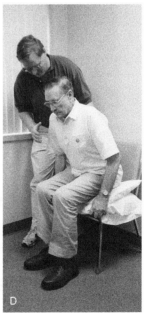

FIGURE 5-17. Have the patient accomplish the sit-to-stand maneuver from chairs of varying heights. Once the patient has successfully managed the maneuver from a high seat (*A,B*), have the patient practice it from a lower seat (*C,D*).

from chairs with raised seats to enable them to move through normal symmetrical patterns. As this movement becomes easier, lower seat heights should be used to make it more difficult; this will also require the muscles used in this movement sequence to contract differently (Fig. 5-17). Tasks can be made even more difficult by asking patients to stand without using their hands or by having them hold a weighted box in their hands as they stand up.

Climbing stairs is another example of a functional task that can be used to increase strength. If patients have weakness in the muscles of flexion, repeatedly stepping up and down on a step will increase the concentric strength of flexor muscles and the eccentric strength of extensor muscles (Fig. 5-18). This task can be

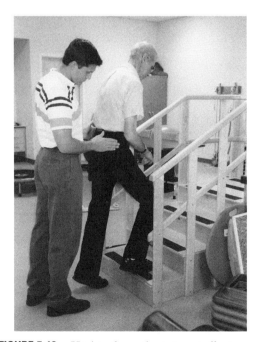

FIGURE 5-18. Having the patient repeatedly step up and down on a step will increase the concentric strength of flexor muscles and the eccentric strength of extensor muscles as he lowers himself down from the step.

made easier or more difficult by allowing or disallowing upper extremity support on handrails and by modifying the height of the step. Adding weight to the involved extremities also makes the task more difficult and strengthens the muscles used in performing the activity.

Whole-task activities are ideal for practice regimens. However, patients who are unable to perform the whole task may have to perform partial-task activities. Progression to whole-task activities should be made as soon as the patient can participate in the task with assistance if needed.

Having the patient repeatedly step up and down with one leg is an example of breaking the whole task of reciprocal stair climbing into its component partial tasks. Stepping forward and back with one leg is another example of a partial task of walking (Fig. 5-19). Practicing this activity repeatedly and then incorporating the whole task of walking into treatment sessions should increase strength and control movement patterns.

It is unclear in the literature whether partial-task activities should be used as a precursor to more functional whole-task activities, or if partial-task activities should be avoided because they are not functional. It is also difficult to determine which partial-task activities carry over to whole-task performance and which whole tasks can and cannot be broken down into partial tasks. Naylor and Briggs (1963) suggest that whole tasks that involve continuous movements (ie, coordination and timing of movements are linked together) and last less than 200 msec may not be appropriate for part-task practice. When movements are more serial, or step-by step in their pattern, part-task practice may be effective. Unfortunately, aside from the information provided by Naylor and Briggs, no research conclusively documents whether partial-task activities are valid. Furthermore, no research reports which functional activities can

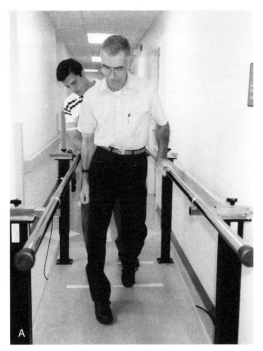 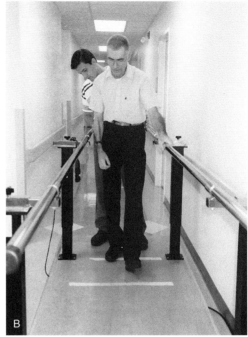

FIGURE 5-19. Having the patient step forward (*A*) and back (*B*) is one way to break the whole task of walking into its component parts.

be broken down into partial tasks and which activities should not be broken down.

Practicing tasks of functional mobility under the guidance of a therapist may enhance movement patterns and muscle strength. Activities that imitate situations patients may face on discharge should be added to the treatment program as soon as possible. This may include designing ambulation exercises in the hospital lobby that simulate ambulation in the patient's home environments (ie, other people moving about in a room and repeatedly stopping and starting ambulation). Whenever possible, therapists should make a visit to the patient's home before discharge to assess the environment and architectural impediments so that they may further modify the treatment program.

Other tasks of functional mobility that should be practiced include rolling, the supine-to-sit and sit-to-stand maneuvers, standing, walking, and climbing the stairs. Examples of functional tasks or recreational activities to be included are throwing a ball, tossing a ring, reaching to a cabinet, reaching on tables for objects, practicing a golf swing, sweeping, vacuuming, hammering, brushing hair/teeth, and opening doors. It is important to use functional tasks that patients were capable of performing before the disability. If patients did not previously play golf or vacuum, then attempting these new tasks may be difficult for the patient after the disability develops. Incorporating functional mobility as part of strength training programs enables therapists to be creative in developing treatment plans. It also allows the therapist to address disabilities that limit a patient's independence.

Other Treatments for Strengthening

Task-oriented activities are not the only activities that can be used in a treatment program to increase strength. The following are examples of specific treatments that have been described in the literature as appropriate to strengthen muscles:

- Therapeutic exercise: AAE, AROM, and ARE with free weights
- Proprioceptive neuromuscular facilitation (PNF)
- Isokinetic training
- Electric stimulation
- Biofeedback
- Isotonic weight machines
- Therapeutic ball
- Endurance training

Therapeutic Exercise: AAE, AROM, and ARE With Free Weights

Therapeutic exercise programs that incorporate the normal movement patterns of muscles and joints can be designed for patients. We recommend that these exercises be performed in a functional position such as sitting or standing whenever possible. This will give the patient practice in maintaining posture during functional movement or exercise. Programs may be modified to include gravity-eliminated positions, active assistance, gravity positions, and free weights based on the patient's abilities. Free weights have been used in several studies to increase the strength of weak muscles (Aitkens, McCrory, Kilmer, & Bernauer, 1993; Inaba, Edberg, Montgomery, & Gillis, 1973; Judge, Underwood, & Gennosa, 1993; Kilmer, McCrory, Wright, Aitkens, & Bernauer, 1994; Milner-

Brown, 1993; Milner-Brown & Miller, 1988; Thompson, 1994).

When designing therapeutic exercise programs for patients, remember to start at levels where they can accomplish the task. To increase muscle strength, progress them into positions where gravity resists movement as soon as possible.

Proprioceptive Neuromuscular Facilitation (PNF)

The theoretical basis for PNF is discussed in Chapter 4. See Display 5-2 for a brief description of diagonal movements and Figure 5-20 for photographic representations of those movements.

In the text that follows, we present the verbal commands that would accompany each of the diagonal movements as well as treatment techniques. Readers should be aware that PNF relies on external stimulation to activate motor control. This is not what occurs in real life because facilitation techniques are not provided in daily activities. As with therapeutic exercise, we advocate performing the PNF diagonals sitting or standing.

Suggested verbal commands for moving the upper extremity through diagonals may include the following:

- For D1 flexion and extension: ''Close your hand and pull up and across your body; open your hand and push down and away from your body.''
- For D2 flexion and extension: ''Open your hand and pull up and away from your body; close your hand, pull down and across your body.''

Suggested verbal commands for moving the lower extremity through diagonals may include:

- For D1 flexion and extension: ''Point your toes up; pull up and across your body; point your toes down, push down and away from your body.''
- For D2 flexion and extension: ''Point your toes up, pull up and away from

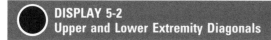

DISPLAY 5-2
Upper and Lower Extremity Diagonals

Upper Extremity Diagonals

D1 flexion	shoulder flexion, adduction, external rotation, supination, wrist and finger flexion
D1 extension	shoulder extension, abduction, internal rotation, pronation, wrist and finger extension
D2 flexion	shoulder flexion, abduction, external rotation, supination, wrist and finger extension
D2 extension	shoulder extension, adduction, internal rotation, pronation, wrist and finger flexion

Lower Extremity Diagonals

D1 flexion	hip flexion, adduction, external rotation, ankle inversion and dorsiflexion
D1 extension	hip extension, abduction, internal rotation, ankle eversion and plantar flexion
D2 flexion	hip flexion, abduction, internal rotation, ankle eversion and dorsiflexion
D2 extension	hip extension, adduction, external rotation, ankle inversion and plantar flexion

* Note: The description of lower extremity diagonals is with knee extension; diagonals can also be performed with knee flexion.

your body; point your toes down, push down and across your body."

When performing diagonals, the first step is positioning the extremities so that the muscles are lengthened. Provide graded resistance as patients move through the diagonals. At the end range, antagonist muscles are lengthened and thus ready to contract in the opposite direction. For example, in upper extremity D1 flexion the muscles of flexion, adduction, and lateral rotation are lengthened in the beginning and shortened at the end range. D1 extension begins in this end range of D1 flexion with the muscles of extension, abduction, and medial rotation in a lengthened state.

Treatment Techniques With PNF.   The following techniques have been developed with PNF but could be incorporated in any type of active exercise program.

- Slow reversal: repeated slow movement through the diagonal such as D1 flexion and extension
- Slow reversal hold: repeated slow movement through the diagonal such as D1 flexion/extension with isometric contractions at the end of each movement
- Repeated contractions with quick stretch: one diagonal (eg, D1) with a quick stretch added throughout the range to increase motor unit recruitment.

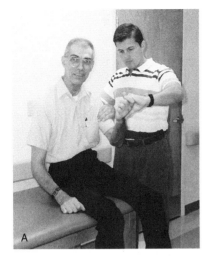
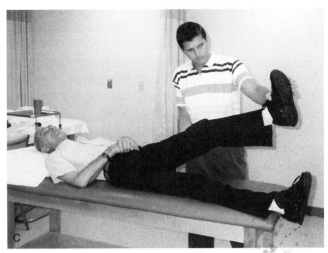
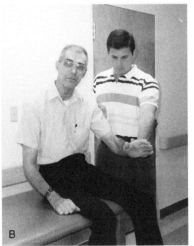
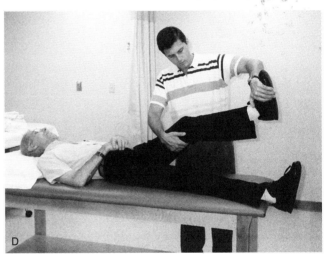

FIGURE 5-20.   PNF diagonals: (*A*) D1 flexion; (*B*) D1 extension; (*C*) D2 flexion; (*D*) D2 extension.

- Agonistic reversals: one diagonal of concentric then eccentric contractions. Eccentric contractions are performed with the therapist pulling the patient out of the diagonal. For example, the patient does D1 flexion concentrically and is then told, "Hold it. Don't let me move you," while the therapist overcomes the isometric contraction and produces lengthening contractions.
- Hold relax active movement: an isometric contraction performed midrange of a diagonal, or at a weak point in the diagonal; this is followed by relaxation while the extremity is passively moved back to the beginning range of the diagonal;

thereafter follows active movement back to or beyond the ROM where the isometric was performed.

In the slow reversal hold technique, diagonal patterns (D1 or D2) are performed with isometric contractions at end ranges. Isometric contractions are held while gentle pressure is applied to move the extremity in the opposite diagonal. Physiologically, this activates muscle spindles that were not activated due to shortening of muscle fibers. Manual contact and gentle resistance activate additional sensory information to increase muscle activation.

A similar principle is at work with repeated contractions with quick stretch and agonistic reversals. All treatment techniques use some form of external (exteroreceptive) or internal (proprioceptive) sensory information to facilitate muscle activation, which is a component of the reflex model.

Isokinetic Training

This type of strengthening program uses machines that can vary resistance throughout the ROM, while maintaining a set speed of motion. Several different protocols are used that incorporate isometric, concentric, and eccentric contractions. Studies have demonstrated that muscle strength increases when the muscle is exercised in any of these modes of contraction (Einarsson, 1991; McMurdo & Rennie, 1994). However, the current debate is over whether these gains in strength carry over to improved functional mobility.

Some activities for the lower extremities can be performed in weight-bearing positions that enhance a stable posture in standing. Movements performed on isokinetic equipment should be designed to resemble functional movement patterns to enhance the transference of strength to functional tasks.

Strength training spastic muscle does not appear to be detrimental to gait development. However, gait patterns are not enhanced by strength training alone (Giuliani, Light, & Rose, 1993; Rose et al., 1992). In studies by Rose and coworkers (1992) and Giuliani and colleagues (1993), isokinetic strength training was conducted on lower extremities that displayed spasticity. Gait training was not part of the treatment protocol but was one of the outcome measures. A change in gait was not found with the strength training program, and neither were detriments in function.

Electric Stimulation

Electric stimulation was discussed earlier in the section on strength training patients with flaccidity. It has been demonstrated to increase muscle strength, especially when used in conjunction with some form of therapeutic exercise (Abel-Moty et al., 1993; Delitto & Snyder-Mackler, 1990). We advocate the use of electric stimulation with functional tasks, such as gait training, to address weakness in the anterior tibialis. Protocols for application of electric stimulation vary within facilities.

Biofeedback

Electromyographic biofeedback is the process by which muscle potentials are transformed into auditory or visual cues in an attempt to increase or decrease voluntary muscle activity. To increase muscle activity, biofeedback can be used to assist the patient in recruiting more motor units, increasing the rate at which those motor units are fired, or both. To achieve this goal, the threshold of auditory or visual cues (or both) should be placed at a low or minimal setting. The threshold can be increased as the patient is able to recruit more motor units, increase the rate of firing, or both. Thresholds should be set so that patients can succeed at the required task, even as they are continually provided with visual cues, auditory cues, or both (Rosenfalck & Andreassen, 1980; Umphred, 1995).

Placement of biofeedback electrodes is an important consideration. When treating weak muscle, electrodes should be placed as far apart as possible so that even low muscle activity will be sensed. As the muscle becomes stronger, specific areas of the muscle group can be targeted by placing the electrodes closer together over those targeted areas (Rosenfalck & Andreassen, 1980; Umphred, 1995).

Biofeedback can be used to selectively recruit muscles that are antagonistic to the hyperactive muscles. By recruiting such muscle groups, the patient is able to actively stretch shortened, hypertonic muscle groups by contracting the antagonistic muscle.

With neurologically involved patients, EMG biofeedback is typically applied in a proximal-to-distal progression. Recruitment of proximal muscles precedes recruitment of distal muscle groups, regardless of whether recruitment is in the upper or lower extremities. It is also best to attempt to recruit muscle groups to perform functional activities (Rosenfalck & Andreassen, 1980; Umphred, 1995).

Isotonic Weight Machines

Isotonic weight machines are found in most outpatient physical therapy clinics. We have advanced far beyond the days of the N-K table for knee extension, and now have devices to strengthen all major muscle groups. Just as with free weights, isotonic machines are effective in strengthening muscles. Many activities are performed in non–weight-bearing positions, so transference of strength to functional tasks is questionable.

Therapeutic Balls

Therapeutic balls can be used for a variety of activities to increase postural stability, upper extremity strength, balance, righting, and equilibrium reactions. Patients can sit statically on balls or rock gently to address postural stability as well as balance reactions. Rising to stand from sitting on a ball (whether large or small) will increase lower extremity strength while also incorporating postural reactions. The difficulty of the task can be made greater by moving to a smaller ball from a larger ball. Throwing a therapy ball will increase upper extremity strength and address postural stability and balance reactions. These are examples of simple activities that can be performed with therapeutic balls. Continuing education courses offer a variety of treatment applications that can be used in this area.

Endurance Training

Muscles that fatigue after a few submaximal contractions require endurance training. This type of training will not increase muscle strength but will enable muscle to sustain activity over longer periods of time. Low-resistance, high-repetition exercise will increase muscle endurance. This can be performed with functional tasks, free weights, isokinetic machines, or isotonic devices. Endurance training is time consuming, so selecting an activity or several activities that patients enjoy performing is critical. Walking on flat surfaces or on treadmills, stair climbing, using exercise bikes (especially upper and lower extremity bikes), rowing machines, or simulated cross-country skiing increases endurance and may be more enjoyable than lifting light weights.

Case Study

Treatment of the Disability

Results of the assessment of disabilities and impairments:

- Rolling to right—independent.
- Rolling to left—moderate assistance to protract shoulder and advance right hip forward.
- Supine-to-sit maneuver—moderate assistance, unable to use right arm to push up, and unable to bear weight on the right arm. Left leg is used to push right leg off the side of the bed.
- Stable sitting—requires minimal assistance to maintain sitting, which is asymmetrical. Patient also supports self with left upper extremity.
- Sit-to-stand maneuver and standing— requires maximal assistance, the patient does not appear to bear weight on the involved lower extremity, and leans excessively toward the involved side.
- Ambulation is not attempted due to the difficulty of coming to a standing posture.
- AROM—limited in right upper and lower extremities, with appearance of synergistic movement as the patient attempts isolated movement.
- PROM—within normal limits and no resistance to passive ROM felt.

- Sensory—localization and proprioception intact.
- Balance assessment—negative for vertigo, nausea, or nystagmus with positional changes.

At the bedside, demonstrate a technique of rolling to the left side that will reinforce previously learned movement strategies of rolling that the patient used when rolling to the right. Instruct Mr. Jones to use his noninvolved upper extremity to assist in shoulder protraction of the involved arm if needed. You may have to assist in placing the right hip and knee in flexion to enable joint alignment for pushing into hip extension if that was the strategy used. Joint approximation through the hip joint can be provided occasionally to facilitate firing of hip extensors (Fig. 5-21).

Repeat rolling activities two to three times toward the involved and noninvolved sides. After practicing rolling, have the patient stay in side-lying, and begin to address side-lying to sitting at the edge of the bed. Again, have Mr. Jones practice this on both sides. Provide assistance as needed.

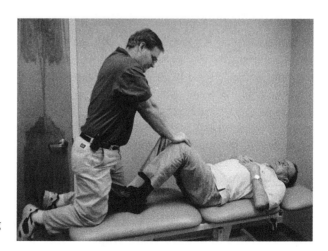

FIGURE 5-21. Place the patient in a hook-lying posture and provide joint approximation.

Once Mr. Jones is sitting, work on stable symmetrical sitting postures. If an unstable posture exists, place the involved upper extremity out to the side of the body in a weight-bearing position. Provide manual approximation or stabilize the limb as needed. Decrease your support and use the patient's upper extremities as soon as possible to enable activation of trunk musculature. As this is obtained, withdraw your support on the patient's arm and work on having him assume an unsupported, symmetrical sitting posture.

Visual feedback from a mirror often helps the patient correct postural abnormalities due to weakness or somatosensory loss. The sit-to-stand maneuver should be practiced (with the assistance of two people if needed) to maintain stable upright postures. To facilitate the patient's learned movement of the task without assistance, consider including some of the modifications described in the section on assessing the disability. The progression of treatment should continue to ambulation as soon as possible.

Gait training programs can be broken into several smaller partial-task components if needed. Shifting the weight from side to side and forward and backward will activate the muscles of stance in the involved lower extremity. Stepping forward with the involved limb, weight-shifting forward and then backward, and stepping back with the involved limb activates muscles of both the stance and swing phases (Fig. 5-22). Stepping forward with the noninvolved limb activates weight shift and the muscles of the stance phase of the involved limb. Whole-task practice of ambulation must be included in the treatment program for the patient to relearn the motor sequence.

Depending on the setting in which Mr. Jones is receiving treatment, therapeutic exercises for upper and lower extremities can be initiated. If treatment is initially in an acute care facility, the emphasis should be on functional movements with instruction of these activities to appropriate family caregivers. If he is in a medical rehabilitation unit or subacute facility, therapeutic exercises for all extremities can and should be part of his functional treatment program. Whenever possible, exercise should be performed in sitting or standing to activate trunk muscles in upright postures, and to train the muscles of the involved extremities to work in functional postures.

INCREASING RANGE OF MOTION

Limitations in ROM may contribute to a decrease in active movement and performance of functional tasks. Treatments to increase joint ROM resulting from soft tissue restrictions include: moist heat, PROM, positioning, and contract relax exercises. Moist heat can be applied before stretching exercises are performed to increase muscle elasticity. Performing light repetitive exercises, such as riding a stationary bike, is another way to increase muscle temperature to increase elasticity.

Passive ROM performed to increase joint range should be slow, with a prolonged holding of the extremity at the end range to stretch tight muscles. For example, with tight hamstrings, the limb should be moved into hip flexion until resistance is met. At this point, the limb should be maintained in maximum hip flexion for a minimum of 30 seconds, then tension released by slightly lowering the limb into hip extension.

Positioning of extremities provides prolonged stretch on tight muscles. For example, to address tight wrist flexors, which are evident

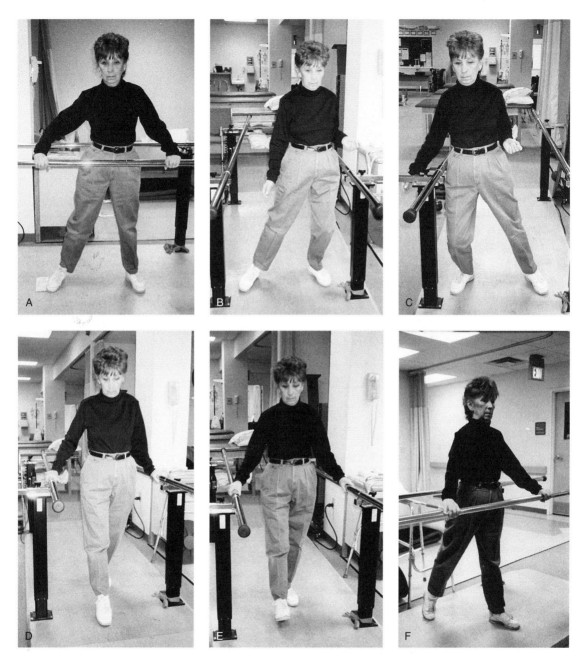

FIGURE 5-22. Patient assumes a wide base of support in (*A*) standing; (*B,C*) weight-shifting; (*D*) transfer to a narrow base of support; (*E,F*) stepping forward and back.

in hemiplegia, position the wrist passively in as much extension as possible, with the patient bearing weight through the extremity in seated or standing positions (see Fig. 5-23). As patients lean forward and bear weight through their arms, they produce prolonged stretch on wrist flexors.

The technique of contract relax can be performed in a variety of manners to produce muscle elongation. One technique involves an isometric contraction of the muscle positioned at its greatest length followed by passive lengthening. Another technique requires that the muscle be positioned in the same manner, but with isometric contractions of the antagonist muscle, followed by passive lengthening.

Limitations in ROM must be addressed to achieve optimal strength of muscle in functional movement patterns.

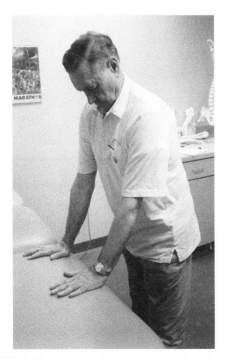

FIGURE 5-23. Patient demonstrates weight-bearing through the extended wrist from a standing position.

SUMMARY

- Exercising muscle in isolated, nonfunctional movements will result in increased muscle strength, but it may not contribute to improved patient function.
- Task-oriented activities should be the emphasis of treatment programs to ensure maximal functional mobility in our patients.
- Weakness, defined as the inability to generate normal levels of muscle force, can result from a disruption of inadequate corticospinal activation, disruption of impulses through alpha motor neurons, synaptic dysfunction, or damage within the muscle tissue.
- Weakness may limit patients' ability to perform tasks of functional mobility by interfering with their ability to maintain their centers of gravity and postural symmetry.
- The presence of abnormal muscle tone or synergy may impair normal movement. Emphasis in treatment should be on strengthening agonist and antagonist muscles together.
- A task-oriented approach to strengthening should be used in patients with flaccidity, synergy, spasticity, or weakness.
- The systems model and task-oriented model are the theoretical frameworks on which the evaluation and treatment program for the impairment of weakness is structured.

REFERENCES

Abel-Moty, E, Fishbain, DA, Goldberg, M, Cutler, R, Zaki, AM, Khalil, TM, Peppard, T, Rosomoff, RS, & Rosomoff, HL. (1994). Functional electrical stimulation treatment of postradiculopathy associated muscle weakness. *Archives of Physical Medicine and Rehabilitation, 75,* 680–686.

Aitkens, SG, McCrory, MA, Kilmer, DD, & Bernauer, EM. (1993). Moderate resistance exercise program: Its effect in slowly progressive neuromuscular disease. *Archives of Physical Medicine and Rehabilitation, 74,* 711–715.

Berta Bobath Assessment and Treatment. (1982). *An adult with hemiplegia.* Funded by the Administration on Aging and the NDT Instructors Group. University of Maryland, Department of Physical Therapy, School of Medicine. Copyright 1982.

Bohannon, RW. (1989). Is the measurement of muscle strength appropriate in patients with brain lesions? A special communication. *Physical Therapy, 69*(3), 225–236.

Bohannon, RW, & Smith, MB. (1987a). Interrater reliability of a modified Ashworth Scale of muscle spasticity. *Physical Therapy, 67*(2), 206–207.

Bohannon, RW, & Smith, MB. (1987b). Upper extremity strength deficits in hemiplegic stroke patients: Relationship between admission and discharge assessment and time since onset. *Archives of Physical Medicine and Rehabilitation, 68,* 155–157.

Brouwer, BJ, Ambury, P. (1994). Upper extremity weight-bearing effect on corticospinal excitability following stroke. *Archives of Physical Medicine and Rehabilitation, 75,* 861–866.

Cress, ME, Johnson, J, & Agre, JC. (1991). Isokinetic strength testing in older women: A comparison of two systems. *Journal Orthopedic and Sports Physical Therapy, 13*(4), 199–202.

Craik, RL. (1991). Abnormalities of motor behavior. In *Contemporary management of motor control problems.* Proceedings of the II Step Conference. Foundation for Physical Therapy, Alexandria, VA.

Daniels, L, & Worthingham, C. (1986). *Muscle testing: Techniques of manual examination* (5th ed.). Philadelphia: Saunders.

Danneskiold-Samsoe, B, Kofod, V, Munter, J, Grimby, G, Schnohr, P, & Jensen, G. (1984). Muscle strength and functional capacity in 78–81-year-old men and women. *Journal of Applied Physiology, 52,* 310–314.

Dantes, M, & McComas, AJ. (1991). The extent and time-course of motoneurone involvement in amyotrophic later sclerosis. *Muscle and Nerve, 14,* 416–421.

Delitto, A, & Snyder-Mackler, LS. (1990). Two theories of muscle strength augmentation using percutaneous electrical stimulation. *Physical Therapy, 70,* 158–164.

Demeurisse, G, Demol, O, & Robaye, E. (1980). Motor evaluation in vascular hemiplegia. *European Neurology, 19,* 382–389.

Einarsson, G. (1991). Muscle conditioning in late poliomyelitis. *Archives of Physical Medicine and Rehabilitation, 72,* 11–14.

Falkel, J. (1978). Plantar flexor strength testing using the Cybex isokinetic dynamometer. *Physical Therapy, 58*(7), 847–850.

Fisher, NM, Gresham, GE, Abrams, M, Hicks, J, Horrigan, D, & Pendergast, DR. (1993). Quantitative effects of physical therapy on muscular and functional performance in subjects with osteoarthritis of the knees. *Archives of Physical Medicine and Rehabilitation, 74,* 840–847.

Flanagan, EM. (1966). Methods for facilitation and inhibition of motor activity. *American Journal of Physical Medicine, 46*(1), 1006–1011.

Gentile, AM. (1987). Skill acquisition: Action, movement, and neuromotor processes. In JH Carr & RB Shepherd (Eds.). *Movement science, foundations for physical therapy in rehabilitation.* Rockville, MD: Aspen.

Giuliani, CA, Light, KE, & Rose, DK. (1993). The effect of an isokinetic exercise program on gait patterns in patients with hemiparesis. *Neurology Report, 17,* 23.

Glendinning, DS, & Enoka, RM. (1994). Motor unit behavior in Parkinson's disease. *Physical Therapy, 74*(1), 61–70.

Gordon, T, & Mao, J. (1994). Muscle atrophy and procedures for training after spinal cord injury. *Physical Therapy, 74,* 50–60.

Graves, JE, Pollock, ML, Carpenter, DM, Leggett, SH, Jones, A, MacMillan, M, & Fulton, M. (1990). Quantitative assessment of full range-of-motion isometric lumbar extension strength. *Spine, 15*(4), 289–294.

Grimby, G, Aniansson, A, Hedberg, M, Henning, GB, Grandgard, V, & Kvist, H. (1992). Training can improve muscle strength and endurance in 78- to 84-year old men. *Journal of Applied Physiology, 73*(6), 2517–2523.

Guyton, AC. (1996). *Textbook of medical physiology* (9th ed.). Philadelphia: Saunders.

Haley, SM, & Inacio, CA. (1990). Evaluation of spasticity and its effect on motor function. In MB Glenn & J Whyte (Eds.). *The practical management of spasticity in children and adults.* Philadelphia: Lea & Febiger.

Hamrin, E, Eklund, G, Hillgren, AK, Borges, O, Hall, J, & Hellstrom, O. (1982). Muscle strength and balance in post-stroke patients. *Upsula Journal of Medicine and Science, 87,* 11–26.

Hasson, SM. (1994). *Clinical exercise physiology*. St. Louis: Mosby-Year Book.

Hasue, M, Fujiwara, M, & Kikuchi, S. (1980). A new method of quantitative measurement of abdominal and back muscle strength. *Spine, 5*(2), 143–148.

Heller, A, Wade, DT, Wood, VA, Sunderland, A, Hewer, RL, & Ward, E. (1987). Arm function after stroke: Measurement and recovery over the first three months. *Journal of Neurology, Neurosurgery, and Psychiatry, 50,* 714–719.

Hufschmidt, A, & Mauritz, K-H. (1985). Chronic transformation of muscle in spasticity: A peripheral contribution to increased tone. *Journal of Neurology, Neurosurgery, and Psychiatry, 48,* 676–685.

Inaba, M, Edberg, E, Montgomery, J, & Gillis, MK. (1973). Effectiveness of functional training, active exercise, and resistive exercise for patients with hemiplegia. *Physical Therapy, 53,* 28–35.

Judge, JO, Underwood, M, & Gennosa, T. (1993). Exercise to improve gait velocity in older persons. *Archives of Physical Medicine and Rehabilitation, 74,* 400–406.

Kendall, FP, McCreary, EK, & Provance, PG. (1993). *Muscles, testing and function* (4th ed.). Philadelphia: Williams & Wilkins.

Kilmer, DD, McCrory, MA, Wright, NC, Aitkens, SG, & Bernauer, EM. (1994). The effect of a high resistance exercise program in slowly progressive neuromuscular disease. *Archives of Physical Medicine and Rehabilitation, 75,* 560–563.

Kisner, C, & Colby, LA. (1990). *Therapeutic exercise, foundations and techniques*. Philadelphia: Davis.

Kleyweg, RP, Frans, GA, Meche, VD, & Schmitz, PI. (1991). Interobserver agreement in the assessment of muscle strength and functional abilities in Guillain-Barre syndrome. *Muscle and Nerve, 14,* 1103–1109.

Larsson, L, Grimby, G, & Karlsson, J. (1979). Muscle strength and speed of movement in relation to age and muscle morphology. *Journal of Applied Physiology, 46*(3), 451–456.

Lenman, JAR. (1959). A clinical and experimental study of the effects of exercise on motor weakness in neurological disease. *Journal of Neurology, Neurosurgery, and Psychiatry, 22,* 182–194.

Leonard, CT. (1993). H-reflex and surface electromyographic testing to quantity progress in the neurologic patient (pp. 39–43). Presented at the 1993 Combined Sections Meeting of the American Physical Therapy Association.

Lewis, KS, & Mueller, WM. (1993). Intrathecal baclofen for severe spasticity secondary to spinal cord injury. *Annals of Pharmacotherapeutics, 27*(6), 767–774.

Light, KE. (1996). Clients with spasticity: To strengthen or not to strengthen. *Neurology Report, 15*(1), 19–20.

Lord, JP, Aitkens, SG, McCrory, MA, & Bernauer, EM. (1992). Isometric and isokinetic measurement of hamstring and quadriceps strength. *Archives of Physical Medicine and Rehabilitation, 73,* 324–330.

McCartney, N, Moroz, D, Garner, SH, & McComas, AJ. (1988). The effects of strength training in patients with selected neuromuscular disorders. *Medicine and Science in Sports and Exercise, 20*(4), 362–368.

McComas, AJ. (1991). [Invited Review]. Motor unit estimation: Methods, results, and present status. *Muscle and Nerve, 14,* 585–597.

McMurdo, MET, & Rennie, LM. (1994). Improvements in quadriceps strength with regular seated exercise in the institutionalized elderly. *Archives of Physical Medicine and Rehabilitation, 75,* 600–603.

Millington, PJ, Myklebust, BM, & Shambes, GM. (1992). Biomechanical analysis of the sit-to-stand motion in elderly persons. *Archives of Physical Medicine and Rehabilitation, 73,* 609–617.

Milner-Brown, HS. (1993). Muscle strengthening in a post-polio subject through a high-resistance weight-training program. *Archives of Physical Medicine and Rehabilitation, 74,* 1165–1167.

Milner-Brown, HS, Mellenthin, M, & Miller, RG. (1986). Quantifying human muscle strength, endurance, and fatigue. *Archives of Physical Medicine and Rehabilitation, 67,* 530–535.

Milner-Brown, HS, & Miller, RG. (1989). Increased muscular fatigue in patients with neurogenic muscle weakness: Quantification and pathophysiology. *Archives of Physical Medicine and Rehabilitation, 70,* 361–366.

Naylor, J, & Briggs, G. (1963). Effects of task complexity and task organization on the relative efficiency of part and whole training methods. *Journal of Experimental Psychology, 65,* 217.

Newton, M, & Waddell, G. (1993). Trunk strength testing with Iso-machines. Part I: Review of a decade of scientific evidence. *Spine, 18*(7), 801–811.

Nicholas, JJ, Robinson, LR, Logan, A, & Robertson, R. (1989). Isokinetic testing in young nonathletic able-bodied subjects. *Archives of Physical Medicine and Rehabilitation, 70,* 210–213.

Peach, PE. (1990). Overwork weakness with evidence of muscle damage in a patient with residual paralysis from polio. *Archives of Physical Medicine and Rehabilitation, 71,* 248–250.

Pedersen, SW, & Oberg, B. (1993). Dynamic strength in Parkinson's disease. *European Neurology, 33,* 97–102.

Perry, J. (1992). *Gait analysis, normal and pathological function.* Thorofare, NJ: Slack.

Perry, J, Mulroy, SJ, & Renwick, SE. (1993). The relationship of lower extremity strength and gait parameters in patients with post-polio syndrome. *Archives of Physical Medicine and Rehabilitation, 74,* 165–169.

Pitetti, KH. (1990). A reliable isokinetic strength test for arm and leg musculature for mildly mentally retarded adults. *Archives of Physical Medicine and Rehabilitation, 71,* 669–672.

Ringsberg, K. (1993). Muscle strength differences in urban and rural populations in Sweden. *Archives of Physical Medicine and Rehabilitation, 74,* 1315–1318.

Rose, DK, Giuliani, CA, & Light, KE. (1992). The immediate effects of isokinetic exercise on temporal-distance characteristics of self-selected and fast hemiplegic gait (pp. 37–42). Paper presented at Combined Sections Meeting, American Physical Therapy Association.

Rosenfalck, A, & Andreassen, S. (1980). Impaired regulation of force and firing pattern of single motor units in patients with spasticity. *Journal of Neurology, Neurosurgery, and Psychiatry, 43,* 907–916.

Rothstein, JM, Lamb, RL, & Mayhew, TP. (1987). Clinical uses of isokinetic measurements. *Physical Therapy, 67,* 1840–1844.

Rothstein, J. (1989). Commentary. *Physical Therapy, 69,* 237–240.

Schenkman, M, Berger, RA, Riley, PO, Mann, RW, & Hodge, WA. (1990). Whole body movements during rising to standing from sitting. *Physical Therapy, 70*(10), 638–648.

Sunderland, A, Tinson, D, Bradley, L, & Hewer, RL. (1989). Arm function after stroke. An evaluation of grip strength as a measure of recovery and a prognostic indicator. *Journal of Neurology, Neurosurgery, and Psychiatry, 52,* 1267–1272.

Suomi, R, Surburg, PR, & Lecius, P. (1993). Reliability of isokinetic and isometric measurement of leg strength on men with mental retardation. *Archives of Physical Medicine and Rehabilitation, 74,* 848–852.

Thompson, LV. (1994). Effects of age and training on skeletal muscle physiology and performance. *Physical Therapy, 74,* 71–81.

Umphred, DA. (1995). *Neurological rehabilitation.* St. Louis: Mosby-Year Book.

Vignos, PJ. (1983). Physical models of rehabilitation in neuromuscular disease. *Muscle and Nerve, 6,* 323–338.

SUGGESTED READINGS

Bohannon, RW. (1987). Relationship between static strength and various other measures in hemiparetic stroke patients. *International Rehabilitation Medicine, 8*(3), 125–128.

Thirty-eight stroke patients had the strength of different muscles measured. Relationships between strength and other variables (eg, sex, weight, age, side of paresis, time since onset) were calculated for each muscle. Results showed that the paretic side was correlated with the strength of only four nonparetic muscle groups, time since onset was unrelated to strength, and final strenth was always correlated with initial strength on the paretic side.

Connor, NP, & Abbs, JH. (1991). Task-dependent variations in Parkinsonian motor impairments. *Brain, 114,* 321–332.

Patients with Parkinson's disease and controls were compared on the performance of single, rapid, visually guided movements; equivalent movements associated with a single speech syllable; and well learned speech movements produced in a natural sequence. Parkinson's disease subjects produced similar deficits for visually guided jaw lowering. However, analogous jaw movements during sequential speech tasks were unimpaired on these measures.

Fowler, WM, & Taylor M. (1982). Rehabilitation management of muscular dystrophy and related disorders: I. The role of exercise. *Archives of Physical Medicine and Rehabilitation, 63,* 319–321.

This manuscript reviews the work capacity of individuals with motor unit diseases and the effect of exercise training in humans and animals with neuromuscular disorders. This review illustrated that exercise is not harmful and may be beneficial in patients with motor unit diseases, particularly if started early in the course of the disease, when muscle fiber degeneration is minimal, and carried out at submaximal levels.

Fries, W, Danek, A, Scheidtmann, K, & Hamburger, C. (1993). Motor recovery following capsular stroke. *Brain, 116,* 369–382.

The functional anatomy of motor recovery was studied by assessing motor function in 23 patients who had suffered from capsular stroke. Lesions of the anterior or posterior limb of the internal capsule led to an initially severe motor impairment followed by an excellent recovery. Conversely, lesions of the posterior limb of the internal capsule in combination with damage to the lateral thalamus compromised motor outcome. Small capsular lesions also disrupted the output of functionally and anatomically distinct motor areas selectively.

Lord, SR, & Castell. S. (1994). Physical activity program for older persons: Effect on balance, strength, neuromuscular control, and reaction time. *Archives of Physical Medicine and Rehabilitation, 75,* 648–652.

Forty-four elderly subjects were assessed for quadriceps strength, reaction time, neuromuscular control, and body sway before and after a 10-week exercise program. At the end of the exercise program, subjects showed improved quadriceps strength, reaction time, and body sway. Control nonexerciser subjects did not show improvements in any of these variables.

Nugent, JA, Schurr, KA, & Adams, RD. (1994). Dose-response relationship between amount of weight-bearing exercise and walking outcome following cerebrovascular accident. *Archives of Physical Medicine and Rehabilitation, 75,* 399–402.

This study used a weight-bearing exercise designed to strengthen leg extensor muscle to supplement a motor relearning approach for stroke patients. Two groups of patients were studied—those who could bear weight on their involved lower extremity and step forward with their other leg, and those who could not bear weight on the involved lower extremity. For the first group, a dose-response relationship was found between an increasing number of repetitions of this weight-bearing exercise and improved walking as measured on the Motor Assessment Scale for stroke.

For the second group, no relationship was noted. All patients, however, who practiced the exercise achieved independent walking for at lease 3 meters.

Palmer, SS, Mortimer, JA, Webster, DD, Bistevins, R, & Dickinson, GL. (1986). Exercise therapy for Parkinson's disease. *Archives of Physical Medicine and Rehabilitation, 67,* 741–745.

Outcomes of two 12-week exercise programs were assessed by measurements of motor signs, grip strength, motor coordination and speed, and neurophysiologic determinations of long-latency stretch responses in two groups of patients with Parkinson's disease. Outcomes of these two different exercise programs were similar. Most patients in both groups improved in gait, tremor, grip strength, and motor coordination on tasks requiring fine control. There was a decline in one task involving whole body control, and muscle rigidity was unchanged.

Perry, J. (1992). *Gait analysis, normal and pathological function.* Thorofare, NJ: Slack.

Perry, an orthopaedic surgeon and physical therapist, has examined gait extensively. The results of her work and those of her colleagues are presented in this seminal text. Information found therein served as the basis for most of the information on gait abnormalities due to weakness presented in this chapter.

Taub, E, Miller, NE, Novack, TA, Cook, EW, Fleming, WC, Nepomuceno, CS, Connell, JS, & Crago, JE. (1993). Technique to improve chronic motor deficit after stroke. *Archives of Physical Medicine and Rehabilitation, 74,* 347–354.

The noninvolved upper extremities of stroke patients were restrained in a sling during waking hours for 14 days. On 10 of those days, patients practiced using their impaired upper extremities for 6 hours. An attention-comparison group received procedures designed to focus attention on use of the impaired upper extremities. Those who were restrained improved on motor functions. Improvements were also noted for the restraint group in the life situation, and these gains were maintained during a 2-year follow-up period. The control group showed improvement in only one measure, and this was lost in the follow-up period.

CHAPTER 6

Sensory and Perceptual Dysfunction

MARGARET FRYE

LEARNING OBJECTIVES

After reading this chapter, you should be able to:

1. Discuss the ways in which sensory and perceptual dysfunctions are implicated in neurological impairments.
2. Explain the ways in which anatomic lesions may produce impairments.
3. Discuss how to assess disabilities when sensory and perceptual impairments are present.
4. Understand the treatment concepts associated with sensory and perceptual dysfunctions.

This chapter discusses the sensory and perceptual dysfunctions generally associated with neurological impairments. The assessment and treatment of these dysfunctions, and their associated disabilities, are discussed in general terms.

Physical therapists do not specifically treat perceptual deficits. However, in many patients perceptual problems occur in conjunction with mobility problems. Under these circumstances, it is important for physical therapists to understand the perceptual problems and the impact they have on functional mobility. To enhance treatment and decrease both patient and therapist frustration, physical therapists should become aware of perceptual deficits and incorporate techniques used to treat these deficits into tasks of functional mobility.

Patients with perceptual deficits will benefit from treatment by other professionals, such as occupational therapists and speech and language pathologists. Physical therapists should consult with these professionals as needed to enhance treatment or consider cotreatment with occupational therapists if such opportunities exist.

IMPAIRMENT: SENSORY AND PERCEPTUAL DYSFUNCTION

Appropriate integration, organization, and interpretation of stimuli (eg, visual, auditory, tactile, kinesthetic) are necessary for normal interaction within the environment. The ability to perform tasks of functional mobility relies on the reception, organization, integration, and interpretation of sensory information. Without these abilities, one cannot generate an appropriate response to a need or request to perform a functional task.

Proper functioning of the human sensory systems relies on the basic principles of information processing and organization. All sensory modalities have different sensory receptors, but each has in common exposure to physical stimuli, conversion of the stimuli into nerve impulses, and response(s) to the original stimuli, otherwise referred to as perception of the sensation. Perceptions of physical stimuli differ because the nervous system is able to interpret certain pieces of sensory information based on past experiences while ignoring other pieces of sensory information.

For example, sensory processing allows the brain to produce mental constructs for such things as colors, sounds, smells, and tastes. These constructs, or perceptions, do not exist outside the nervous system. Thus, perceptions are not directly recorded from the world around us, but are rather constructed internally according to the innate rules and constraints imposed by the nervous system's capabilities.

ANATOMY OVERVIEW

As discussed in Chapter 2, the somatosensory system can be divided into the protopathic, phylogenetically older, and less specific spinothalamic system that is organized to respond to stimuli for protective responses, and the epicritic, phylogenetically newer, and more specific lemniscal system that possesses discriminative properties to somatosensation. The following is a brief overview of sensory anatomy.

Lemniscal System

The lemniscal system is involved with transmission of touch, proprioception, and kinesthesia. Receptors of the lemniscal system are located in skin, joints, soft tissue, and other body tissues. Lemniscal receptors are encapsulated and may include Merkel's discs, Meissner's corpuscles, Pacinian corpuscles, Ruffini's corpuscles, muscle spindles, and Golgi tendon organ. Neural signals produced by receptor stimulation cause action potentials that are transmitted to axons of the peripheral nerve that relates information about the stimulus. This is referred to as **neural encoding.**

The terminal endings of lemniscal receptors transduce stimulus energy to their axons, which transmit action potentials to the central nervous system. Somatosensory information is transmitted along large, **myelinated** peripheral nerves that possess high conduction speeds that allow for quick responses to stimuli. Dorsal root ganglia contain cell bodies of these large, myelinated neurons, which project their central processes to the spinal cord through dorsal roots. These central processes ascend the cord in dorsal columns (ie, fasciculus gracilis and fasciculus cuneatus) until they synapse in the medulla on neurons in gracile and cuneate nuclei.

Axons of these second order neurons then cross **midline** and ascend in the medial lemniscus to the ventral posterior lateral nucleus of the thalamus, where they synapse on third-order, thalamocortical fibers. Thalamocortical fibers reach the primary somatosensory cortex (ie, the postcentral gyrus of the parietal lobe) via the posterior limb of the internal capsule.

Somatosensation from the face is transmitted via cranial nerve V (trigeminal). Cell bodies of cranial nerve V are large, myelinated neurons located in the trigeminal ganglia. Peripheral endings of these neurons receive somatosensation, which is transmitted centrally to project to ipsilateral chief sensory nuclei, located bilaterally in the mid-pons.

Axons whose cell bodies are located in chief sensory nuclei ascend bilaterally via the ventral trigeminal tract (contralaterally) and the dorsal trigeminal tract (ipsilaterally), to the ventral posterior medial nucleus of the thalamus, where third-order neurons project somatotopically near the Sylvian fissure.

Proprioceptive information from the face reaches the CNS via the peripheral processes whose cell bodies are located in the mesencephalic nucleus. Central processes from the mesencephalic nucleus project to the motor nucleus of V for **myotatic reflexes** and to the cerebellum for proprioception.

Spinothalamic System

The spinothalamic system includes the lateral and anterior spinothalamic tracts and is involved with perception of pain, temperature, light touch, sexual sensations, noxious stimuli, and primitive protective responses. Receptors are nonencapsulated, or free nerve endings, which are found throughout the body. Information transmitted via free nerve endings travels along small, slow-conducting, unmyelinated fibers.

Like the lemniscal system, cell bodies of primary neurons of the spinothalamic system are located in dorsal root ganglia. Unlike the lem-

niscal system, central processes project through dorsal roots into the spinal cord and synapse on second-order neurons in the dorsal horn. Second-order neurons then decussate in the spinal cord and ascend contralaterally as the lateral and anterior spinothalamic tracts, continuing through the brainstem where they synapse in the ventral posterior lateral nucleus of the thalamus. From the thalamus, axons of third-order neurons project through the posterior limb of the internal capsule to the postcentral gyrus in the parietal lobe of the cerebrum.

Dorsal Spinocerebellar Tract

Some proprioceptive and discriminative touch information enters the spinal cord and synapses in Clarke's column, a continuous column of cells running from T1 to L2 or L3. From Clarke's column, large axons ascend ipsilaterally and **posterolaterally** in the spinal cord in what is known as the dorsal spinocerebellar tract (DSCT). Axons in the DSCT reach the ipsilateral cerebellum via the inferior cerebellar peduncle. The DSCT carries information concerned with fine coordination of posture and kinesthetic facts from limb muscles. However, this information does not reach conscious levels in the parietal lobe for integration of sensory information.

Ventral Spinocerebellar Tract

The ventral spinocerebellar tract (VSCT) is concerned with coordinated movements and posture from the lower extremities. Fibers of the VSCT have their cell bodies located in dorsal root ganglia and receive signals from Golgi tendon organs in the lower extremities. Cells of origin of the ventral spinocerebellar tract are found in the spinal cord and extend from coccygeal levels to upper lumbar levels.

The VSCT is a double crossing tract. From the dorsal horn of the spinal cord, fibers decussate and ascend contralaterally. At the level of the pons, most fibers decussate back in the superior cerebellar peduncle to terminate in the cerebellum.

Lesions

Lesions at different sites along sensory pathways will obviously produce different problems. The farther the lesion from the cell body, the more likely the neuron will survive the injury, and the greater the chance of reinnervation without an appreciable loss of sensation. Crush injuries to axons provide the most common example of this type of injury. However, the closer the lesion site is to the cell body of the sensory neuron, the more likely the neuron will die. In this case, the loss of cutaneous sensation from the neuron will be permanent.

Surgically induced dorsal root lesions, which are sometimes performed to relieve intractable pain or to reduce severe spasticity, can cause diminished sensory input. For example, a **dorsal rhizotomy**, surgical transection of spinal nerve rootlettes, can result in diminished abilities in the sensory modalities of proprioception, discriminative touch, pain and temperature sensation, and loss of reflexes mediated at those levels. Loss of cutaneous sensation has significant functional consequences when dorsal roots from multiple cord levels are involved. For example, surgical lesions of the dorsal roots of the brachial plexus (ie, C5–T1) result in significant losses in cutaneous sensation. Furthermore, information from stretch receptors from C5 to T1 is lost, resulting in tone changes in the muscles innervated by the alpha motor neurons originating from those cord levels. Assuming alpha motor neurons remain intact, motor activity is still possible. However, in this example, the upper extremity may be impaired from a functional perspective due to loss of sensory input. This loss of cutaneous, proprioceptive, and kinesthetic sensation has an impact on the level of skill with which movements are performed.

Lesions involving the lemniscal system, whether they occur in peripheral nerve fibers, dorsal columns, or the medial lemniscus, result in diminished or absent discriminative touch and kinesthetic sense. The loss of these sensory powers is especially noticeable in the distal extremities. The loss of proprioception in the lower extremities noted with lemniscal lesions can result in dysfunctions of balance, coordination, gait, or all three.

Lesions associated with the lateral spinothalamic tract produce contralateral loss of pain and the ability to detect thermal changes. *Light touch* is carried by the spinothalamic tract; it would be lost if this tract were lesioned. However, *touch* is carried in the posterior columns of the spinal cord, in the lemniscal system. As a result, it would remain intact. Lesions of the spinocerebellar tracts, both ventral and dorsal, will produce diminished information to the cerebellum. Generally, patients would display ipsilateral deficits in posture and kinesthesia from limb muscles.

Lesions located in the thalamus are functional extensions of lesions seen in the ascending tracts. That is, a lesion in the **ventral posterolateral (VPL) nucleus** of the thalamus, which receives sensory information from the body, will produce the same consequences as lesions in the lemniscal and spinothalamic systems. A lesion in the **ventral posteromedial (VPM) nucleus** of the thalamus, which receives sensory information from the face, will produce results that are similar to those caused by lesions in the trigeminothalamic tracts (ie, loss of discriminative touch and the ability to detect pain and temperature from the face). Conversely, lesions in the cerebellum may produce motor deficits resulting from diminished sensory information to the cerebellum.

Like lesions in the thalamus, lesions of the sensory cortex will result in losses of the following senses, from both the body and the face: proprioception, kinesthesia, discriminative touch, pain, light touch, and temperature. However, the potential for harm is greater with sensory cortex lesions because they interfere with the cortical integration of various inputs, as well as with stimuli perception. Patients with cortical lesions will be unable to identify the location of light touch, discriminate objects placed in their hands, or distinguish between a one-point stimulus and a two-point stimulus (eg, the prick of a single pin or the prick of two pins).

ASSESSING THE DISABILITY

Sensory and perceptual problems will become evident through observation of functional activities. Patients with sensory and perceptual deficits may find it difficult or impossible to navigate environments or successfully manipulate their surroundings to accomplish functional tasks. Therapists must accurately identify the sensory or perceptual problem(s) that affect the patient's task performance. Through the analysis of activities and tasks, therapists become aware of those skills needed to successfully complete the task(s). Information from the analysis, observation of the performance of the task, and identification of the breakdown within the performance provide therapists with clues to the underlying deficit(s).

Observation of more than one functional task is necessary to enhance the therapist's ability to identify deficits as specifically sensory or perceptual in nature. Perceptually impaired patients will display similar characteristics in different tasks. For example, patients with left unilateral neglect will consistently have difficulty attending to stimuli presented on their left sides. This deficit will typically manifest in awkward ambulation or clumsy wheelchair propulsion because patients will consistently bump into objects in the environment located to their left. If, however, individuals do not display left-side neglect during other tasks, such as eating or dressing, then their difficulty with ambulation or wheelchair propulsion is probably due to a deficit other than unilateral neglect. Other deficits that may fit this example are apraxia, visual field deficits, or problems with spatial relations.

Once numerous functional tasks have been observed and related sensory and perceptual problems have been identified, a more specific assessment can be completed to confirm the deficit. The following section addresses four sensory and perceptual disorders: spatial relations disorders, body scheme disorders, apraxia, and agnosia. Each perceptual disorder will be addressed in a general sense. For example, the effects of apraxia on functional mobility are discussed, but the different types of apraxia and their effects on movement are not differentiated.

- *Spatial Relation Disorders.* Patients with spatial relations disorders will have difficulty perceiving the spatial orientation of objects in relation to each other or in relation to themselves. These deficits can be a significant detriment to their ability to effectively and safely move through the environment, either by ambulation or by wheelchair. Patients may bump into or fall over objects.
- *Body Scheme Disorders.* Patients with body scheme disorders may be unable to effectively and safely move their bodies, either spontaneously or in response to verbal cues from the therapist, due to a decrease in awareness of their own bodies. These patients may have difficulty maintaining static positions, such as static sit and static stand. Patients who are unable to acknowledge or attend to their own body parts may also have diffi-

culty maintaining the position of those body parts or moving those body parts in a goal-oriented pattern.

- *Apraxia.* Apraxia will typically cause difficulty with many tasks of functional mobility, specifically sequenced motor activities. The ability to maintain static positions should not be affected by apraxia, but patients may find it difficult or impossible to move into the static position. Transfers and assuming a sitting posture from the supine position are two good examples of sequenced motor activities. A patient with apraxia may be able to maintain a static stance but unable to properly sequence the motor actions necessary to rise from a sitting posture.

- *Agnosia.* Patients with **agnosia** (inability to recognize objects) will have difficulty recognizing and interpreting objects in the environment. They should not have problems with functional mobility. Agnosia may make it difficult for patients to locate objects, read signs, or recognize their therapists, but these deficits typically do not affect functional mobility.

  Somatognosia is an exception. **Somatognosia** is the lack of awareness of body structure and the inability to recognize one's own body parts and their relationships to each other (Zoltan, Siev, & Freishtat, 1986). Somatognosia is considered a body scheme disorder and its effect on functional mobility was described previously in the section on body scheme disorder.

Each area of functional mobility will be discussed, as in previous chapters. However, only a few examples of specific perceptual deficits and their effects on functional mobility are discussed. The reader must be aware that these are only examples and that each patient will perform differently depending on the specific motor, sensory, and perceptual deficits that exist.

Rolling

Unilateral neglect has a negative impact on all tasks that require the body to move and function as a whole unit. Individuals with unilateral neglect have a very difficult time incorporating their neglected sides into movements such as rolling. Perhaps this is because these patients no longer perceive their neglected sides as part of their bodies.

Patients with right-left discrimination problems will become confused if given directions to roll that include right and left references. For example, instructions to "... pick up your right hand with your left hand and roll to the right, pushing with your left foot" may fail to elicit a response from the patient, not because the motor requirements of rolling are difficult to master, but because the patient is unable to follow the directions.

Supine-to-Sit Maneuver

Patients with **ideational apraxia** (inability to correlate purpose and accomplishment of tasks) may have difficulty planning and executing the sequenced movements necessary to move from a supine posture to sitting. This is especially true for persons with hemiplegia, who must learn to assist their affected sides or incorporate their affected sides into movement sequences.

Patients with somatognosia have decreased awareness of body structure and may have difficulty recognizing their own body parts. This body scheme deficit is a huge detriment when attempting to move the entire body. Patients with this deficit have difficulty locating body parts and maneuvering body parts during functional mobility tasks. They may omit entire body parts from movement sequences. For example, the patient may not slide a neglected lower extremity off the bed when moving from side-lying to sitting due to decreased awareness of that extremity. The patient may also be unaware of what is causing discomfort or hindering the movement.

Static Sit and Static Stand

Generally, perceptual deficits affect the patient's ability to interpret and interact with the environment. Not many perceptual deficits interfere with the patient's ability to maintain static positions. A body scheme disorder such as unilateral neglect is, however, a notable exception. Patients with unilateral neglect have difficulty attending to stimuli presented on their neglected side. The neglected side typically presents with motor, and possibly sensory, deficits. The combination of these three deficit areas can interfere with the patient's ability to maintain static positions.

Perceptual neglect results in a decreased ability to attend to the affected side. When perceptual deficits are combined with motor deficits, patients will demonstrate difficulty maintaining symmetrical postures. They will lean or fall to the affected side. Commonly, patients are completely unaware that they are falling. Patients may lean excessively on another individual, or on a wheelchair arm rest, but remain unaware that they are not independently maintaining upright, symmetrical positions. Even when questioned regarding their perception of their own postures, patients with these deficits report feeling as if they are sitting or standing symmetrically.

Sit-to-Stand Maneuver

A patient with unilateral neglect may have difficulty standing up from a seated position due to decreased awareness of the neglected side.

These individuals typically have perceptual neglect in conjunction with motor deficits on the involved side. For example, patients with left neglect usually have left hemiparesis or hemiplegia as a result of right hemispheric damage. Neglect of the left side makes improving or compensating for motor deficits difficult. If patients have difficulty attending to the left side, they will certainly have difficulty attending to or compensating for the motor deficit. This difficulty can be observed as they attempt to move from sitting to standing.

Commonly, physical therapists verbally cue patients to move from sitting to standing by bearing their weight through both upper extremities, leaning the head and shoulders forward, and extending the hips and knees. Patients with left unilateral neglect typically will be unable to effectively bear weight through their affected extremities (even with proper assistance from the therapist) and will lean excessively to the left. In performing this task, they are unaware that they are leaning to the left or at risk for falls. This difficulty in moving from sitting to standing is a combination of the unilateral neglect and motor deficits. Patients without unilateral neglect are able to attend to motor deficits and are more successful at incorporating their affected sides into the sit-to-stand movement sequence.

Transfers

Patients with deficits in spatial relations may demonstrate difficulty with transfers. They have difficulty perceiving their own spatial orientation in relation to other objects. This deficit may render patients unable to properly position their wheelchairs for safe transfers. They may, likewise, have difficulty pivoting in the proper direction and orienting the body correctly to sit on the targeted surface.

Ideational apraxia, when present, is commonly seen in the task of transferring from a bed to a chair. Safe, independent transfers require patients to plan and execute numerous motor actions in their proper sequence. Patients with ideational apraxia may demonstrate difficulty starting the transfer and may show incomplete movements, such as not coming to a complete stand, or disorganized movements, such as coming to a complete stand and immediately sitting before pivoting toward the chair.

Ambulation

A patient with deficits in spatial relations, including how the body is positioned in space, may not be able to ambulate safely through crowds. Even though objects in a room are visible to these patients, their perceptual deficits can alter their ability to comprehend where objects are in relation to their own bodies, as well as in relation to other objects. As a result, patients are at risk for walking into, or tripping and falling over, objects.

Patients with ideational apraxia and motor deficits may demonstrate difficulty ambulating with assistive devices because they are unable to properly organize their movements. They may have the necessary skills to carry out this task, but without the ability to plan the sequenced actions of first advancing the walker, then one lower extremity, and then the other lower extremity, they are unlikely to accomplish the motor task before them.

Climbing Stairs

Patients with deficits in depth perception may be either completely unable to climb stairs or, at the very least, unable to climb them safely. This deficit causes difficulty in perceiving and judging changes in the planes of various surfaces. Patients may be unaware of changes in surfaces or unable to quickly judge distances between steps. They are, therefore, at risk for falling. Tape of different colors may be placed on each step to assist patients in the perceptual processing needed to safely locate the next level.

Case Study

•••

Mr. Smith was admitted to the neurology service of the acute care hospital in his hometown with left-sided weakness and slurred speech. A computed tomography scan showed a large infarct in the right inferior parietal lobe. Bedside physical therapy evaluation was ordered.

•••

Assessing the Disability

•••

As you introduce yourself and explain your function to the patient, be aware of Mr. Smith's ability to maintain eye contact. As you move around his room, can he visually track you on the right and left side? Does he look at you as you assess his left extremities?

Ask Mr. Smith to roll from side to side. Do his left extremities move naturally with his body or do they lag behind? If he is unable to roll to the right, ask him to grasp his left upper extremity with his right hand. Can Mr. Smith locate his left upper extremity, either with his right upper extremity or visually? You may have to assist Mr. Smith with grasping his right upper extremity. Note if Mr. Smith maintains his right hand grasp on his left upper extremity during the rolling sequence. Some patients let go of their affected extremity (during the task) and allow it to fall. Mr. Smith may be unaware that his left upper extremity has been left behind as he rolls to the right.

As Mr. Smith rolls from side to side (even with your assistance), does he appear to be aware of the position of his limbs? If his left upper extremity becomes caught under him, does he realize it, complain of pain, or both?

In moving from the left side-lying posture to a sitting position, does Mr. Smith use his left extremities to assist with the movement, or does his left lower extremity fall off his bed? Does his left upper extremity hang at his side, or does it spontaneously assist with movement and balance?

Once sitting, can Mr. Smith maintain a midline position? If he cannot, in which direction does he lean? Ask Mr. Smith if he feels as if he is sitting up straight. Also, ask him if his feet are flat on the floor. Notice if he can correctly answer without looking at his feet.

Next, direct Mr. Smith to stand up from sitting. Take note of the sequence of movements used. Does the left upper extremity spontaneously push off the edge of the bed? Can he extend his left hip and knee to attain and maintain a symmetrical standing position? Can Mr. Smith achieve a standing position, with or without your assistance?

Note the quality of the standing position. Is the left upper extremity properly positioned for standing? Are the lower extremities bearing weight equally? Are the trunk and head both upright in the midline position? The inability to achieve and maintain a symmetrical sitting or standing posture may be due to sensory impairment, balance dysfunction, muscle weakness or a combination of these deficits.

Results of Assessment of Functional Mobility

- Rolling to the left—independent, but he rolls onto his left upper extremity without being aware of it.

- Rolling to the right—needs moderate assistance to locate his left upper extremity, protract his left shoulder, and advance his left hip forward. Patient also drops his left upper extremity during rolling, allowing it to fall onto the bed.
- Supine-to-sit maneuver—needs moderate assistance; unable to push up with his left upper extremity. He requires assistance to advance his left lower extremity off the bed.
- Stable sitting—patient requires moderate assistance to maintain sitting position. Patient sits with increased weight-bearing on his right hip. His trunk is laterally flexed to the left, yet he is unaware of his asymmetry. Mr. Smith is also unable to tell if his left foot is flat on the floor without looking at it.
- Sit-to-stand maneuver and standing—patient requires maximal assistance to move into and maintain a standing posture. His position is asymmetrical and he leans to the left but is unaware of his asymmetry.
- Ambulation—was not assessed due to Mr. Smith's inability to stand.

ASSESSING THE IMPAIRMENT

This section is divided into two parts: testing for sensory impairments, and testing for perceptual impairments. The sensory tests described are discriminative touch and pressure, static joint position, dynamic joint position, stereognosis, tactile localization, two-point discrimination, and recognition of textures. The perceptual tests are performed to determine the presence of spatial relation disorders, body scheme disorders, apraxia, and agnosia.

Sensation

The tools that may be used to assess sensory impairment include:

- Pinwheels—to assess sharp sensation
- Cotton—to assess light touch
- Protractor—to assess two-point discrimination
- Any number of instruments to apply pressure to the skin—to assess pressure sense
- Small objects that can be placed in the palm of the hand—to assess stereognosis

Sensory testing is performed bilaterally so that comparisons can be made between the involved and noninvolved sides. When sensory testing indicates the absence of an impairment, sensation is referred to as being *normal* or *intact*. However, when sensory impairments are noted, they may be said to be *diminished*, *absent*, or *exaggerated*. Results of sensory tests may also be rated as inaccurate when repeated or mimicked movements are used to assess joint position or movement (ie, proprioception or kinesthesia). When this occurs, the number of accurate responses should be documented. For example, a movement that was successfully completed 4 of 10 times would be rated 4/10.

Assessing the integrity of the dorsal column-medial lemniscus system may begin with the patient in a comfortable position, such as sitting or lying supine. Modalities carried in this system are then tested.

Discriminative Touch and Pressure

The senses of discriminative touch and pressure can be assessed by the examiner's moving his or her finger(s) across the skin, by applying pressure with the finger(s) into skin surfaces, or both.

Proprioception—Static Joint Position

Static joint position can be assessed by placing the patient's *involved* extremities in various positions and having the patient match or copy these positions with the *noninvolved* extremities.

Loss of proprioception in the lower extremities noted with lemniscal lesions can result in balance, coordination, and gait dysfunctions, either singly or in combination. Maintaining balance is a complex interaction of many neuromuscular and musculoskeletal systems. The inability to maintain balance may result in falls, dizziness, or apprehension about movement. See Chapters 7 and 8 for further information concerning the assessment of coordination and balance dysfunctions.

Kinesthesia—Dynamic Joint Position

Dynamic joint position can be assessed by slowly moving the patient's *involved* extremities and having the patient simultaneously match or copy this movement with the *noninvolved* extremities. Readers should be aware that even those who have not suffered from a neurological lesion have some difficulty with these activities. Therefore, when viewing patients as they perform these movements, be cognizant that some movement error will undoubtedly occur.

Stereognosis

Placing various objects (eg, rubber bands, paper clips, coins) into the palm of patients' hands and having them identify these objects with their eyes closed tests their ability to perceive the size, shape, and texture of objects.

Tactile Localization

Tactile localization can be measured in a couple of ways. The therapist can touch different areas of the patient's body while the patient's eyes are closed, and (1) have patients verbally identify where they were touched, or (2) have them touch with their finger the exact point where they were touched.

Two-Point Discrimination

Two-point discrimination may be assessed using a protractor. By gradually decreasing the distance between the two tips, one is able to assess the patient's ability to distinguish between two points. Areas of the body responsible for fine, subtle movements, such as the fingertips, are able to discern distances as small as 1 to 2 mm. Other areas, such as the back, are less sensitive to the two points of stimulation. This is logical when you consider the number of sensory receptors in the fingers and hand versus those in the back.

Recognition of Textures

Recognition of textures can be assessed by moving different objects with different textures across the skin. Sand paper, soft towels, sponges, and cotton are just some of the stimuli that can be used.

Perception

Before the assessment of visual perceptual skills, therapists must first rule out, or be aware of, impairments in gross visual skills. Gross visual skills include visual attention, visual scanning, saccadic eye movements, and visual fields.

Visual attention is the ability to obtain and maintain visual fixation (Zoltan et al., 1986). Adults should be able to maintain visual attention to a specific stimulus for 20 seconds (Zoltan et al., 1986). This visual skill is necessary for the completion of many tasks, such as hammering a nail, inserting a key into a lock, and pouring liquid into a cup. Without adequate visual attention, the individual would probably have difficulty hitting the nail with the hammer, placing the key in the lock, or pouring the liquid without spilling it.

Visual scanning is the ability to gaze up, down, and laterally (Zoltan, 1990). **Saccades** are sequenced rapid eye movements. The eyes must move rapidly across varied distances and localize on specific, typically stationary, stimuli, such as the words on a page.

For saccadic eye movements to be efficient, individuals must localize specific stimuli (Zoltan et al., 1986) and not attend to peripheral vision. Deficits in visual skills may render individuals incapable of participating in visual perceptual assessments. They, likewise, may be confused with visual perceptual deficits. This confusion may occur because the functional manifestations of a deficit in gross visual skills may be similar to a perceptual deficit.

For example, left **homonymous hemianopsia** (loss of vision on one side of the visual field) is a visual field deficit producing blindness in the nasal half of the right eye and the temporal half of the left eye, resulting in the inability to see to the left of midline (Zoltan et al., 1986). This visual field deficit may be confused with left unilateral neglect (Van Deusen, 1993) because the functional presentation of these deficits is similar.

In the case of the left homonymous hemianopsia, patients are unable to see to the left of midline and can easily be taught to compensate for the deficit by turning their heads to the left. Patients with unilateral neglect are unable to attend to stimuli presented on the left and cannot compensate for the deficit by turning their heads (Van Deusen, 1993). Although visual field deficits and unilateral neglect may occur simultaneously, this is not always the case. Clinicians must be able to distinguish between sensory problems and perceptual problems.

Intact gross visual skills are the foundation for visual perceptual skills. The ability to see the environment accurately is paramount to appropriately perceiving and interpreting information.

The following are perceptual deficits commonly seen in a variety of neurologically involved patients. The deficits discussed are associated with spatial relations disorders, one of which is a spatial relations deficit. Assessment tests for each deficit are also described.

Spatial Relations Disorders

Figure–Ground Deficit. A figure–ground deficit is the inability to perceive a specific stimulus as distinct from its background (Fig. 6-1). Clinically, this deficit may be seen as the inability to find a white shirt on an unmade bed or the difficulty in finding a spoon in a crowded kitchen drawer. Figure–ground deficits are informally assessed by asking the patient to identify objects or shapes hidden within a larger picture (DeRenzi & Scotti, 1970). This deficit is formally assessed through the Ayres Figure-Ground test (Zoltan, 1990). This test was originally designed for children, but it is also a reliable, useful tool for an adult population with brain damage (Baum, 1981).

Depth Perception Deficit. A depth perception deficit expresses itself as difficulty determining the relative distance between objects, figures, or landmarks and oneself. This deficit also involves difficulty perceiving changes in the planes of surfaces (American Occupational Therapy Association, 1994). Patients with this deficit may attempt to fit through spaces that are too small. They may also be unable to safely negotiate a curb or set of stairs because of their inability to perceive differences in the planes of surfaces or accurately judge distances between the surfaces.

One way to evaluate depth perception is to hold two pencils in front of the patient at eye level and at different distances from the face. One pencil is slowly moved toward the other and the patient is instructed to indicate when the pencils are parallel (Trombly, 1994). Patients with depth perception deficits will have

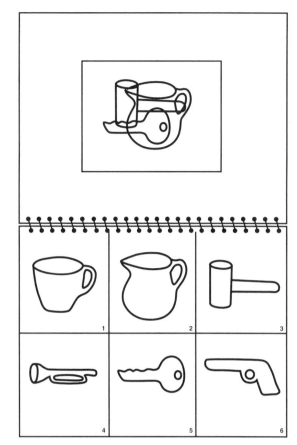

FIGURE 6-1. Sample page from the California figure–ground perception test. (Zoltan, B. [1996]. *Vision, perception, and cognition: A manual for the evaluation and treatment of the neurologically impaired adult.* Thorofare, NY: Slack, Inc.).

difficulty determining when the pencils are parallel because they have difficulty determining the relative distance between the objects and themselves.

Spatial Relations Deficit. Any difficulty or inability to perceive one's own spatial orientation in relation to other objects is referred to as a *spatial relations deficit* (Zoltan et al., 1968). This deficit may produce disabilities in ambulation, or maneuvering a wheelchair through a crowded room, or properly positioning a wheelchair for a safe transfer (Quintana, 1989). Patients may have difficulty properly orienting clothing in relation to their bodies, and may have difficulty dressing themselves.

Position in Space Deficit. A patient who has difficulty interpreting the concepts of in/out, up/down, and front/behind has a deficit of position in space (Quintana, 1989). This deficit can be clinically observed through the patient's inability to comprehend statements such as, ". . . your socks are in the drawer, under your shirt."

Deficits in spatial relations and spatial position are sometimes referred to as **visual spatial agnosia** (Quintana, 1989). Both deficits may be informally assessed by having the patient copy block designs (eg, peg board designs) or position colored blocks on command (eg, place the red block in front of the green block) (Zoltan et al., 1986).

The Space Visualization Test, a subtest of the Sensory Integration and Praxis Test (Ayres, 1987), may be used to assess these deficits, but this tool is standardized for children only. The Cross Test may also be used to test spatial relations deficits. This is a nonstandardized test that requires patients to duplicate a cross on a blank piece of paper just as it appears on the stimulus. Patient scores are determined by placing a transparent copy of the stimulus over the patient's drawing and measuring the distance between the bisected point of the patient's cross and that of the stimulus (Pehoski, 1970).

Topographical Disorientation. *Topographical disorientation* is the inability to understand and remember the relationship of places to one another (Van Deusen, 1993). Patients with this disorder have difficulty finding their way in previously known or present environments. Typically, patients in inpatient settings are unable to find their way to and from therapy even after being shown its location on numerous occasions.

Topographical disorientation is most commonly seen in conjunction with other deficits in the spatial relations syndrome. If other visual spatial problems are not found, these patients are probably getting lost as a result of other deficits, such as attention problems, memory problems, or confusion (Zoltan, 1990).

There is no standardized evaluation for topographical disorientation (Quintana, 1989). This disorder is usually identified functionally by observing patients find their way from one place to another. The ability to draw maps of familiar places or describe familiar routes has also been used to assess topographical disorientation (Brain, 1941; Paterson & Zangwill, 1944).

Body Scheme Disorders

The following are body scheme disorders commonly seen in neurologically involved patients. Assessment tests for each deficit are described.

Somatognosia. **Somatognosia** is the lack of awareness of body structure and the inability to recognize one's own body parts and where they are in relation to each other (Zoltan et al., 1986) (Fig. 6-2). Patients with this deficit may be unable to dress themselves independently because they can no longer understand how their own body parts relate to each other. Patients may have difficulty moving their contralateral limbs, and they may not be able to differentiate their own body parts from those of the therapist (Selecki & Herron, 1965).

Somatognosia is typically evaluated with nonstandardized assessments. These assessments include having patients point to body parts on command or by imitation and instructing patients to draw a person (Zoltan et al., 1986) or complete puzzles of the body (Quintana, 1989).

Right–Left Discrimination. A right–left discrimination deficit is the inability to understand the

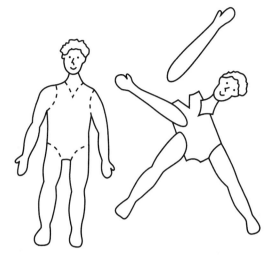

FIGURE 6-2. (*Left*) A human figure puzzle. (*Right*) The puzzle as put together by a patient with somatognosia. (Zoltan, B. [1996]. *Vision, perception, and cognition: A manual for the evaluation and treatment of the neurologically impaired adult.* Thorofare, NY: Slack, Inc.).

concepts of right and left (Quintana, 1989). Patients with this deficit have difficulty identifying their own right–left body parts. The deficit may also include an inability to discriminate between the examiner's right and left sides (Zoltan et al., 1986).

Right–left discrimination can be evaluated with the standardized Right/Left Orientation Test (Benton, Hamsher, Varney, & Spreen, 1983). This 20-item standardized test requires patients to point to lateralized body parts on command. A total score of less than 17 correct answers is considered indicative of right–left disorientation. This deficit can also be assessed through nonstandardized means. Most commonly, patients are asked to identify body parts on command (Quintana, 1989). Commands such as, ''Point to your right eye,'' or, ''Show me your left hand,'' are typically given. More complex directions can also be given, such as,

''Touch your left knee with your right hand'' (Trombly, 1995).

Unilateral Neglect.   The failure to respond or orient to stimuli presented contralateral to the side of a brain lesion (Heilman, Watson, & Valenstein, 1985) is known as **unilateral neglect** (Fig. 6-3). This deficit most commonly occurs following right hemisphere damage, and it results in left-side neglect. Left hemisphere damage can also cause neglect, but of the right side. However, this deficit is usually less severe (Quintana, 1989) than left-side neglect.

Severe deficits will affect most daily tasks such that patients will attend and respond only to stimuli presented on the noninvolved side. Thus, a patient with left neglect will eat only food presented to the right of midline, shave the right side of his face, and dress the right side of the body. Patients will bump into obstacles located to the left side.

Unilateral neglect is assessed with a variety of nonstandardized tools. These include cancel-

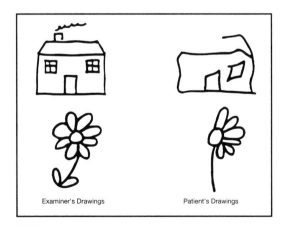

Examiner's Drawings   Patient's Drawings

FIGURE 6-3.   Examples of impaired performance on a copy test given to a patient with unilateral neglect. (Zoltan, B. [1996]. *Vision, perception, and cognition: A manual for the evaluation and treatment of the neurologically impaired adult.* Thorofare, NY: Slack, Inc.).

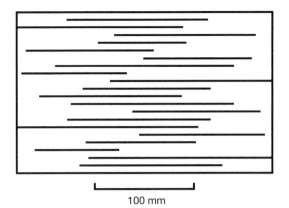

FIGURE 6-4. Schenkenberg line bisection test. (Trombly, C.A. [1995]. *Occupational therapy for physical dysfunction* [4th ed.]. Baltimore: Williams & Wilkins. From Schenkenberg, T., Bradford, D.C., and Ajax, E.T. (1980). Line bisection and unilateral visual neglect in patients with neurologic impairment. *Neurology,* 30:509–517.)

lation and reading tasks, as well as instructions to draw a person and a clock (Quintana, 1989).

The Schenkenberg Line Bisection Test (Schenkenberg, Bradford, & Ajax, 1980) is a standardized test for unilateral neglect consisting of 20 lines of various lengths (Fig. 6-4). Patients are asked to bisect the lines by drawing a pencil mark through the center of each line. Patients can make only one mark on each line and cannot move the paper. Six of the lines are located primarily to the left side of the page, six lines are on the right, and six lines are in the middle. The top and bottom lines are used for instruction and do not affect the score. The distances between the actual center of the line and where the patient's marks appear are measured in millimeters (Quintana, 1989).

Individuals with left neglect will have the greatest difficulty bisecting the lines located on the left. Patients with severe left neglect may omit the lines on the left. The lines in the middle will typically be bisected toward the right half of the line. Patients with left neglect will be most accurate at bisecting the lines on the right.

Apraxia

Apraxia is the inability to carry out purposeful, skilled movements even though sensation, motor function, and coordination are intact (Zoltan et al., 1986). The types of apraxia discussed are constructional, dressing, ideomotor, and ideational.

Constructional Apraxia. The inability to produce designs in two or three dimensions by copying, drawing, or constructing (Zoltan et al., 1986) is known as **constructional apraxia** (Figs. 6-5, 6-6, and 6-7). The deficit becomes apparent during tasks that require patients to organize or arrange component parts into final products, such as setting a table or making a bed.

Patients with either right or left hemispheric damage can display this form of apraxia. Vast differences in the performance of constructional tasks have led many researchers to believe that the underlying basis for constructional apraxia differs according to the side on which the lesion is located (Benton, 1967; Piercy, Hecaen, & Ajureaguerra, 1960). Constructional apraxia in patients with right hemispheric damage is felt to be due to visual or spatial disorders, whereas left hemispheric damage results in the

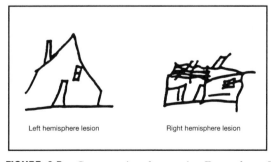

Left hemisphere lesion   Right hemisphere lesion

FIGURE 6-5. Constructional apraxia: Examples of impaired performance in drawing a house. (Zoltan, B. [1996]. *Vision, perception, and cognition: A manual for the evaluation and treatment of the neurologically impaired adult.* Thorofare, NY: Slack, Inc.).

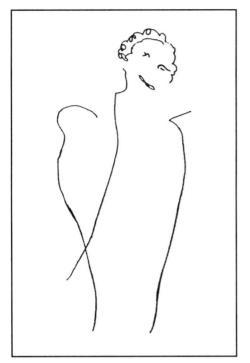

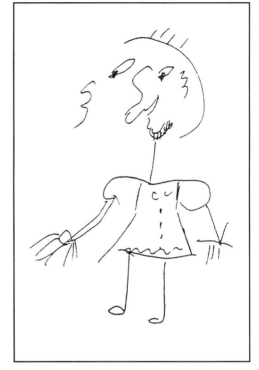

FIGURE 6-6. Constructional apraxia: Drawing of a person by a patient with left-brain damage. (Trombly, C.A. [1995]. *Occupational therapy for physical dysfunction* [4th ed.]. Baltimore: Williams & Wilkins).

FIGURE 6-7. Constructional apraxia: Drawing of a person by a patient with right-brain damage. (Trombly, C.A. [1995]. *Occupational therapy for physical dysfunction* [4th ed.]. Baltimore: Williams & Wilkins).

conceptual planning disorders that make it impossible to perform constructional tasks (Zoltan et al., 1986).

Constructional apraxia should be evaluated through both graphic and assembly tasks (Benton et al., 1983). Commonly used graphic assessments are copying geometric shapes and drawing a house or flower (Quintana, 1989). Individuals with constructional apraxia are unable to properly complete these designs. Lesions of the left hemisphere typically result in drawings that are oversimplified, have few details, and contain improperly drawn angles (Zoltan et al., 1986) (see Fig. 6-6). Drawings of patients with right hemispheric damage, on the other hand, tend to be complex and show disorganized spatial relationships (see Fig. 6-7).

Constructional apraxia can be assessed with nonstandardized block designs. Patients are required to build block designs from pictures of block designs or by copying a block design built by the therapist. The designs patients are required to build are typically of increasing difficulty. The difficulty of the block designs can be enhanced by increasing the number of blocks in the design and moving construction from two to three dimensions. Individuals with constructional apraxia will find it difficult or impossible to copy block designs correctly. Greater difficulty will be seen with the more complex block designs.

Dressing Apraxia. *Dressing apraxia* is the inability to dress oneself. The deficit may be due to constructional apraxia, visual or spatial disorganization, or unilateral neglect (Quintana, 1989). When the underlying cause of dressing apraxia is constructional apraxia, patients display an inability to appropriately assemble or orient clothing to apply it properly to the body. Clothing may be applied in an inappropriate order (eg, shoes before socks) or in an inappropriate place (eg, shirt may be pulled on over the feet). Patients may also have difficulty positioning a pullover shirt so that its head, front, back, and sleeves are appropriately placed once the shirt is pulled over the head.

Unilateral neglect may also cause dressing apraxia. In this case, patients typically do not dress the involved side of the body. These patients may realize that they have been unsuccessful with the task but may remain completely unaware that the reason they cannot finish the task is because the neglected side of the body is completely undressed.

Ideomotor Apraxia.   The inability to carry out purposeful movement on command is known as **ideomotor apraxia** (Quintana, 1989). Individuals with ideomotor apraxia may respond to the command "Lock your wheelchair" with inadequate or clumsy movement, although they could be observed to lock the wheelchair spontaneously, without being asked to do so. Another typical example is the inability to follow the command, "Show me how you would answer a phone." Again, the patient could answer a ringing phone without difficulty. Due to the nature of the deficit, ideomotor apraxia can only be observed during evaluation or over a period of time with the spontaneous demonstration of tasks.

Ideational Apraxia.   Ideational apraxia is a more serious deficit and can be observed during tasks of functional mobility. **Ideational apraxia** results in difficulty performing sequenced motor acts and is believed to be caused by a disruption in the conceptual organization of movement (Quintana, 1989). Patients have difficulty

with selecting and sequencing the appropriate movements for task completion. Patients with hemiplegia who have this deficit may have difficulty with planning the sequenced motions necessary to perform functional activities (eg, ambulate with a wide-based quad cane, propel a wheelchair with their unaffected upper and lower extremities, roll in bed, or perform a sit-to-stand maneuver).

The deficit may also manifest during eating. Patients will be completely bewildered by utensils or use them incorrectly (eg, they may attempt to use a fork in a bowl of soup or a cup of coffee) (Quintana, 1989). Patients may not eat the food but simply move the food around on the plate. Generally, these patients possess the appropriate capabilities but are unable to properly organize and sequence those movements for successful task completion.

Ideational and ideomotor apraxia can be evaluated with the Goodglass and Kaplan Test of Apraxia (Goodglass & Kaplan, 1972). This is a nonstandardized test that requires patients to perform common movements. Patients are first asked to perform movements on command, such as "Show me how to use a toothbrush." If they are unable to do this task, they are then asked to imitate the therapist brushing his or her teeth. If they are still unsuccessful, they are given the toothbrush and asked to demonstrate its use.

Agnosia

Agnosia is the inability to recognize or perceive familiar objects in the absence of impairments of the primary senses. Agnosia may occur in one or all of the following sensory areas: visual, tactile, proprioceptive, and auditory (Zoltan et al., 1986). For example, visual agnosia is the inability to recognize familiar objects even though visual acuity remains intact (Van Deusen, 1993). Individuals with this deficit can, however, recognize familiar objects by touch when vision is occluded (Gregory & Aitkin,

1971). Different visual object and tactile agnosias are addressed here.

Visual Object Agnosia

Simultanognosia. **Simultanognosia** is the decreased ability to perceive and interpret stimuli as a whole. For example, patients with this disorder are able to identify specific letters of the alphabet although they are unable to read words made up of identifiable letters (Zoltan et al., 1986). These patients have difficulty following signs to and from therapy or reading written exercise programs.

Prosopagnosia. Facial agnosia, formally known as **prosopagnosia**, is the inability to recognize familiar faces or distinctive characteristics of unfamiliar faces (Van Deusen, 1993). Patients with this deficit can learn to recognize others by their voices or how they walk.

Metamorphosia. The visual distortion of objects such that things appear much larger or smaller than their actual size (Zoltan et al., 1986) is known as **metamorphosia**. Patients may perceive a wheelchair to be larger or smaller than its actual size. This perceptual distortion may cause the patient anxiety.

Tactile Agnosia

Astereognosis. Tactile agnosia, or **astereognosis** is the inability to recognize objects by touch even though tactile, thermal, and proprioceptive functions remain intact (Zoltan et al., 1986). Patients with this deficit may have difficulty reaching into a bag or pocket and retrieving specific objects by using tactile information only.

Agnosias are generally evaluated through nonstandard assessments. Patients are asked to identify objects using only the sensory modality in question. When evaluating visual object agnosia, patients must identify objects by using vision only.

Case Study

• •

Mr. Smith is independent in rolling to the left, but he rolled onto his left upper extremity without being aware of it. When rolling to the right, he required moderate assistance to locate his left upper extremity, protract his left shoulder, and advance his left hip forward. He also dropped his left upper extremity during rolling, allowing it to fall onto the bed. In moving from a supine position to a sitting position, Mr. Smith needed moderate assistance and was unable to push up with his left upper extremity. He also required assistance to advance his left lower extremity off the bed.

This patient required moderate assistance to maintain a stable sitting position. He also sat with increased weight-bearing on his right hip; his trunk was laterally flexed to the left, yet he was unaware of his asymmetry. Mr. Smith was also unable to tell if his left foot was flat on the floor without looking at it.

This patient required maximal assistance to move into and maintain a standing posture. His standing position was asymmetrical and he leaned to the left, but he was unaware of his asymmetry. Ambulation was not assessed because Mr. Smith was unable to stand.

• •

Assessing the Impairment

• •

Difficulties noted during Mr. Smith's performance of functional mobility may be due, in part, to sensory and perceptual problems. Muscle weakness and balance dysfunction may be responsible for many of the noted mobility problems, but his performance also indicates the presence of sensory and perceptual problems. Specifically, Mr. Smith's performance of the tasks of functional mobility suggests deficits in proprioception and the ability to sense pressure, as well as left unilateral neglect.

During rolling to the left, muscle weakness may cause the left upper extremity to become trapped under his trunk in left side-lying, but Mr. Smith's lack of awareness of this position is probably due to sensory problems, perceptual problems, or both. Similarly, once in a stable sitting position, Mr. Smith was unable to accurately report the position of his left lower extremity. Mr. Smith's inability to properly position his left lower extremity may be due to muscle weakness, but his inability to perceive the position of his lower extremity is probably due to sensory problems, perceptual problems, or both.

Lack of awareness of affected extremities during movement suggests sensory deficits and unilateral neglect. If Mr. Smith does not know that his upper extremity is trapped under his trunk, he probably lacks the sensation of deep pressure. If a patient cannot describe where his limbs are in space without visual cues, he probably lacks proprioception. A full sensory evaluation of his extremities should be completed.

Mr. Smith's performance also suggests unilateral neglect. During the rolling sequence, he had difficulty locating his left upper extremity and was unable to hold onto his left upper extremity throughout the movement. Although muscle weakness may be the reason the left shoulder cannot protract and flex to actively assist with the rolling motion, decreased sensa-

tion and left neglect are probably the causes of the general inattention to, or lack of awareness of, the left upper extremity.

When Mr. Smith was positioned in a stable sitting position, he displayed an asymmetrical posture with increased weight-bearing on his right hip and left lateral trunk flexion. This asymmetrical posture may be caused by muscle weakness and balance dysfunction, but the patient's inability to recognize his asymmetry may be due to his decreased perception of the left side of his body.

Unilateral neglect can be assessed by having the patient locate objects in the environment. Typically, patients with left neglect have no difficulty finding objects located on the right but are unable to find objects located to the left of midline.

Results of Impairment Testing

- Sensory assessment–patient has diminished light touch, pressure, temperature sense, and proprioception.
- Left unilateral neglect–patient was unable to locate objects placed on his left, but had no difficulty locating objects placed on his right.

TREATMENT OF DEFICITS

In most cases, sensory and perceptual deficits will be seen together rather than separately. However, in this chapter they are discussed separately to assist the reader in understanding the specific treatments prescribed for specific deficits.

Treatment outcomes of sensory and perceptual deficits are variable. The amount of improvement a patient is likely to show depends on the severity of the initial sensory or perceptual problem. If the original problem is moderate or slight, then look for vast improvements in function over time. Severe initial problems tend to be associated with lingering or permanent sensory and perceptual deficits. In these severe cases, the goal of treatment is to teach patients to compensate for their deficits.

Sensory

Initially, most treatments for sensory deficits should be performed with the patient's eyes open for visual feedback. When patients become comfortable and treatments become easier, they should be allowed to close their eyes to remove visual feedback. This will increase the difficulty of the task.

One treatment for proprioception deficits includes repeated active and passive joint positioning with the eyes closed. This is achieved by placing the patient's involved extremities in various positions within the range of motion for the affected joint. Treatment outcomes can be assessed easily by having patients match or copy those joint positions with their noninvolved extremities. When inaccuracy occurs, ask the patient to visually inspect and then reposition the noninvolved extremity to match the involved extremity.

The treatment for kinesthetic deficits is similar, but involves active and passive movement of the involved extremities within the available ranges of motion for the joints being assessed. Treatment outcomes can be assessed easily by having patients exactly copy the movement with their noninvolved extremities while the involved extremities are being moved. Again, treatment should be performed first with the eyes open, and then with the eyes closed to increase difficulty of the activity.

Treatment to improve stereognosis can include placing various objects into the palms of the patients' hands. Have them keep their eyes open and feel the objects to get a sense of their textures and shapes. When patients are able to identify objects correctly with their eyes open, have them close their eyes and ask them again to identify the same or similar objects.

To improve tactile localization, simply touch different areas of the patient's body and either have them identify where they were touched or have them touch with their index finger the exact point where you originally touched them.

To improve discriminative touch, gently rub different objects with different textures across the surface of the patient's skin. Objects should possess varying textures (eg, hard, soft, rough, smooth). Patients should look at the objects as needed to increase feedback.

Treating patients with somatosensory loss may include use of the external environment or additional stimuli to increase their awareness of their extremities. At times, changing the external environment or stimulus may increase awareness, or assist in retraining the patient to perceive the environment.

Having patients who rely too heavily on visual cues stand on stable surfaces while distorting their incoming visual cues (such as having them look through a prism) is helpful for retraining their perceptions. This activity requires patients to use available somatosensory information rather than visual feedback.

To increase somatosensory input for trunk alignment, position patients in midline, with their backs against a chair or wall. The wall or back of a chair provides additional sensory information on trunk alignment. You may place a mirror a few yards directly in front of the patient to provide access to the visual cues needed to maintain midline posture. Once the patient processes these cues, withdraw them as well as the wall and chair stimuli.

Having patients stand without shoes or socks may also be useful in increasing input through their feet. Patients need to maintain upright postures without additional sensory cues to perform tasks of functional mobility.

Patients who rely on hard, smooth surfaces for somatosensory feedback should practice walking on irregular or soft surfaces. Walking barefoot changes the surface stimuli used in ambulation.

A force plate may be used to provide patients with biofeedback during weight shift. This has been beneficial in patients with hemiparesis (Perry, 1992; Umphred, 1995) In this activity, patients begin with static standing and equal weight distribution, then move from standing to sitting (and from sitting to standing) while their weight is equally distributed. Therapists may then instruct the patient to shift the weight laterally from limb to limb, or anteriorly and posteriorly with the involved limb forward and then behind. This may be followed by having the patient step in place.

Patients who display loss of somatosensory input may have weights placed on their ankles or on their assistive devices to increase sensory stimulation. There is no evidence to support the efficacy of this technique, but anecdotal reports from patients and therapists support its use (Umphred, 1995).

Overuse of visual compensation in sensory-deprived conditions should also be addressed in treatment programs. To decrease reliance on visual input, therapists may place blinders on patients, or blindfold them, and then assist them into positions where their static or dynamic balance will be challenged. This forces patients to use whatever somatosensory feedback is available.

Conversely, for patients who are unable to use somatosensory processing, mirrors may be used to integrate visual input to achieve midline sitting or stance. Mirrors should be withdrawn as soon as patients develop appropriate compensatory CNS strategies for maintaining midline without visual feedback.

Perceptual

Treatment of perceptual deficits varies depending on the particular impairment. Factors that must be considered include visual input; external stimuli; shortening of tasks within the range of perception, with gradual movement into impaired areas; and the use of other sensory modalities to compensate for the deficit, (eg, with vertical disorientation, one may use touch to increase awareness of alignment).

Generally, physical therapists do not treat specific perceptual deficits. They may, however, enhance their treatment and goal achievement through understanding perceptual deficits and how these deficits affect the patient's functional mobility. The physical therapist should incorporate techniques used in the treatment of perceptual deficits during tasks of functional mobility. This will enhance the patient's ability to interpret and appropriately interact with the environment, thereby facilitating success in movement.

Techniques used in the treatment of perceptual deficits include:

1. Structuring of tasks within the patient's range of perception, with gradual movement into impaired areas
2. Use of external stimuli to compensate for a deficit
3. Use of other sensory modalities to compensate for the deficit

Tasks should be structured within the patient's range of perception and gradually moved into impaired areas. A patient with ideational apraxia will have difficulty performing sequenced motor acts. In treating the functional mobility problems initially, request sequenced motor actions within the patient's capabilities. Gradually demand increasingly complex sequenced motor actions. For example, transfers require numerous motor skills that must be performed in a specific order.

Typical directions for a transfer may begin with a sequence of three motor actions: (1) ''Lock the chair,'' (2) ''Place both feet flat on the floor,'' and (3) ''Bring your hips forward in the chair.'' Patients who are unable to sequence these three actions would be unable to successfully complete this task as directed. However, if directions were given one step at a time, these patients might then be able to perform these individual motor skills. Therapists should treat functional mobility problems while gradually requesting increased numbers of motor skills for the completion of complex tasks.

External stimuli can be used to compensate for a deficit. In treating a patient with left unilateral neglect, place brightly colored tape on necessary items located to the left of midline. These items may include the left lock, the left armrest, and the left footrest of the wheelchair. This will enhance the patient's ability to attend to the left side and increase awareness of functional mobility.

Other sensory modalities may need to be added to compensate for the deficit. Patients with unilateral neglect or somatognosia will have difficulty attending to or identifying their own body parts. Typically, these deficits have a negative impact on the patient's ability to participate in or successfully complete tasks of functional mobility. The therapist can verbally cue the patient to look at the moving body part. This may enhance movement by increasing the patient's attention to the neglected side. Alternatively, the visual feedback may increase the patient's ability to recognize body parts.

The following are examples of techniques that may be used in the treatment of tasks of functional mobility when perceptual deficits are present.

Rolling

Patients with unilateral neglect may be unable to locate and therefore grasp their affected hand to roll toward their noninvolved side. In this case, therapists should instruct patients to touch the neck with the unaffected hand, after which the unaffected hand should be moved over to locate the affected shoulder. Finally, have the patient slide the unaffected hand down the affected arm until the affected hand is reached.

Patients should clasp their hands or hold their affected wrists with their unaffected hands. This position will enable both upper extremities to be incorporated in the task of rolling.

Supine-to-Sit Maneuver

The ability to incorporate the affected sides of the body into each step of this task requires that patients plan and execute new movements. This is difficult for patients with ideational apraxia because they are unable to plan or conceptually organize new motions, although they possess the sensory, coordination, and motor functions necessary to complete the task. This is due to their inability to plan or conceptually organize new motions.

When working with patients with apraxia to develop movement strategies for moving from a supine position to sitting provide concise and consistent one-step directions. Be sure to allow patients enough time to attempt the movement. If patients are unable to perform the motion, or if the motion is incomplete, assist them in completing the motion and simultaneously provide verbal cues or directions on how to complete the task.

Ambulation

Patients with deficits in spatial relations and spatial position are not safe ambulating through crowded spaces. Initially, ambulation should be practiced in open spaces. To improve a patient's ability to safely negotiate obstacles, gradually add objects to the pathways and assist the patient with safe completion of the route. Before patients attempt to ambulate around objects, point out objects and verbally assist them with mapping out a safe route.

Climbing Stairs

When working with patients with deficits in depth perception, first orient them to the existence of stairs. This measure is for their own safety. Then, if possible, have patients feel the distance between steps. They can use their hands, feet, or a cane. Also inform patients of the number of steps and whether or not all steps are the same distance apart. Placing pieces of tape of different colors on each step may help patients identify the next level of each step.

Case Study

From the disability and impairment assessment, it is apparent that Mr. Smith suffers from diminished proprioception and discriminative touch, as well as left-side neglect.

Generally, when treating patients like Mr. Smith, you should position yourself on the left side of the patient. One of your treatment goals would be to increase the patient's ability to attend to the neglected side. Having everyone who enters the room consistently approach Mr. Smith from the left side will force him to attend to stimuli on the left. This may prompt him to become more aware of the left side of the environment and the left side of his body.

Throughout the treatment, consistently draw the patient's attention to the left. This includes consistently asking Mr.

Smith to look at his left extremities during all of the functional mobility tasks. This technique will assist the patient with attending to his left side. It will also help to prevent the neglected limbs from being injured.

- Rolling: Ask the patient to locate his left upper extremity. A bright watch band or hospital identification band on the left wrist would assist the patient with visually locating and attending to the left upper extremity. As the patient attempts to roll, give verbal cues such as, ''Don't drop your left hand.'' The patient rolls by flexing his shoulder and hip that is opposite to the direction of the roll.

- Supine-to-sit maneuver: As Mr. Smith moves from lying supine to lying on his left to sitting, you will need to continually ask him to look at and attempt to push up with his left upper extremity. Without these cues, Mr. Smith may attempt to pull up with his right upper extremity or roll onto his back and push up with his right upper extremity.

  You could position Mr. Smith in a side-sitting position so that he can bear weight on his left upper extremity with his shoulder protracted, abducted, externally rotated, and his elbow flexed. Weight-bearing provides proprioceptive input that is effective in treatment of both proprioceptive deficits and unilateral neglect.

- Stable sitting: Again, focus the patient's attention on the left side of the body. You can do this by asking questions such as, ''Where is your left leg?'' and ''Is your left foot flat on the floor?'' The use of a full-length mirror can be helpful for a patient who is sitting asymmetrically but is unaware of his asymmetry. If the full-length mirror is placed directly in front of the patient, he will be able to see the asymmetry that he cannot otherwise perceive. This visual assistance helps the patient achieve and maintain a more symmetrical posture.

• •

Having the patient bear weight on the left upper extremity while sitting increases proprioceptive input and increases his attention to the left upper extremity. Weight-shifting activities in sitting (eg, anteroposterior) would provide proprioceptive input to the left lower extremity as well.

Because this patient is unable to maintain a symmetrical sitting position, or attend to his left extremities, moving from a sitting to standing posture, standing, and ambulation will be difficult. These functional positions and activities should be attempted to stimulate appropriate motor and sensory responses.

• •

SUMMARY

• Because perceptual and sensory dysfunctions frequently occur in conjunction with mobility problems, physical therapists must incorporate treatments for them into tasks of functional mobility.
• Lesions at different sites along sensory pathways will produce different impairments. The closer the lesion to the cell body of the sensory neuron, the greater the likelihood of neuronal death. The farther the lesion from the cell body, the greater the chances that the neuron will survive the injury.
• Lesions involving the lemniscal system lead to decreases in or an absence of the senses of discriminative touch and kinesthesia, especially in the distal extremities. Loss of proprioception in the lower extremities results in balance, coordination, and gait dysfunctions.
• Sensory cortex lesions result in losses of proprioception, kinesthesia, discriminative touch, pain, light touch, and temperature.
• Sensory and perceptual deficits are assessed by observation of functional activities. More than one functional task should be observed to increase the chances of identifying the deficit. The sensory modalities assessed are sensation, discriminative touch and pressure, proprioception, kinesthesia, stereognosis, tactile localization, two-point discrimination, and recognition of textures. The perceptual deficits studied include those of figure-ground and depth perception, spatial relations and spatial positions, topographical orientation, body scheme, somatognosia, left-right discrimination, unilateral neglect, and various apraxias and agnosias.
• The amount of improvement a patient with perceptual or sensory deficits shows depends on the severity of the initial problem. In severe cases, the goal of treatment is to compensate for the deficits.

REFERENCES

American Occupational Therapy Association. (1994). Uniform terminology for occupational therapy. *American Journal of Occupational Therapy*, *48*, 1049–1054.

Ayres, A. J. (1987). *Sensory integration and praxis test.* Los Angeles: Western Psychological Services.

Baum, B. (1981). *The establishment of reliability and validity of perceptual evaluation on a sample of adult head trauma patients.* Unpublished master's thesis, University of Southern California.

Benton, A. L. (1967). Constructional apraxia and the minor hemisphere, *Confina Neurologica, 29,* 1–16.

Benton, A. L., Hamsher, K. deS., Varney, N. K., & Spreen, O. (1983). *Contributions to neuropsychological assessment–A clinical manual.* New York: Oxford University Press.

Brain, W. R. (1941). Visual disorientation with special reference to lesions of the right cerebral hemisphere. *Brain, 64,* 244–272.

DeRenzi, E., & Scotti, G. (1970). Autopagnosia: Fiction or reality. *Archives of Neurology, 23,* 121–132.

Goodglass, H, & Kaplan, E. (1972). *The assessment of aphasia and related disorders.* Philadelphia: Lea & Febiger.

Gregory, M. E., & Aitkin, J. A. (1971). Assessment of parietal lobe function in hemiplegia. *Occupational Therapy, 34,* 9–17.

Heilman, K. M., Watson, R. T., & Valenstein, E. (1985). Neglect and related disorders. In K. M. Heilman & E. Valenstein (Eds.). *Clinical neuropsychology.* New York: Oxford University Press.

Paterson, A, & Zangwill, O. L. (1944). Disorders of visual space perception associated with lesions of the right cerebral hemisphere. *Brain, 67,* 331–358.

Pehoski, C. (197). *Analysis of perceptual dysfunction and dressing in adult hemiplegics.* Unpublished master's thesis, Sargent College, Boston University.

Perry, J. (1992). *Gait analysis, normal and pathological function.* Thorofare NJ: Slack.

Piercy, M., Hecaen, H., & Ajureaguerra, J. (1960). Constructional apraxia associated with unilateral cerebral lesions–left and right sided cases compared. *Brain, 83,* 225–242.

Quintana, L. A. (1989). Cognitive and perceptual evaluation and treatment. In C. A. Trombly (Ed.). *Occupational therapy for physical dysfunction* (3rd ed.). Baltimore: Williams & Wilkins.

Schenkenberg, T., Bradford, D. C., & Ajax, E. T. (1980). Line bisection and unilateral visual neglect in patients with neurologic impairment. *Neurology, 30,* 509–517.

Selecki, B. R., & Herron, J. T. (1965). Disturbances of the verbal body image: A particular syndrome of sensory aphasia. *Journal of Nervous and Mental Disease, 141,* 42–51.

Trombly, C. A. (1995). *Occupational therapy for physical dysfunction* (4th ed.). Baltimore: Williams & Wilkins.

Umphred, D. A. (1995). *Neurological rehabilitation.* St. Louis: Mosby-Year Book.

Van Deusen, J. (1993). *Body image and perceptual dysfunction in adults.* Philadelphia: Saunders.

Zoltan, B. (1990). Evaluation of visual, perceptual, and perceptual motor deficits. In L. W. Pedretti & B. Zoltan (Eds.). *Occupational therapy practice skill for physical dysfunction* (3rd ed.). St. Louis: Mosby-Year Book.

Zoltan, B., Siev, E., & Freishtat, B. (1986). *The adult stroke patient.* Thorofare, NJ: Slack.

• •

SUGGESTED READINGS

Carpenter, M. B. (1991). *Core text of neuroanatomy* (4th ed.). Baltimore: Williams & Wilkins.

This popular, easy-to-read, and thorough neuroanatomy text covers such neuroanatomic topics as gross morphology of the central nervous system, ascending and descending tracts, blood supply, and the meninges. It also separately considers the different sections of the central nervous system.

Cohen, H. (Ed.). (1993). *Neuroscience rehabilitation.* Philadelphia: Lippincott.

This neuroanatomy text writes to rehabilitation therapists as its audience. Its descriptions of neuroanatomy are complete, with an emphasis on clinical situations.

Guyton, A. C. (1991). *Basic neuroscience–anatomy and physiology* (2nd ed.). Philadelphia: Saunders.

This basic, but extensive, neuroscience text is divided into seven sections that cover, among other topics, gross anatomy of the central and peripheral nervous systems, the cytoarchitecture of the nervous system, synapses, and neurotransmission. There are separate sections on general sensory, special sensory, and motor anatomy. The final six chapters discuss neural control of certain body functions (eg, contraction of skeletal muscle and control of heart functions).

Kandel, E. R., Schwartz, J. H., & Jessel, T. M. (1995). *Essentials of neural science and behavior.* East Norwalk, CT: Appleton & Lange.

This is an extensive text that provides considerable information on the cellular mechanics of neuroscience, including neurotransmission. There is abundant material on such neural topics as cognition, perception, language, learning, and memory.

Van Deusen, J. (1993). *Body image and perceptual dysfunction in adults.* Philadelphia: Saunders.

A textbook for rehabilitation professionals that focuses on the dysfunctions that result from deficits in visual perception, somesthetic discrimination, and body image. Each chapter concerns a different diagnostic category and the assessment and treatment of the perception and body image deficits associated with that diagnosis. Each topic is enhanced with case studies related to the content of body image or perceptual dysfunction.

Zoltan, B. (1996). *Vision, perception, and cognition: A manual for the evaluation and treatment of the neurologically impaired adult.* Thorofare, NJ: Slack.

This book is used extensively by occupational therapy clinicians and educators. It outlines the theoretical basis for visual, perceptual, and cognitive deficits along with specific evaluations and treatment techniques for each deficit.

Incoordination

LEARNING OBJECTIVES

After reading this chapter, you should be able to:

1. Describe how coordinated movement requires the integration of information from the sensory cortex, motor cortex, cerebellum, and basal ganglia.
2. Analyze how functional mobility may be impaired by incoordination, especially when combined with a balance dysfunction.
3. Identify the clinical tests that can be performed to indicate the presence of a coordination deficit, and the standardized tests that can be used to assist in quantifying the functional limitations evident with the incoordination.
4. Discuss the treatment of incoordination specifically related to functional tasks limited by the impairment.
5. Discuss how the practice of functional tasks can be improved by shortening the range of movement, decreasing the rate of movement, and adding sensory cues, visual cues, or both.

Coordinated movements occur when muscles work together to produce smooth, controlled, accurate movements. Coordination deficits occur when muscles fail to fire in sequence, or when the central nervous system (CNS) is unable to direct movement activities accurately. Lack of coordination can impair the quality of movement or be so severe that it limits movement altogether. Coordinated movements require adequate strength and range of motion (ROM) to complete a particular task.

Lack of coordination may occur with CNS lesions or with muscle weakness. In CNS lesions, several movement dysfunctions may occur such as movement decomposition and dysmetria. In **movement decomposition,** there is a breakdown of movements between multiple joints (eg, the movements between shoulder, elbow, wrist, and hand), which then move in segments, not as one fluid movement. **Dysmetria** is characterized by overshooting or reaching beyond the target. This activity is sometimes referred to as past-pointing.

Coordination deficits from muscle weakness are typically associated with slow movement and inadequate muscle strength. Without the necessary muscle strength, the stability of proximal joints cannot be maintained and accurate movements cannot occur. For example, weak shoulder musculature can limit the ability to reach for a cup in a cabinet. The inability to maintain an isometric contraction at 90° shoulder flexion while the elbow, wrist, and hand move to reach for the cup can produce awkward movements.

●●●●●●●●●●●●●●●●●●●●●●●●●●●●●●●●●●
IMPAIRMENT: INCOORDINATION

Coordination is a measure of the quality of movement, and as such, it requires adequate strength and ROM as the foundation for movement. Incoordination occurs when the firing rates of muscles are disrupted, resulting in loss of smooth reciprocal movement, or when the CNS loses its ability to direct movement activity that requires accuracy.

Motor Control

When addressing motor control problems, it is possible to treat strength and quality of movement at the same time. However, the initial emphasis should be on strengthening the muscle if that impairment is a factor in the movement dysfunction.

For example, patients with stroke often have diminished motor recovery in an upper extremity, which may limit their ability to reach for a cup placed on a table. To complete this task, the patient may place the involved extremity on the table and attempt to protract the shoulder and extend the elbow, wrist, and hand toward the cup. During this activity, the patient must also aim for the cup and complete the task of opening and closing the hand to grasp the cup. Two coordinated movements must occur in this task. Hand–eye coordination is needed when aiming for the cup, and the finger flexors and extensors must be activated in a coordinated fashion to grasp the cup.

Reaching for a cup also requires coordination of multiple body segments (the shoulder must be protracted, the elbow extended, and the wrist and hand alternately extended and flexed.) Placing the arm on the table and opening and closing the hand is a simpler task that incorporates many of these movements. However, this task is not goal-directed, nor does it address the multiple joint activity required for the task of reaching for a cup. It also fails to incorporate strengthening activities of other muscles. In the task of reaching for a cup, sequencing of shoulder activity must be timed with elbow, wrist, and hand activity.

If patients are having difficulty with this whole task, it can be broken down into single segments, such as protracting the shoulder, extending the elbow, or opening and closing the hand. Single segments can be practiced, first emphasizing strengthening, then increasing speed and range of movement to build coordination. Other movement segments can then be added, building on what has previously been attained.

Timing and Accuracy

Coordination entails accuracy in reaching targets, as well as the ability to carry out complex motor activities with smooth reciprocal movement patterns. Touching one's fingertips to one's nose tests accuracy in reaching targets. Performing repetitive, reciprocal activities, such as supination and pronation, opening and closing the hands, and tapping the feet, requires activation and deactivation of agonist and antagonist muscles.

To complete these tasks in a coordinated fashion, muscle activation must be timed to enable contraction of agonist muscle(s), then inhibition to enable antagonist muscle(s) to move the joint in the opposite direction. Inability to perform this task may occur only when patients attempt to perform it quickly, because patients learn to compensate by moving slowing and using synergistic muscles. Remember, in synergistic movement, muscles work together to produce motion by contracting to compensate for any weakness in the primary muscle that performs the joint movement.

ANATOMY OVERVIEW

Control of coordinated movements occurs at spinal and supraspinal levels within the CNS. Spinal cord control occurs via reflexes mediated through group Ia and Ib afferents which enter the CNS through dorsal roots. Some afferents synapse directly on motor neurons, but the majority indirectly influence motor neuron activity by synapsing on interneurons, which are the building blocks of spinal reflexes.

Interneurons coordinate spinal reflex timing through interneuronal circuits, such as divergence, convergence, presynaptic inhibition, and reverberating circuits. Divergence occurs when the output of one neuron affects two or more neurons, whereas convergence is concerned with the termination of more than one neural input onto a single neuron (Cohen, 1993). During **presynaptic inhibition,** the neurotransmitter is not released due to the depolarization of the nerve terminal by a second neural input (Cohen, 1993). In **reverberating circuits,** axon collaterals re-excite the same neuron through excitatory interneurons (Kandel, Schwartz, & Jessel, 1991). Inhibitory interneurons associated with group Ia afferents coordinate muscle activity via reciprocal innervation. Group Ib afferents from receptors, such as **Golgi tendon organs (GTOs)** may synapse on inhibitory interneurons that reflexively inhibit homonymous muscles, synergistic muscles, or both, to contribute to smooth, coordinated movements.

Coordination results from tremendous synaptic activity within the CNS. This activity includes processing sensory information and integrating information from the cerebellum, parietal lobe, and motor cortex (including motor strip, prefrontal, and supplemental motor area) (Kandel et al., 1991). Continuous feedback and reassessment on how the task was completed is provided by the cerebellum. Neurons in the motor cortex receive information on body position and movement speed, as well as more detailed proprioceptive input from the muscles to which they project, from joint receptors, or from the skin that overlies such muscle. These same neurons also receive sensory information from corticocortical fibers from the somatic sensory cortex or from the thalamus.

The cerebellum is the center for balance and coordinated activity. It functions by comparing motor activities, compensating for motor tasks, and learning new motor programs (Kandel et al., 1991). In the role of comparator, the cerebellum modifies motor programs based on sensory input and motor output. As a compensator, it performs predictive compensatory modifications of reflexes in anticipation of movement. It sets stretch and other reflexes through its connections with subcortical nuclei (eg, red nucleus) (Kandel et al., 1991). The cerebellum learns new motor programs or memorizes simple motor programs that can be added to develop complex tasks (Kandel et al., 1991). Figure 7-1 shows the relationships between the integration of information from the sensory cortex, the peripheral system (eg, vestibular system, dorsal columns, and spinocerebellum tracts), and the motor cortex.

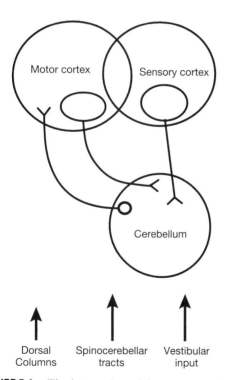

FIGURE 7-1. The integration of the sensory and motor cortex and the peripheral nervous system.

The basal ganglia also contribute to the development of smooth, coordinated activity by communicating directly with the motor cortex through a complex looping pattern within the basal ganglia nuclei. Figure 7-2 shows the relationships between basal ganglia and motor cortex.

Coordinated movement patterns are activated with the transmission of impulses along corticospinal tracts. The movement patterns that are produced are the result of multiple **program generators,** neuronally encoded ''commands'' that can elicit patterned movements such as locomotion and respiration (Cohen, 1993). These program generators work at all levels of the **neuraxis,** eg, the spinal cord, cerebellum, and basal ganglia (Cohen, 1993).

To initiate movement, these program generators select the necessary movement patterns to enable us to carry out motor tasks. The basic motor plan from the program generator is modified to meet the demands of the environment. It is the job of the corticospinal tracts to recruit sufficient numbers of alpha motor neurons to activate muscles and to generate the appropriate forces needed to accomplish intended tasks.

Lesions

Damage to areas that contribute to the execution of smooth, coordinated movement may result in some type of impairment in the quality of movement. The symptoms most often displayed involve the timing of muscle activation, sequencing of muscles, accuracy of movement, or the addition of involuntary movement as a result of the muscles firing spontaneously.

Specific symptoms seen with cerebellar lesions include movement decomposition (also referred to as *asynergy*), dysmetria, hypotonia, **asthenia, dysdiadochokinesia,** tremor, and speech and eye movement disorders (Kandel et al., 1991). Basal ganglia lesions may produce

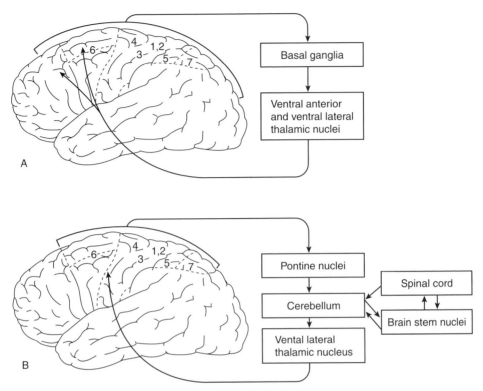

FIGURE 7-2. (*A*) Subcortical connections of the basal ganglia. (*B*) Subcortical cerebellar connections.

bradykinesia, **rigidity,** tremor, akinesia, chorea, athetosis, **hemiballismus,** and **dystonia** (Kandel et al., 1991).

The dorsal columns and spinocerebellar tracts transmit a significant amount of peripheral sensory information along the spinal cord to the cortex and cerebellum. Lesions in the spinal cord that affect sensory tracts typically result in diminished sensory feedback and may result in proprioceptive loss, wide base of stance, gait dysmetria, balance and equilibrium problems, and slowing of voluntary movements. The presence of these clinical signs will limit the patient's ability to execute smooth, coordinated movements.

Patients with muscle weakness resulting from lesions of the CNS may also demonstrate lack of coordination. Lack of strength can prevent patients from performing certain tasks and may also result in poor movement quality. Two prerequisites for performing coordinated tasks are adequate strength to perform the activity and adequate ROM to move through the required movement. Deficiencies in either area should be addressed first to improve the quality of movement or coordination.

The quality of movement may also be limited if muscular imbalance is present, either from weakness, abnormal muscle tone, or muscle shortening. The patient in Figure 7-3*A* demon-

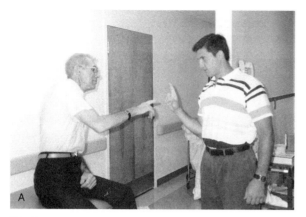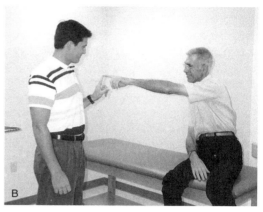

FIGURE 7-3. (*A*) Patient is unsuccessful at a task of coordination. (*B*) Patient successfully performs task of coordination.

strates difficulty performing a coordinated task because a synergistic pattern generated by inadequate cortical activation of muscles (weakness) interferes with the coordinated movements of joints. The predominance of shortened flexor muscles and the weakness of extensor muscles limits his ability to protract his shoulder, extend his elbow, and reach for the target. The quantity of movement in his right arm must be addressed before testing or treating coordination problem(s).

ASSESSING THE DISABILITY

Assessment of the disability allows examiners to determine which functional activities are difficult or impossible for patients to perform because of an underlying impairment. Disabilities associated with incoordination may range from the inability to perform tasks requiring fine coordination, to ataxic gait patterns. Patients with incoordination may have difficulty with dressing, daily hygiene activities such as brushing their hair or teeth, or using utensils to cut food.

Most patients with incoordination can perform the gross movements needed for bed mobility and transfers, although they may have difficulty standing without a wide base and may display ataxia with any movement.

Functional movements described in previous chapters are again discussed here to illustrate how incoordination may limit or interfere with movement abilities. The reader will note that the impairments described in this text are interrelated in that they contribute to similar limitations in functional mobility. Henceforth, the need to perform specific impairment testing after a disability has been identified.

The alternative movement strategies presented in the next section refer to movements outside of the normative movements described in Chapter 3.

Rolling

Rolling may not be limited with incoordination unless the patient displays severe ataxia of the trunk. Most positions in lying (ie, supine, prone, and side-lying postures) are stable for patients with incoordination because they are fully supported by the bed or mat surface. When moving out of the stable posture, patients may display ataxia of the extremities or may attempt to limit movement of an extremity due to the presence of chorea.

Supine-to-Sitting Maneuver

Patients with incoordination dysfunctions will not have difficulty moving from supine to sitting unless ataxia of the trunk or choreoathetoid movements are present. During the dynamic phases of this task, patients may exhibit slow, deliberate movements as they try to maintain stability to decrease ataxia of the trunk or extremities.

Stable Sitting Posture

Stable sitting posture is assessed with the feet flat on the floor and the arms and hands at the sides of the trunk or on the thighs. Therapists should look for symmetry, or lack thereof, and trunk stability in this position. Patients with ataxia of the trunk may have difficulty maintaining this posture. The addition of dynamic movements to enable functional tasks to be performed (ie, donning socks and shoes or putting on a shirt) may be limited in patients with ataxia or chorea.

Sit-to-Stand Maneuver

Coordination is required for all aspects of sit-to-stand movements. During the dynamic phases of this task, patients may exhibit a wide base of stance and slow, deliberate movements as they try to maintain stable postures. Careful assessment of this movement must be performed to identify the specific impairments that may have led to the observed dysfunction. Was

it somatosensory or vestibular in nature? Did it arise from incoordination or was it attributable to muscle weakness? When coordination deficits are accompanied by balance dysfunction, patients may use alternative movement strategies when standing up from sitting. They may, for example, use their upper extremities to support themselves or accomplish the push-off, and they may adopt a wide base of stance in standing.

Stable Standing Posture

Body symmetry and the ability to maintain this position should be evaluated while patients are standing unsupported. The examiner should look for a wide base of stance, the presence of body sway, flexing the posture to lower center of gravity, or all three. In addition, the patient with incoordination may not want to release hand support if chorea is present, and may display truncal ataxia in this stable posture.

Transfers

Patients performing pivot transfers are required to stand, pivot, and then sit in chairs placed close to those in which they were sitting. A lateral transfer with continuous hand support is an alternative movement strategy used with incoordination to diminish tremor or ataxia in the arms or trunk. A wide base of support, slow deliberate movements, truncalataxia, and chorea may also be displayed during this test.

Ambulation

Initiation of gait from a static posture requires that the weight be shifted so that the center of gravity changes and that unilateral support on the lower extremities be altered. Shuffling of the feet or ataxic movement patterns may be seen during gait. This may result from diminished somatosensory feedback or problems with motor activation and timing.

Two common types of *ataxic* gaits are spinal ataxia and cerebellar ataxia. Spinal or sensory ataxia is characterized by gait patterns with broad bases of stance and flailing movements of the feet. Heels strike the ground first, followed by slapping of the feet. It is characteristic of patients to watch their feet while walking to compensate for loss of sensory awareness in their lower extremities. This gait pattern is thought to result from the disruption of sensory pathways in the spinal cord, as seen with tabes dorsalis or multiple sclerosis. In milder cases, the patient may ambulate normally if allowed to walk with the eyes open. However, gait problems such as staggering, unsteadiness, and the inability to walk may occur when the eyes are closed (Rothstein, Roy, & Wolf, 1990).

Cerebellar ataxia results in gait deviations that are equally severe when patients walk with their eyes open or closed. This gait pattern is of a wide base, unsteady, and irregular. Patients stagger and are unable to walk in tandem or follow straight lines. As the name indicates, this form of ataxia is associated with lesions of the cerebellum. If lesions are localized to one hemisphere, there is persistent deviation or swaying toward the affected side (Rothstein et al., 1990).

Climbing Stairs

Ascending stairs requires that patients shift weight from one leg to the other, as well as lift them alternately onto the steps. The complexity of this task may result in increased ataxic movements. Many patients rely on handrails during this maneuver to compensate for instability and incoordination. Therapists should assess patients with less hand support and observe their ability to move their extremities in a coordinated pattern. Patients may rely on visual input to assist with placement of each foot on the stair; they may, likewise, widen the base of stance to increase stability and decrease ataxia.

Case Study

....

Mr. Black is seen in the outpatient physical therapy clinic for evaluation and treatment of clumsiness and ataxia. The patient reports he sustained a mild stroke a month ago that required hospitalization for 5 days. He experienced left-sided weakness, which resolved within 4 days. He continues to experience difficulty buttoning his shirt, putting on and zippering his pants, cutting food with a knife and fork, and reaching for objects. He is ambulating with a walker independently, but is unable to drive his car.

....

Assessing the Disability

....

Because Mr. Black reports independent ambulation with a walker, evaluation of gait is a good place to begin. Observe his posture, ability to balance while advancing the walker forward, placement of the walker on the floor, ability to shift weight to initiate the toe-off and swing phase, components of the swing phase, heel strike, and the stance phase. Is there any asymmetry of movement? Are movements smooth and reciprocal? Are tremors or added movements noted with volitional activity? Is the patient able to place the walker and his feet in appropriate positions for safe and effective ambulation?

Changes in the gait cycle or asymmetrical movement may suggest weakness, balance disturbance, antalgia, or incoordination. Jerky movements or tremulous activity superimposed on volitional movement suggest incoordination. Inappropriate placement of the walker, feet, or both may suggest balance dysfunction, incoordination, somatosensory loss, or a visual disturbance.

Assess ambulation in the parallel bars with one hand support and then no hand support. How does his gait change with reduced hand support? Does balance become impaired? Are movements more ataxic? Are components of the swing and stance phases altered with diminished hand support? What is the speed of movement without hand support? Does it increase or slow down?

Changes in gait with reduced hand support suggest lower extremity weakness, painful weight-bearing, balance dysfunction, or incoordination. An increase in ataxic movements, changes in components of the gait cycle with reduced hand support, or both suggest balance deficits or incoordination, as does any slowing of movement.

Assess Mr. Black's ability to lower himself into a chair and then return to standing. Is this movement performed symmetrically, or is one side doing most of the work? Is this a controlled smooth movement, or does the patient "plop" into the chair? In sitting, is he able to maintain a stable sitting posture with and without movement? On returning to standing, are movements symmetrical and coordinated, or asymmetrical and disjointed. Is hand support used to achieve standing? Once the patient is standing, is hand support needed to maintain standing?

The patient's asymmetrical movement and his inability to lower himself into the chair indicate weakness or a problem in the timing and sequencing of muscle activation. Stable sitting and standing with and without dynamic movement indicate that balance may be intact. These movements also show that the patient has adequate strength in his trunk and lower extremities. To confirm that balance is not a problem, the patient should be able to perform these movements with his eyes closed. Evidence of disjointed or jerky movement patterns suggest incoordination. Hand support throughout the movement pattern and on standing suggests a balance deficit or weakness in the lower extremities.

As Mr. Black progresses to stair climbing, observe his pattern of movement. Does he step reciprocally or lead continuously with one leg? If he steps reciprocally, are patterns of movement symmetrical between both legs, or does one leg display exaggerated or excessive movement?

If the patient does not engage in reciprocal stair climbing, assess his ability to perform this task. Observe the timing and sequencing of movements, as well as Mr. Black's ability to lift his body up the stairs with each leg (strength). Reduce hand support on handrails and observe any change in movement patterns. Lack of a reciprocal gait on stairs and asymmetry of movement suggests weakness or incoordination. Exaggerated or excessive movement or difficulty with timing and sequencing of muscle activity suggest incoordination. Reducing hand support challenges balance and may also indicate weakness or incoordination.

It could be assumed that bed mobility and supine-to-sit maneuvers are accomplished safely and efficiently because the patient is independent in ambulation with a walker. However, it is best to assess the movement patterns to determine if any additional movement deficits exist.

Results of Assessment

The assessment of functional mobility revealed that bed mobility, sitting, sit-to-stand, standing, ambulation with a walker, and nonreciprocal stair climbing were all independent. Some ataxia was noted in the left lower extremity with ambulation and stair climbing, which was performed nonreciprocally and favored the right leg. Ambulation in the parallel bars with one hand support revealed increased ataxia in the left lower extremity and a wider base of support. The patient was unable to ambulate without one hand support. Attempts at stair climbing with a reciprocal pattern required one hand support (the patient preferred two hands); the patient was slower in movement and had increased ataxia in the left lower extremity.

ASSESSING THE IMPAIRMENT: INCOORDINATION

Coordination should be assessed bilaterally for reciprocal motion, the sequencing of multiple joints, movement accuracy, and fixation (or postural holding). Tests for coordination assume that:

- Isolated selective movements are possible
- Strength is adequate
- ROM is adequate

Make sure the tasks of functional mobility that are performed to assess coordination include movements that require the patient to alter the range and speed of movement. During the course of these tasks, patients should be able to maintain smooth, reciprocal muscle activation and move accurately without involuntary contractions or muscle activity. If abnormalities are found, their presence and frequency of occurrence must be documented. For example, if patients display dysmetria and **intention tremor** in four of five trials of the finger-to-nose

test, we know that they touch their own nose in a coordinated pattern only once.

Assessment of coordination may also include timed tests. Patients may be evaluated to see how many repetitions of a given activity they can perform in a given time frame. The time required to complete a task accurately and successfully can also be recorded.

Clinical Tests to Assess Coordination

The tests described below are used in a clinical assessment of coordination; however, validity, reliability, and normative values for these clinical tests are unknown. Abnormalities in the performance of these tests suggest the presence of incoordination. Patients should perform these tests twice: first with the eyes open, then with the eyes closed. The latter variation allows the therapist to determine how accurate movement is without visual input. Patients should perform all movement patterns in both sitting and standing positions. Standing for any of these tests will challenge the patient's balance, especially when the eyes are closed.

Finger-to-Nose Test

Beginning with the arms abducted from the body, the patient touches the tip of the nose with an index finger. Have the patient slowly repeat this test five times, then perform it as quickly as possible five more times. Observe the five trials of movement for accuracy and the presence of any tremor activity (Mayo, Sullivan, & Swaine, 1991; O'Neil et al., 1992; Swaine & Sullivan, 1992, 1993; Wilson, Pollock, Kaplin, Law, & Faris, 1992). Record the number of times out of five that the task is completed accurately (eg, 4/5 times) at a slow speed and a faster speed.

Finger-to-Nose and Examiner's Finger

This is a modification of the finger-to-nose test. Patients reach out and touch the examiner's finger after touching their own nose (O'Neil et al., 1992). As with the finger-to-nose test, patients should repeat this test slowly and then quickly while the therapist observes for accuracy, tremor, and dysmetria.

Figure 7-3B, shown earlier, depicts a patient successfully performing this test with his noninvolved extremity. In Figure 7-3A, the patient is unable to perform this test with his involved extremity due to muscle imbalance. Be sure to record the number of times the task is performed successfully.

Drawing Numbers or Alphabet With Finger or Toes

Ask patients to write on a chalk board or a piece of paper or have them use their fingers to draw letters of the alphabet or numbers in the air. To assess the lower extremities, have patients draw letters or numbers on the floor with their toes or with a pencil placed between their toes. You may also instruct them to trace circles you have drawn on the floor (Olgiati, Burgunder, & Mumenthaler, 1988).

In all of these tests, observe the patient's ability to move through patterns and to trace or draw letters and numbers accurately. Documentation should include information on the patient's ability to complete the task without ataxic or tremulous movements, as well as their accuracy in the task.

Heel-to-Shin or Heel-to-Ankle Maneuver

Have the patient place a heel on the opposite shin, knee, or ankle. The movement is deemed abnormal if the patient points past or misses the targeted body parts, displays tremulous activity, or exhibits ataxia (Mayo et al, 1991; O'Neil et al.,

1992). This test is similar to Frenkel's exercises, which are described later in this chapter. Figure 7-4 shows a patient performing this test with the noninvolved extremity.

Tracking Test With or Without a Computer

The age of technology has introduced computer programs that display screens with various objects, both stationary and movable, that patients track using joysticks (Behbehani et al., 1990; Smith & Kondraske, 1987). The speed at which objects move can be varied, as can the pattern in which the objects move.

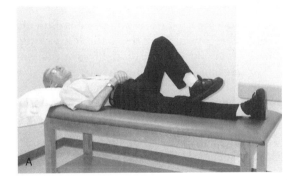

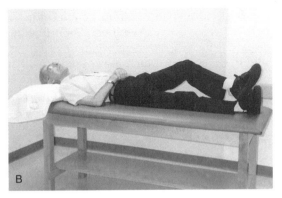

FIGURE 7-4. Patient performs the heel-to-shin (*A*) and the heel-to-ankle (*B*) maneuvers with the noninvolved leg.

Behbehani and colleagues (1990) compared the responses of normal subjects and those of patients diagnosed with multiple sclerosis, Parkinson's disease, and myasthenia gravis to the following two patterns: a random step from a horizontal line, and a phase plane plot of any shape within two coordinates of an *x* and *y* plane. They reported variations in both the random step and phase plane that were descriptive of the different pathologic conditions (Behbehani et al., 1990).

If a computer program is not available, ask the patient to track your index finger with his or her own as you move your hand in front of the patient in different patterns. In this test the patient attempts to mirror your movements.

Writing

Writing is a functionally important skill, but using it as a measure of coordination is difficult. Comparing samples of the patient's writings from before and after the disability is one means of quantifying change. This may be impossible to detect in patients with hemiplegia who have learned to compensate with their nondominant, uninvolved extremity (Wade, 1989).

Gross Movement Patterns

Bilateral shoulder flexion, abduction, or both may be performed to assess movement composition between two extremities. Abnormalities displayed include slower movement of the involved extremities, which also overshoot their normal ROM. Documentation with this test should include abnormal movements, presence of ataxia or tremor, and the patient's abilities or inabilities to perform the bilateral movement pattern at slow or fast speeds.

Rapid Alternating Movements

Rapid alternating movements involve bilateral activities of any extremity joint and alternate foot tapping or hand tapping on the knees. The

most commonly tested bilateral activity is the rapid alternation of supination and pronation. All of these activities can be performed with both extremities moving in the same or opposite directions.

Initially testing alternating movements in the same direction is usually easiest for patients to comprehend. Therapists should observe for reciprocal movement patterns at various speeds and smooth rhythmic movements without ataxia or tremulous movements. The presence or absence of these abnormalities should be documented, as should the inability to execute smooth reciprocal movements at varying speeds.

Standardized Tests to Measure Coordination

The standardized tests listed below have been shown to assess manual dexterity and coordination (Desrosiers, Bravo, Hebert, Dutil, & Mercier, 1994; Jebsen, Taylor, Trieschmann, Trotter, & Howard, 1969; Sullivan, Winstein, & Pohl, 1993; Sunderland et al., 1992; Wade, 1989, 1992; Williamson & Leiper, 1993). These tests are different from the clinical tests described previously in that they are based on functional tasks or activities. They have also been tested for validity and reliability (see Appendix B).

Fitt's Tapping Test

Several investigators (Sullivan et al., 1993; Williamson & Leiper, 1993) have used the Fitt's Tapping Test to assess coordination or dexterity. Patients are asked to depress a tap key, continuously, and as quickly as possible, within a specific time. The size of the tap key can be varied. Smaller keys result in slower tapping rates from most normal subjects. The use of nondominant extremities and increasing age also contribute to slower tapping rates.

One concern that has been raised with this test is that it fails to consider the patient's motivation. If patients do not try their best at this task, they may receive lower scores. This may wrongly suggest impaired dexterity (Sullivan et al., 1993; Wade, 1989; Williamson & Leiper, 1993), thus making this test appear unreliable (Wade, 1992).

Frenchay Arm Test

This test originally consisted of 25 test items. It was shortened to five items to increase its clinical applicability. The Frenchay Arm Test is based on five functional movement patterns:

1. Stabilizing a ruler on paper with the involved hand while drawing a line with the noninvolved hand
2. Grasping a cylinder 12 mm in diameter and 5 cm long, lifting it at least 30 cm above a table, and then replacing it on the table without dropping the cylinder
3. Picking up a half-filled glass of water, taking a drink from the glass, and then returning it to the table without spilling
4. Removing a sprung clothespin from a dowel mounted on a block
5. Combing or imitating the process of combing hair, being sure to reach the top and back of the head

The placement of the glass, cylinder, or dowel on the table is specified in the test directions to increase testing consistency. Patients are given three trials to perform each task successfully. For each task, examiners record a one if the task is completed successfully and a zero if patients are unable to complete the task (Sullivan et al., 1993; Sunderland et al., 1991; Wade, 1989, 1992; Williamson & Leiper, 1993).

Rivermead Test

The Rivermead Motor Assessment consists of three sections: gross function, leg and trunk function, and arm function. The test for arm function consists of nine activities that assess coordination:

- Picking up and releasing a tennis ball
- Picking up and releasing a pencil
- Picking up a piece of paper and releasing it for five repetitions
- Cutting putty with a knife and fork and placing pieces on a mat set on the side
- Standing in place and bouncing a large ball five times
- Opposing the thumb and forefinger 14 times within 10 seconds
- Alternating supination and pronation of the hand 20 times in 10 seconds
- Tying a string around the neck with the bow in the back
- Performing 'pat-a-cake' seven times in 15 seconds

The Rivermead is scored exactly like the Frenchay test (ie, the numeral one represents the ability, and zero represents the inability, to perform the tasks) (Wade, 1992). This test was reliable within one point (Wade, 1992).

Peg Tests

Two commonly used peg tests are the nine-hole and the 10-hole peg tests. The nine-hole peg test measures the time it takes patients to pick up and place nine dowels into nine corresponding holes (Fig. 7-5). The timed trial can also include removal of pegs from holes.

The 10-hole peg test requires patients to transfer 10 pegs from one row of holes to another. The variable measured is the time required to complete the task (Wade, 1989, 1992).

Box and Block Test

This test requires patients to transfer 2.5-cm^2 cubes from a full box into an empty box. In performing this activity patients must move their arms across a 15 × 2 cm barrier that is

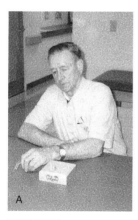 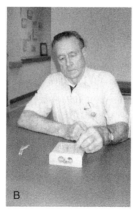

FIGURE 7-5. Patient performs the nine-hole peg test.

placed between the two boxes. The amount of time required to transfer all the cubes is recorded (Desrosiers et al., 1994; Mathiowetz, Volland, Kashman, & Weber, 1985). The box and block test has been used to study motor loss in patients with multiple sclerosis (Wade, 1992).

Jebsen Hand Function Test

The Jebsen test consists of seven timed test items:

- Writing a 24-letter sentence
- Turning over five 3 × 5 inch cards
- Placing six small common objects (eg, paper clips, pennies) into an empty coffee can
- Using a teaspoon to pick up five kidney beans and place in an empty can
- Stacking four wooden checkers
- Moving large light objects (eg, large empty cans) to an area on the table
- Moving large heavy objects (eg, 1-lb cans) to an area on the table

All tests are performed one after the other, and each test is timed for comparison against normative data (Jebsen et al., 1969).

Tests of Higher Functional Coordination

Therapists may also assess patients' ability to perform higher skilled motor activities while maintaining balance. Examples of functional activities that examiners may observe patients performing include:

- Reaching into a cabinet for a cup
- Walking (specifically their gait pattern)
- Marching to cadence
- Walking on heels or toes
- Walking clockwise and counterclockwise
- Walking on uneven ground
- Dressing in sitting and standing
- Buttoning or zippering in sitting and standing
- Feeding activities

In observing these activities, examiners record the patient's success rate and document any noticeable deviations, including the rate of movement and any limitations in ranges of movement. In Figure 7-6, the patient is successful in performing the task with his noninvolved extremity; however, his muscle imbalance prevents him from performing the task with his involved extremity. In this case, documentation should state that coordination could not be tested due to limited extremity ROM and strength, which should have been previously assessed.

Case Study

Mr. Black's disability was assessed previously, and the potential impairments of weakness, balance dysfunction, somatosensory loss, incoordination, or some combination thereof were identified. The assessment of functional mobility revealed

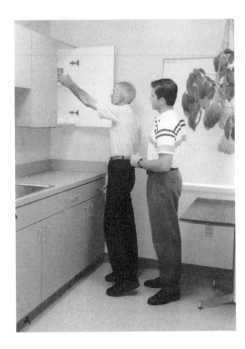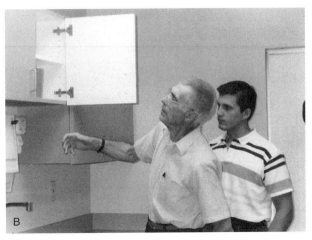

FIGURE 7-6. (*A*) Patient successfully reaches for a cup in a cabinet with his noninvolved arm. (*B*) The same patient reaches unsuccessfully with his involved arm due to muscle imbalance.

that bed mobility, sitting, sit-to-stand, standing, ambulation with a walker, and nonreciprocal stair climbing were all independent. Ataxia was noted in the left lower extremity with ambulation and stair climbing, especially when performed with one hand support and with a reciprocal pattern for stair climbing. Weakness in the trunk could be ruled out because Mr. Black displayed stable sitting and standing with and without dynamic movement. Balance may also be intact as evidenced by the ability to sit and stand statically and dynamically. However, these tasks should also be tested with the eyes closed. Reciprocal stair climbing would be an indicator of adequate strength in the lower extremities. However, the patient displays increased ataxia with this movement.

Assessing the Impairment

Assess lower extremity strength with manual muscle testing. Muscle grades less than fair (3/5) could contribute to disability. To assess balance, have the patient close the eyes while you perform the Romberg test (see Chap. 8). If the Romberg test is positive, assess the dorsal column/medial lemniscus system and spinocerebellum tracts to assess proprioception and kinesthesia. A positive test for the loss of proprioception in the lower extremities indicates that the loss of somatosensation may be causing the ataxia seen in the patient's gait and stair climbing. If strength, sensation, and balance are intact, assess coordination.

Test coordination of the lower extremities in sitting first, then progress to standing. Have the patient perform alternating dorsiflexion and plantar flexion, and observe for symmetry of movement. Observe the unilateral performance of the heel-toe movement pattern as the patient does it slowly and then as fast as possible. Compare the movement pattern bilaterally. Ask Mr. Black to trace letters or numbers on the floor. Observe his posture during this activity and movement of the entire lower extremity. Are movements exaggerated?

Have Mr. Black repeat these same tasks in standing position. Next, have him walk between the parallel bars, either on his heels or toes, in a pattern. You may accomplish this by having him step on "footprints" placed on the floor or through a floor ladder. Difficulty with any of these tasks indicates a problem with timing, the sequencing of muscle activity, and accuracy of movement.

Because Mr. Black reported difficulty buttoning his shirt, zippering his pants, cutting his food, and reaching for objects, assess his upper extremity function using the Rivermead Motor Assessment. Difficulty performing these tasks with adequate strength and ROM indicates a problem with coordination.

Results of Assessment of Impairments

Strength, ROM, sensation, and balance were intact. In the Romberg test (eyes closed) the patient displayed increased postural sway but no loss of balance. The patient did display ataxic movement with the left extremities in all tests of coordination, especially when moving the extremities through a large range. Coordination was improved when moving at a slower speed and through smaller ROMs, such as dorsiflexion and plantar flexion in sitting. However, asymme-

try of movement was noted when the right and left leg moved through this motion simultaneously and at an increasing rate.

TREATMENT OF INCOORDINATION

This section describes the treatment activities that may be used clinically to treat incoordination. Based on the assessment of disabilities, therapists should incorporate treatment that is task oriented and focuses on the impairments contributing to the disabilities. For example, if sensory loss is a factor in the lack of coordination, sensory cues should be added to the functional tasks practiced. Specific exercises to treat incoordination are also presented in this section.

Functional Activities

To improve the coordinated movements of functional tasks, it is imperative that the patient repeat those tasks. The key to improving coordination is to vary the distance and speed of the movement to enable successful completion of the task and gradually retrain muscle activity.

For example, the task of picking up a cup from a table should be performed slowly and within a shortened range to enable the patient to perform the movement successfully. Cups should be large enough for patients to grasp, and the targets on which cups should be replaced should also be within shortened ranges. To improve the performance and coordination of functional tasks, have patients place cups on the table at distances that are farther and farther away from them. Target placements should include having patients bring the cups to their mouths to simulate taking a drink. The rate of movement patterns should be increased, with the therapist cuing patients verbally to move faster.

Sensory Cues

Functional activities limited by incoordination can be enhanced with practice of the tasks and the use of added sensory cues. The most powerful sensory cue that can improve coordination is visual feedback. Provide visual feedback early in treatment sessions to facilitate the successful performance of tasks. Gradually withdraw visual feedback to enable normal sensory processing to be used in the performance of tasks. Cuing patients to watch what they are doing may enhance accuracy, but it will not eliminate ataxic or tremulous movements.

To address ataxic movements, add weights to the extremities to increase peripheral sensory feedback. There is no evidence to support the efficacy of this technique, but anecdotal reports from patients and therapists support its use (Lucy & Hayes, 1985). For reaching activities that involve an upper extremity, apply weights to the patient's wrists. To decrease lower extremity ataxia, attach weights to the patient's ankles (Fig. 7-7). If patients experience difficulty moving assistive devices due to ataxia, the device may be weighted as well. The more severe the ataxic movements, the greater the weight that should be added. The goal is to gradually decrease the amount of weight applied while maintaining improved quality of movement.

Muscle Weakness or Instability

When incoordination is combined with muscle weakness or proximal joint instability, instability must be addressed to enable improved quality of movement in functional tasks. Often, it may be the proximal joint instability that produces incoordination. Stability may be increased with the following techniques:

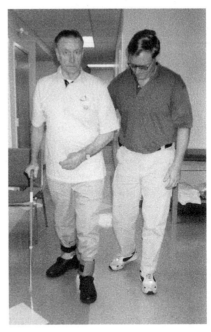

FIGURE 7-7. Patient walks with weights attached to his lower extremities.

- Isometric holding contractions of the extremities in mid or lengthened ranges
- Weight-bearing activities through proximal joints (eg, standing, kneeling, sitting on mats and weight-bearing through the involved upper extremities)
- Proprioceptive neuromuscular facilitation (PNF) with and without rhythmical stabilization (see Chap. 5)
- Tasks emphasizing movement and control of proximal components versus distal manipulation

Distal manipulation of objects (such as picking up a fork) may be preceded either by postural activation or external positioning of proximal joints to provide a stabilizing framework for the movement. This is an important point to consider when working with hemiplegic patients. It has been suggested that preparatory movements for posture may not be the result of a central motor program, but rather a hierarchically organized motor pattern that responds to proprioceptive and exteroceptive feedback (Diener, Bacher, Guschlbauer, Thomas, & Dichgans, 1993). In patients with hemiplegia, accomplishing stabilizing postural responses with varied proprioceptive feedback may be one way of activating muscles. Some researchers (Stuberg & Harbourne, 1994) have suggested that distal and proximal control can be addressed at the same time, even though the stability of proximal joints is needed for distal manipulation.

Walking is a good example of a functional activity where lack of proximal stability can result in impaired placement of the feet. A patient with hemiplegia may display some instability in the involved hip and a foreshortening of steps taken with the noninvolved limb. In this case, the patient consciously takes smaller steps out of fear that the involved lower extremity will be unable to support the body's weight. Patients with this problem can practice weight-bearing activities through the involved limbs to increase the stability of proximal joints to enable normal swing phase and placement of the opposing extremities. Patients who display weakness and incoordination in the lower extremities must increase strength and stability before coordination can be improved.

Patients with multiple sclerosis may have a variety of impairments based on where the demyelination occurs within the CNS. It is common for these patients to have generalized fatigue, which can restrict their daily functional mobility. Patients with multiple sclerosis who display weakness and incoordination in both lower extremities can perform strengthening activities to increase stability and perform coordination activities to improve placement. These patients often follow a treatment program that includes performing standing therapeutic exercises in parallel bars (Fig. 7-8).

As patients actively move one extremity through certain ranges, they must bear weight through the opposite extremity. Targets may be used for the moving limb to ensure full active ROM and accuracy in foot placement. The patient performs a series of active hip flexion exercises, followed by abduction, then extension exercises for each leg. This encourages weight-shifting onto the supporting limb, a functional component of gait. Performing this task in standing emphasizes the stability needed in the lower extremities. It also challenges the patient to maintain the posture against gravity.

Reaching for objects placed in cabinets is another way to increase weight-shifting and weight-bearing to improve proximal stability (see Fig. 7-6). This activity has the added benefit of requiring patients to coordinate their movements when reaching for objects placed in cabinets. Successful completion of these tasks often demands that the patient rely on sensory cues such as looking at targets or adding weights to the upper extremities.

Other activities that can be used to increase coordination during gait include braiding activities, side-stepping, walking within square tiles on the floor, walking on foot patterns placed on the floor, walking through a floor ladder, or walking over canes placed on the floor (Fig. 7-9). These activities address both balance and coordination.

Patients who need assistance with balance, or who have severe ataxic movements, can be assisted by therapists' placing their hands on each greater trochanter and compressing (Fig. 7-10). This is an anecdotal treatment technique that may increase proximal stability to enable better balance and decrease ataxic movements. The neurophysiologic theory of movement on which this is based is the reflex model, and the therapeutic technique is joint compression. Manual contact by the therapist in this area also allows patients to use their arms or trunk for

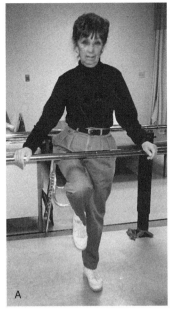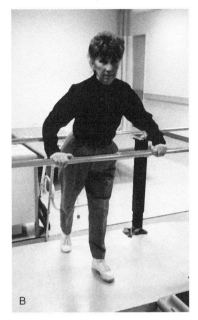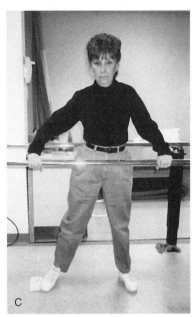

FIGURE 7-8. Patient performs standing therapeutic exercises between parallel bars: (*A*) repeated hip flexion; (*B*) hip extension; (*C*) abduction to a marker placed on the floor.

normal equilibrium reactions that may occur with walking.

Coordination Exercise

Frenkel's exercises were designed to enable voluntary relearning of movement through repetition and retraining of functional patterns. Frenkel's exercises are performed while patients are supine, sitting, or standing. Patients should perform each activity slowly using visual input to help control movements. The exercises, as described by Caliet, cited in Licht (1965), are:

- In supine, have the patient perform the following movements:

1. Flexion and extension of each leg at the knee and hip joints; abduction and adduction with knees flexed; later, abduction and adduction with knees extended
2. Flexion and extension of one knee at a time, with heel raised from the bed
3. Knee flexed and heel placed on some definite part of the opposite limb; for example, on the patella, or the middle of the leg, with the ankle and toe, then changing positions
4. Knee flexed, heel placed on the knee of the opposite leg, heel of flexed leg gliding down the tibia to the ankle joint and back to the knee
5. Flexion and extension of both legs, together with knees and ankles held close together

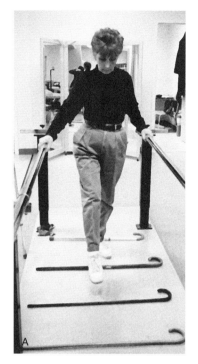 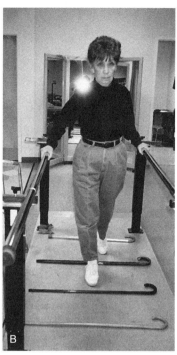

FIGURE 7-9.   (*A,B*) Patient engages in gait training by walking over canes while holding onto parallel bars. Progression of this should be to one hand support, then no hand support.

6. Flexion of one lower extremity during extension of the other (reciprocal movement; Fig. 7-11)
7. Flexion or extension of one leg during adduction and abduction of the other

- When performing these movements becomes easy, patients should perform them with their eyes closed.
- In sitting:

8. Try to place the heel of the foot into the therapist's hand (Fig. 7-12). The therapist changes the position of his or her hand after each attempt.
9. Maintain sitting unsupported for several minutes.
10. Raise each knee alternately and place each foot firmly on the ground on a traced footprint. This task may be performed in sitting or standing position.
11. Rise from a chair and then sit again holding knees together.
12. Place feet forward and backward on a straight line, then repeat on a zig-zagged line. This task may be performed sitting or standing.

- During walking:

13. Walk between two parallel lines.
14. Walk on foot tracings placed on the floor.

Chapter 5 provides additional exercises that may be performed to address muscle weakness displayed by patients with incoordination. Use of the PNF diagonals produces smooth reciprocal movement patterns that may aid in relearn-

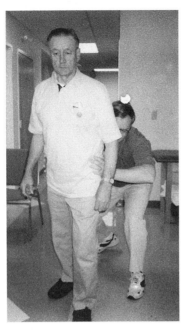

FIGURE 7-10. Manual approximation of the hips by physical therapist.

- Practice writing.
- Don and doff shirt and slacks.
- Brush teeth, comb hair.
- Pick up small objects from table (eg, coins, paper clips).
- Repeatedly step up and down steps of varying heights.

Case Study

••

Mr. Black's impairment and disability have been assessed. Treatment of his disability is now discussed.

••

Treatment of Mr. Black

••

Treatment should focus on practicing tasks that are difficult for the patient to perform. Initially, modifications should be made in activities to decrease the range and speed of movement. Sensory cues (especially visual feedback) can be used ini-

ing sequential movements. Techniques of rhythmic stabilization and slow reversal hold can address dysmetria through learned control of proximal joints. However, the reader is reminded that the goal in rehabilitation is efficient and safe functional mobility, and this can only be achieved with practice of the tasks that present disabilities. Incorporation of exercise can be advantageous to the improved quality of movement when combined with task-oriented treatment.

Functional activities for testing coordination may be used as treatments to improve the patient's ability to complete quality movements. Practicing the following tasks while modifying the speed and range of movement can enhance the patient's coordinated performance of tasks.

Tasks to practice as treatment include:

- Draw numbers or alphabet on paper.

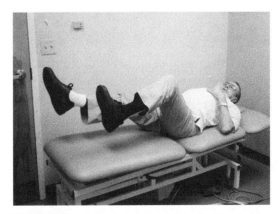

FIGURE 7-11. Patient performs Frenkel's exercise, practicing flexion of one leg and simultaneous extension of the other leg.

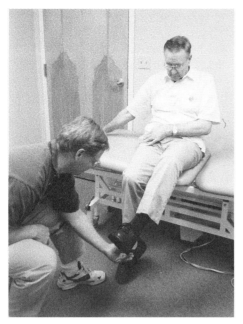

FIGURE 7-12. During Frenkel's exercise, the patient tries to place his heel in the therapist's hand.

tially to increase the accuracy of the movement. Weights can be added to the extremities to provide added sensory feedback to improve motor performance. As soon as possible, added sensory feedback should be eliminated from the task.

Examples of activities that may be appropriate for Mr. Black are buttoning a shirt, zippering jackets, putting on and zippering pants, cutting food with a knife and fork, moving the lower extremities in specific patterns in sitting with a progression to standing as soon as possible. Lower extremity movements may include stepping back and forth over a cane on the floor, stepping on and off a footprint on the floor, walking on footprints placed on the floor, and walking around an obstacle course that requires stepping over as well as around obstacles. All these activities can

initially be modified by adding light weights to the wrists and ankles and emphasizing visual feedback.

During the standing and gait activities, reduce the support provided through the upper extremities by the assistive device. Coordination problems are often accompanied by balance dysfunction (cerebellar involvement), so reducing upper extremity support challenges balance as well. Referrals to an occupational therapist and driver rehabilitation program may be indicated to assist in minimizing or eliminating the difficulty experienced with the activities of daily living, as well as to evaluate Mr. Black's potential eligibility for a driver retraining program.

SUMMARY

- Coordinated movement requires the integration of information from the sensory cortex, motor cortex, cerebellum, and basal ganglia.
- Lack of coordination can occur with weakness, sensory loss, or when the sequence and firing of muscles, and the on and off times of muscle contractions have been interrupted.
- Functional mobility may be impaired with incoordination especially when combined with a balance dysfunction.
- Clinical tests are performed to indicate the presence of a coordination deficit. Standardized tests assist in quantifying the functional limitations evident with the incoordination.
- Treatment of incoordination, like other impairments discussed in this text, should focus on the practice of the functional tasks limited by the impairment.

- Shortened ROM, slower speed of movement, and added sensory cues, visual cues, or both can be incorporated into tasks of functional mobility to improve the quality of the patient's movement.

●●●●●●●●●●●●●●●●●●●●●●●●●●●●●●●●●

REFERENCES

Behbehani, K, Kondraske, GV, Tintner, R, Tindall, RAS, & Imrhan, SN. (1990). Evaluation of quantitative measures of upper extremity speed and coordination in healthy persons and in three patient populations. *Archives of Physical Medicine and Rehabilitation, 71,* 106–111.

Cohen, H. (Ed.). (1993). *Neuroscience for rehabilitation.* Philadelphia: Lippincott.

Desrosiers, J, Bravo, G, Hebert, R, Dutil, E, & Mercier, L. (1994). Validation of the box and block test as a measure of dexterity of elderly people: Reliability, validity, and norm studies. *Archives of Physical Medicine and Rehabilitation, 75,* 751–755.

Diener, HC, Bacher, M, Guschlbauer, B, Thomas, C, & Dichgans, J. (1993). The coordination of posture and voluntary movement in patients with hemiparesis. *Journal of Neurology, 240,* 161–167.

Greenberg, DA, Aminoff, MJ, & Simon, RP. (1993). *Clinical neurology.* East Norwalk, CT: Appleton & Lange.

Jebsen, RH, Taylor, N, Trieschmann, RB, Trotter, MJ, & Howard, LA. (1969). An objective and standardized test of hand function. *Archives of Physical Medicine and Rehabilitation, 50,* 311–319.

Kandel, ER, Schwartz, JH, & Jessel, T. (Eds.) (1991). *Principles of neural science* (3rd ed.). New York: Elsevier.

Licht, S. (1965). *Therapeutic exercise.* New Haven, CT: Elizabeth Licht Publisher.

Lucy, SC, & Hayes, KC. (1985). Postural sway profiles: Normal subjects and subjects with cerebellar ataxia. *Physiotherapy Canada, 37*(3), 140–148.

Mathiowetz, V, Volland, G, Kashman, N, & Weber, K. (1985). Adult norms for the box and blocks test of manual dexterity. *American Journal of Occupational Therapy, 39,* 386–391.

Mayo, NE, Sullivan, J, & Swaine, B. (1991). Observer variation in assessing neurophysical signs among patients with head injuries. *Archives of Physical Medicine and Rehabilitation, 70*(3), 118–123.

Olgiati, R, Burgunder, JM, & Mumenthaler, M. (1988). Increased energy cost of walking in multiple sclerosis: Effect of spasticity, ataxia, and weakness, *Archives of Physical Medicine and Rehabilitation, 69,* 846–849.

O'Neil, MB, Woodward, M, Sosa, V, Hunter, L, Mulrow, C, Gerety, MB, & Tuley, M. (1992). Physical therapy assessment and treatment protocol for nursing home residents. *Physical Therapy, 72*(8), 596–604.

Rothstein, JM, Roy, SH, & Wolf, SL. (1990). *The rehabilitation specialist's handbook.* Philadelphia: Davis.

Smith, SS, & Kondraske, GV. (1987). Computerized system for quantitative measurement of sensorimotor aspects of human performance. *Physical Therapy, 67*(12), 1860–1866.

Stuberg, W, & Harbourne, R. (1994). Theoretical practice in pediatric physical therapy: Past, present, and future considerations. *Pediatric Physical Therapy, 6*(3), 119–125.

Sullivan, KJ, Winstein, CJ, & Pohl, PS. (1993). Effects of movement direction in aiming movements in healthy subjects and individuals post-stroke. *Neurology Report, 17*(4), 25.

Sunderland, A, Tinson, DJ, Bradley, EL, Fletcher, D, Langton Hewer, R, & Wade, DT. (1992), Enhanced physical therapy improves recovery of arm function after stroke. A randomized controlled trial. *Journal of Neurology, Neurosurgery and Psychiatry, 55,* 530–535.

Swaine, BR, & Sullivan, J. (1992). Relation between clinical and instrumented measures of motor coordination in traumatically brain injured persons. *Archives of Physical Medicine and Rehabilitation, 73,* 55–59.

Swaine, BR, & Sullivan, SJ. (1993). Reliability of the scores for the finger-to-nose test in adults with traumatic brain injury. *Physical Therapy, 73*(2), 71–78.

Wade, DT. (1989). Measuring arm impairment and disability after stroke. *International Disability Studies, 11*(2), 89–92.

Wade, DT. (1992). *Measurement in neurological rehabilitation.* New York: Oxford Medical Publications.

Williamson, GL, & Leiper, CI. (1993). Assessment of speed and accuracy of movement in older adults using Fitts' Tapping Test. *Neurology Report, 17*(4), 25.

Wilson, B, Pollock, N, Kaplin, BJ, Law, M, & Faris, P. (1992). Reliability and construct validity of the clinical observations of motor and postural skills. *American Journal of Occupational Therapy, 46*(9), 775–783.

●●●●●●●●●●●●●●●●●●●●●●●●●●●●●●●●●●●●●●

SUGGESTED READINGS

Blattner, KA. (1988). Friedrich's ataxia: A suggested physical therapy regimen. *Clinical Management in Physical Therapy, 8*(4), 14–15, 30.

This article describes activities and exercise to address the ataxia present in Friedrich's ataxia. In addition to treatment for incoordination, exercises aimed at improving strength, endurance, and ROM and gait training are described.

Cohen, H. (Ed.). (1993). *Neuroscience for rehabilitation.* Philadelphia: Lippincott.

This comprehensive text describes neuroanatomy and neurophysiology. Readers who desire additional information on the anatomy overview presented in this chapter should review this text.

Cruz, VW. (1986). Evaluation of coordination: A clinical model. *Clinical Management in Physical Therapy, 6*(3), 6–9, 10.

An evaluation of coordination is presented in this article. The author describes tests for low-, middle-, and high-level coordination.

Greenberg, DA, Aminoff, MJ, & Simon, RP. (1993) *Clinical neurology.* East Norwalk, CT: Appleton & Lange.

This is an easy-to-read text that describes the clinical signs and symptoms associated with disease or injury of the cerebellum, as well as the sensory and motor pathways.

Morgan, MH. (1975). Ataxia and weights. *Physiotherapy, 61*(11), 332–334.

The effect of weights applied to extremities to decrease ataxia is described in this article. Evidence of improved movement with the addition of weights is demonstrated through photographs of hand movements on infrared film.

Balance Dysfunction

LEARNING OBJECTIVES

After reading this chapter, you should be able to:

1. Identify the various impairments that can contribute to balance dysfunction.
2. Describe how functional movement may be altered when there is difficulty maintaining balance.
3. Explain the various assessment techniques used to determine the specific balance impairment.
4. Describe general tests of balance.
5. Develop treatment strategies appropriate to balance impairment(s).
6. Develop generalized treatment strategies to address balance dysfunction.

The ability to maintain one's center of gravity over a base of support is the most traditional way of conceptualizing balance. However, definitions of balance have broadened considerably in recent years, making it impractical to use the term (Shumway-Cook & Woollacott, 1995) without first specifying and defining the various components on which balance depends.

In this text **balance** is defined as the state of physical equilibrium (maintenance of one's center of gravity) achieved when vestibular, visual, and somatosensory information is integrated in the central nervous system (CNS) and fed through an intact musculoskeletal system.

Underlying constraints to the maintenance of balance include cognitive deficits, musculoskeletal limitations, loss of sensory acuity, sensory organization deficits, neuromuscular coordination deficits, fine motor control impairments, and inabilities to adapt motor responses (Whitney & Borello-France, 1993). **Predictive** or **feedforward deficits,** which are described as the inability to anticipate movement patterns needed for a task resulting in spontaneous or reactive movement versus planned movement, also contribute to **balance dysfunction.** (Predictive and feedforward deficits are frequently seen with damage to the cerebellum.)

Difficulty maintaining balance may result in apprehension about movement or fear of falling. When assessing balance, therapists must perform detailed assessments to determine specific causes of balance dysfunction. The location of the lesion that causes a particular balance dysfunction will determine which treatment program is implemented.

Patients with lesions of the motor cortex, corticospinal tracts, or alpha motor neurons may have weakness that can be treated with strengthening activities. Loss of sensation should be addressed with treatment to enhance existing sensory pathways or compensatory systems such as vision. Dizziness and loss of balance associated with lesions of the vestibular system can be treated with vestibular–ocular exercises and habituation exercises, depending on the specific pathology.

The interrelatedness of all of these systems contributes to the complexity of treating patients with balance dysfunctions. It is common for patients to experience symptoms from both the motor and sensory systems (such as in stroke) or from both the visual and vestibular systems (often seen in multiple sclerosis).

Patients with a variety of neurological diagnoses can have similar impairments and disabilities. For example, patients with stroke, Guillain Barré syndrome, and multiple sclerosis may have difficulty maintaining sitting and standing postures due to weakness. Peripheral lesions that involve the receptors in the inner ear (semicircular canals, utricle, and saccule), the vestibular nerve, or both may produce symptoms of vertigo and nystagmus, which may produce balance dysfunction. The central components of the vestibular system, which encompass the vestibular nuclei in the brain stem and the multitude of connections with the cerebellum, ocular nerves, subcortical nuclei (eg, the reticular formation), can produce similar symptoms to peripheral lesions (Cooke, 1996).

This chapter will guide the entry-level student through an understanding of various impairments that can contribute to balance dysfunction; how functional movement may be altered when there is difficulty maintaining balance; assessment techniques to determine the balance impairment; general tests of balance; and treatment strategies.

IMPAIRMENT: BALANCE DYSFUNCTION

Maintaining balance is a complex interaction of the neuromuscular and musculoskeletal systems. It is important to determine which component of balance is the cause of the dysfunction. Identifying the cause of balance dysfunction guides the therapist in the development of treatment.

For example, a positive Romberg test with the eyes closed suggests a somatosensory problem. A positive Hallpike maneuver suggests a vestibular abnormality. As readers will learn in this chapter, treatment for a somatosensory deficit is different from treatment implemented for balance dysfunction resulting from a vestibular lesion.

To determine the origins of balance dysfunction, first start with a patient history. Determine when problems with balance started. Are problems associated with head movement? Are there limitations in functional mobility? Is vertigo or nausea experienced with movement? Has the patient fallen? If the answer to the last question is yes, what was the patient doing that caused loss of balance?

After the history has been completed, an assessment of functional mobility should be performed, followed by testing of the musculoskeletal and somatosensory systems. This chapter describes the assessment of these two systems to determine the origin of balance dysfunction. If the musculoskeletal system is intact, then range of motion (ROM) and strength are adequate to maintain stable postures. The sensory systems to be assessed include the vestibular, the visual, and the somatosensory. Patients with somatosensory deficits may have learned how to use their vision to compensate for some of their problems. Patients with vestibular dysfunction will require training in specific exercises to enable the CNS to compensate for the loss of function.

An overview of the motor response and integration of sensory information required to maintain balance is presented next. Despite the inherent risk of oversimplification in an overview, our intent is to demonstrate the interrelatedness of the sensory input from the visual, vestibular, and peripheral systems, and how sensory input works with the musculoskeletal system to maintain the body's center of gravity over the base of support.

Motor Response to Balance Perturbation

There is clearly a motor component to maintaining balance or equilibrium. Movement strategies to maintain balance require functional ROM and adequate strength (Horak, 1987). The movement strategies used to maintain body mass in equilibrium include:

- Ankle movement with hip and knee maintained in extension (a distal movement with proximal activity only when the distal movement is not sufficient to maintain balance)
- Hip strategy (proximal movement progressing to distal movement if the knee and ankle are required to move)
- Stepping strategy, realigning the base of support with a stepping movement
- Suspensory strategy, lowering the center of gravity toward the base of support (ie, flexion of the hip, knee, and ankle) (Montgomery & Connolly, 1991)

The ankle strategy is used when a small perturbation (a disturbance in balance), or weight shift, is experienced with the feet on a firm surface (Fig. 8-1) (Montgomery & Connolly, 1991). To experience this, try standing and allowing your weight to shift posteriorly. Immediately you will feel contraction of your anterior tibialis muscles and movement in your ankles.

The hip strategy is seen when a greater force challenges balance (perturbations), or when the support surface for the feet is small (Horak, 1987; Montgomery & Connolly, 1991; Woollacott & Shumway-Cook, 1990). To experience this, try standing on a balance beam in a heel-to-toe stance, or in a heel-to-toe stance on a piece of dense foam. When your balance is chal-

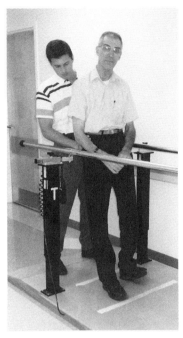

FIGURE 8-1.   Patient demonstrates the ankle strategy, as his weight shifts posteriorly onto the left foot.

strategy. If these players stood up straight, their opponents would easily knock them off their base of support. Maintaining the suspensory strategy, in this case in a low crouch, enables football players to maintain their stability even when 300-pound opponents try to push them off balance.

Sensory System

The sensory component of balance uses vestibular, visual, and somatosensation (Woollacott & Shumway-Cook, 1990). The vestibular system makes the final decision if there is differing information from the other two systems (Newton, 1989).

Vestibular information from the semicircular canals travels to vestibular nuclei in the brain

lenged in this position, your hips will move as a means to attempt to maintain balance.

If the perturbation applied is such that the center of body mass is displaced, then a step, or a series of steps or hops, will occur to realign the base of support and maintain equilibrium (Shumway-Cook & Horak, 1990). This stepping strategy is also seen with unexpected perturbations in quiet standing (Fig. 8-2). The response is either a step across your body to maintain balance, or a step forward or backward depending on the direction of the perturbation.

The suspensory strategy is used during standing or in ambulation to lower the body's center of gravity closer to the base of support, which provides more stability. Individuals lower their centers of gravity by bending their knees (Fig. 8-3). The offensive or defensive linemen of a football team habitually use the suspensory

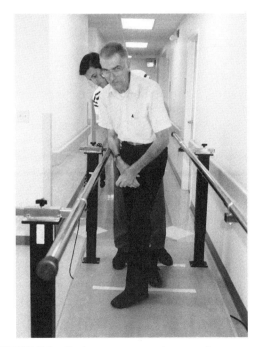

FIGURE 8-2.   Patient resorts to the stepping strategy to realign his base of support and thus maintain equilibrium.

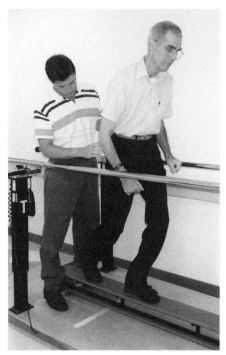

FIGURE 8-3. In the suspensory strategy, the patient bends his knees to lower his center of gravity and thereby increase the stability of his stance.

stem, which can immediately send impulses down the spinal cord via vestibulospinal tracts. Visual input goes both to vestibular nuclei (vestibulo–ocular reflex) and to the cortex. Vision is used most often when impairment of one of the other systems occurs (Stones & Kozma, 1987). Somatosensation represents incoming information from the receptors in the joints and muscles. This information travels to the sensory cortex and cerebellum.

Balance requires integration of sensory information with coordination of many muscles, especially those of the motor strategies involving the hips, knees, and ankles, to maintain the body's center of gravity over its base of support. In quiet standing, proprioception plays the primary role in maintaining this posture. The visual and vestibular systems exercise important but secondary control. Quiet standing is accomplished by a sequence of stereotyped patterns that are mediated from the brain stem and cerebellum, often referred to as "pattern generators" (Umphred, 1990).

Standing on uneven terrain, however, activates visual and vestibular systems to help with movements to maintain balance. Proprioceptive input is reduced or altered when standing in a position of reduced stability, such as in tandem, on a movable surface, or on uneven terrain. The integration of sensory information (proprioceptive input processed in the parietal lobe) alone is unable to distinguish between body motions experienced on a stable support and body motions experienced on an unstable support, such as standing in a boat (Umphred, 1990). The adapation of balance response in this environment is slow and involves the integration of input from all three systems. Walking on ice, through a snow bank, or in a forest are all examples of instances in which the integrated processing of information is accomplished to maintain balance.

ANATOMY OVERVIEW

Major anatomic components for maintaining balance and equilibrium consist of three sensory systems: vestibular, visual, and proprioception. Time to process information from major anatomic components is important when motor responses are needed to maintain balance. Information from proprioceptive systems is processed the fastest (Winstein & Mitz, 1993), followed by visual and vestibular information. Consider the functional consequences that may occur with lesions to these anatomic components (ie, abilities to maintain balance may be compromised) (Winstein & Mitz, 1993).

Proprioceptive input traveling in the dorsal column–medial lemniscus pathway carries touch, vibration, joint position, and joint movement information to the thalamus, where thalamocortical fibers send this information to the sensory cortex. Information processed by touch provides cues on the external environment in which we move (eg, firmness of a surface, uneven terrain).

Proprioceptive information traveling in spinocerebellar tracts carries information from Golgi tendon organs, muscle spindles, and joint and cutaneous receptors to the cerebellum. Sensory information traveling in these tracts is used to develop or modify movement patterns for maintenance of balance, or to enhance movement accuracy and efficiency. Information processed in the cerebellum does not contribute to conscious perception of movement or the awareness of one's own body in space, but rather projects this information to the motor cortex (Kandell, Schwartz, & Jessel, 1991).

The vestibular nuclei integrate information transmitted from the semicircular canals, utricles, and saccules. Sensory information from these receptors travels to the vestibular nuclei via the vestibular division of cranial nerve VIII. Motor responses to this sensory information descend in the spinal cord via the lateral and medial vestibulospinal tracts. Fibers in lateral vestibulospinal tracts descend ipsilaterally through the full length of the cord and directly synapse onto lower motoneurons of extensor muscles controlling the neck, trunk, and knees. Those fibers that travel in medial vestibulospinal tracts descend bilaterally to the cervical and upper thoracic levels.

The synapse of the medial vestibulospinal tract onto lower motor neurons in the cervical and upper thoracic regions is through direct or indirect synapses. An indirect synapse occurs when the tract synapses on an interneuron, which then synapses on the lower motor neuron. The direct synapse does not use an interneuron for communication of information. Lateral and medial vestibulospinal tracts form the

anatomic basis for vestibular influences on balance (Fox & Cohen, 1993).

Visual influences on balance are mediated through visual input to vestibular nuclei. Neurons concerned with eye movements ascend in the medial longitudinal fasciculus (MLF) to the motor nuclei of cranial nerves III, IV, and VI (oculomotor, trochlear and abducens). These projections result in parallel eye movement; that is, the eyes move in the same direction at the same time (Fox & Cohen, 1993). The same fibers that ascend in the MLF also descend to cervical spinal cord levels. These signals are thought to help control neck reflexes such as the vestibulocollic reflex (Fox & Cohen, 1993).

Motor responses to challenges in balance are to bring the center of gravity back over the base of support to regain balance. This was thought (Winstein & Mitz, 1993) to occur via a collection of local stretch reflexes controlling various lower extremity joints. However, it is now well-established (Winstein & Mitz, 1993) that these motor responses are produced by central motor programs that are triggered by proprioceptive, visual, and vestibular stimuli. The exact location of these motor programs in the CNS is unknown. These programs result from activity in such anatomic structures as the cerebellum, basal ganglia, and supplementary motor area in the cerebrum (Winstein & Mitz, 1993).

ASSESSING THE DISABILITY

The first three steps in neurological assessment procedures described in Chapter 3 are observation and assessment for disabilities and impairments. Initial observations enable examiners to gather general information regarding the patient's state of awareness and preliminary observations of the movement dysfunction.

Assessment of the disability allows examiners to determine which functional activities are difficult for patients to perform, or those that patients are unable to perform because of underlying impairments. Disabilities associated with balance dysfunctions may consist of diminished movements. These include daily functional movements such as rolling in bed, moving from a supine position to sitting, rising to standing, ambulation, and climbing stairs. With balance dysfunctions, patients may have the physical ability to perform these activities but lack stability or movement strategies to maintain these new positions. In cases of lesions within the vestibular system, changes in position may cause **vertigo** (a sense of rotation or movement of oneself or of the surroundings) or **nystagmus** (involuntary rapid movement of the eyeball).

A history of falls or disequilibrium indicates the presence of conditions that limit movements that challenge the patient's sense of balance. Walking may be limited to short distances around the house and may include the use of assistive devices for additional support in balance. A decrease in activity may result in other problems (eg, muscle weakness, joint limitation, and depression). Ataxia may be evident during functional mobility because coordinated movements also rely on adequate ROM, strength, somatosensory feedback, and cerebellar integration.

Functional mobility, described in Chapter 3, is again discussed here to illustrate how balance dysfunctions may limit or interfere with movement abilities. Alternative movement strategies refer to movements outside the range of the normative movements described in Chapter 3.

Rolling

The position of supine is a stable posture for most patients with balance dysfunctions because they are fully supported by the surface of the bed or mat, which diminishes the need for a functioning somatosensory, visual, or vestibular system and adequate muscle strength. However, during rolling, patients may display diminished movement for one of two reasons: They may be apprehensive about movement in general or about rolling off the edge of the bed in particular, and they also may be experiencing symptoms of vertigo or nausea with head turning (associated with a vestibular lesion).

Supine-to-Sitting Maneuver

When moving from a position of supine to sitting at the edge of the bed, patients may attempt to use preexisting strategies to accomplish this task. Movement patterns may be slow as they attempt to maintain stable postures during dynamic phases of this movement. On sitting, patients may complain of vertigo or nausea. They may also have nystagmus. These symptoms may imply a lesion in the vestibular system, which is activated with changes in head position.

Stable Sitting Posture

Assessment of a stable sitting posture should include the ability to sit unsupported with a symmetrical posture and to maintain that position. Asymmetrical posture may be seen in patients with weakness or if sensory awareness of the body is distorted. The inability to sit without one or two hand supports may indicate vestibular dysfunction, especially if nystagmus is present with head or eye movement.

Sit-to-Stand Maneuver

Because rising from sitting to standing integrates all aspects of balance, this movement must be closely analyzed to determine which specific impairments lead to dysfunction. The four phases that characterize moving from a sitting posture to standing include the flexion momentum stage, early lift, extension phase, and the stabilizing phase.

The flexion momentum stage activates vestibular receptors and begins to shift the center of gravity forward over the feet. The early lift phase moves patients from stable postures of sitting with wide bases of support to bipedal postures. This requires adequate muscle strength and activation of all components of balance (ie, somatosensory, vestibular, and visual). The extension phase is a continuation of early lift components, with the addition of a higher center of gravity. During early lift, patients may rely on suspensory strategies to assist in maintaining posture. The extension phase moves patients toward upright postures and eliminates suspensory strategies. The stabilizing phase requires the integration of all sensory information and adequate strength to maintain upright static postures.

As with supine-to-sit maneuvers, vestibular symptoms may be present in this task as well. Alternative movement strategies to rise to standing may include slow, deliberate movement; excessive use of the upper extremities for support or push-off; and a wide base of support in standing.

Stable Standing Posture

The assessment of stable standing postures is similar to the assessment of stable sitting postures. When standing unsupported, a patient's body symmetry as well as the ability to maintain position should be evaluated. Asymmetrical posture may be seen in patients with weakness or in those whose sensory awareness of the body is distorted. The inability to stand without one- or two-hand support may indicate weakness in the legs. Head movements in a standing posture may elicit nystagmus, vertigo, or nausea, which would suggest a vestibular problem. Alternative

movement strategies in standing may include wide bases of support, the presence of body sway, flexed postures to lower centers of gravity (suspensory strategy), or all three.

Transfers

The pivot transfer includes moving from a sitting posture to standing (which patients accomplish with the same degree of difficulty as performing sit-to-stand tasks), followed by pivoting and sitting in chairs placed in close proximity to chairs in which the patient had been sitting. An alternative movement strategy may be the use of a lateral transfer versus rising to standing and pivoting. In performing a lateral transfer, hand support can be maintained throughout the transfer for added stability; the flexed posture allows the center of gravity of the body to be closer to the ground; and full upright bipedal stance can be avoided.

Ambulation

Ambulation has been described by some as controlled falling (Whitney & Borello-France, 1993). Initiation of gait from static postures requires weight-shifting that changes the center of gravity and produces alternating unilateral support on the extremities.

Alternative movement strategies in ambulation may include combinations of movements based on the patient's ability to achieve and maintain stabilizing postures. Observing the movement of rising to standing will provide some indication as to how patients will perform with ambulation. Patients may be unable to weight shift or advance a lower extremity due to instability on one-legged support. Shuffling gait patterns may be used to compensate for the inability of one-legged support or to increase somatosensory feedback from the lower extremity. Lack of arm swing and excessive arm abduction are also indicators of balance deficits.

Assessment of balance during ambulation must be performed in the least stabilizing posture that patients can tolerate. For example, if patients walk with a walker, assess them with a wide-base quad cane. If they use a cane, assess ambulation without an assistive device. Assessing ambulation with a stabilizing assistive device may mask problems that patients have with this skilled dynamic activity.

Climbing Stairs

This movement incorporates strategies used in ambulation and rising from sitting positions to standing. Ascending stairs requires weight-shifting and lifting of opposite limbs onto steps. The vestibular and visual systems are activated as patients ascend and descend stairs. Excessive hand support on handrails is a strategy used to compensate for instability during this maneuver. Descending steps is often more difficult than ascending stairs because of the added visual and perceptual input required to accomplish the task.

Assess patients with less hand support and observe their ability to shift the weight, lift or lower the advancing extremity, and bear weight through the opposite extremity. A wider base of support may be used to increase stability before advancing the extremity up or down the stair.

Case Study

Mrs. Jackson was admitted to the hospital 3 days ago complaining of numbness and tingling in both legs and balance problems during walking. Since her admission, she has also developed weakness in her lower extremities. This weakness does not limit her function. Diagnostic tests have not been conclusive for any specific disease process.

Mrs. Jackson states she experienced this once before, but her symptoms were not as severe. She is referred for physical therapy due to problems with ambulation. She is evaluated at bedside. Review of her chart does not reveal any significant past medical or surgical history. There is no evidence of previous problems, although the patient reports a similar incident with milder symptoms.

Assessing the Disability

First, assess bed mobility with this patient. Is she able to roll to both sides and move from supine to sitting on the side of the bed and back? Does she use her lower extremities to roll, either by flexing her hip forward, or by pushing off the bed with her foot? Using the lower extremities would be an indication of ROM and strength. Does rolling or movement from supine to sitting elicit complaints of nausea, vertigo, or nystagmus? These symptoms may indicate a vestibular abnormality.

Next, assess her sitting posture. Does she maintain static sitting unsupported and is her posture symmetrical? Does she appear to be aware of her body in space and maintain her trunk in midline? If static sitting unsupported is intact, then assess dynamic reaching in sitting. Is there loss of balance toward either side when reaching? Do these movements evoke vertigo or nausea?

If these activities elicit alternative movement strategies, note the movements and assess efficiency and safety in performing these activities. If she complains of vertigo or nausea with head position changes, the vestibular system will need to be assessed (described later in this chapter). If she is able to perform all these activities without difficulty, progress to standing activities.

Ask Mrs. Jackson to move from sitting on the bed to standing. Observe how she moves. Does she shift the weight forward over the knees? Is early lift accomplished symmetrically or toward one side? Are upper extremities used to assist in weight shift forward or early lift? Is symmetrical movement evident through extension phases and into standing? Are the upper extremities used during this process? Is full upright stance achieved or does she stay in a slightly flexed stance? Does she complain of vertigo or nausea with this movement? Is she able to stand unsupported and symmetrical or does she use her upper extremities to balance?

Presence of asymmetrical movements suggests unilateral weakness or possibly pain in a weight-bearing extremity. Upper extremity support with symmetrical movement from sitting to standing suggests bilateral weakness or problems with the sensory components of balance. Complaints of nausea or vertigo and presence of nystagmus suggest vestibular abnormalities. Support in standing suggests either balance deficits or weakness in lower extremities which itself may cause balance deficits.

Have Mrs. Jackson attempt dynamic movements if she is able to stand statically unsupported. She may attempt to shift her weight first before reaching with her upper extremities. Ask her to step forward and backward with each leg. Observe the weight shift, her ability to bear weight in a single-limb stance, and the advancement of the opposite leg forward and back.

If Mrs. Jackson demonstrates any difficulty with either of these maneuvers, then the problem could be a painful limb, balance deficit, or weakness. Rule out antalgia as the impairment before progressing with the assessment. Assess her ability to ambulate with the least assistive device possible. Observe the base of support, placement of extremities, step length, speed of movement, and ability to balance while advancing the assistive device. Is ataxia a problem?

Assess stair climbing and the patient's ability to shift weight from one leg to the other, to enable advancing one leg up the step. Perform single-limb stance and advance the opposite limb up a step. Difficulty shifting the weight or attaining single-limb support again could be a problem with antalgic limb, balance deficit, or weakness. Is vision used excessively when movement of the lower extremities occurs? Problems with static or dynamic stance, ambulation, stair climbing, or any combination thereof may indicate balance deficits or weakness. Somatosensory loss would be suspected with ataxic movements of the extremities, use of visual input (ie, looking at the feet during ambulation), or increased body sway with static stance (especially with the eyes closed). Vestibular or visual deficits would be suspected with accompanying nystagmus, vertigo, and nausea.

The assessment of functional mobility revealed the following:

- Bed mobility—independent with normal movement patterns.
- Supine-to-sitting—independent with no complaints of nausea or vertigo.
- Sitting posture—static sitting was symmetrical with no hand support for 60

seconds; dynamic sitting accomplished with reaching to both sides and across midline.

- Sitting-to-standing—slow and deliberate movements to assume weight-bearing on both lower extremities; needed two-hand support on a walker placed in front of her.
- Standing—able to stand statically with two-hand support on the walker for 60 seconds with a symmetrical posture; dynamic standing not assessed because patient was unable to statically stand without hand support.
- Ambulation—with the use of a walker for 50 feet, with contact guard of the therapist; gait pattern slow; used visual input to watch feet; did not pick each foot off the floor; slid each foot forward during ambulation.
- Stair climbing—difficult, requiring vision to watch placement of feet, and some assistance of the therapist in stabilizing patient during single-limb support.

ASSESSING THE IMPAIRMENT: BALANCE DYSFUNCTION

This section is divided into three parts: tests to determine the origin of the impairment (ie, weakness, vestibular, visual, or sensory dysfunction); general balance tests; and laboratory tests.

Assessment techniques that determine origins of impairments help to identify internal systems that may be contributing to balance dysfunctions. General balance testing describes a variety of tests used to quantify patient balance. Laboratory tests are similar to general balance tests but, for the most part, require expensive equipment, or are performed by physicians or specialists in otolaryngology. This part is called "laboratory" because most rehabilitative clinics do not have this equipment, unless they are centers for balance rehabilitation.

As with other chapters on impairments, testing in functional positions or activities is emphasized.

Before performing any tests to determine balance dysfunction, obtain a thorough history from the patient. The history should include the onset of difficulty with balance, dizziness, or vertigo, if symptoms are associated with head movement, and if limitations in functional mobility exist.

Patients often think of dizziness and vertigo as the same, so take time to assess what the patient is experiencing. *Vertigo* is the sensation of rotation or movement of oneself or of one's surroundings. *Dizziness* may be interpreted by the patient as vertigo or as the light-headedness often experienced before syncope (fainting). Indications of hearing loss, tinnitus, double or blurred vision, numbness, weakness, or clumsiness should also be obtained in the history (Borello-France, 1996).

Determining the Origin of the Impairment

When possible, the origins of balance dysfunctions should be identified. In many cases, lesion sites (visual, vestibular, or somatosensory pathways) can be accurately determined, which enables implementation of the optimal treatment approach. Unfortunately, patients who present with multisensory deficits (such as in multiple sclerosis) may not have a localized lesion. The patient with multiple sclerosis may have demyelination within the CNS that results in somatosensory loss, weakness, and visual deficits. All three factors can contribute to a balance dysfunction.

Motor Assessment

The first system to be assessed in determining the origins of balance dysfunctions should be the musculoskeletal system to rule out weakness or limited ROM as a factor in the balance dysfunction. The musculoskeletal assessment should include ROM (especially of the lower extremities), strength, and alignment of body segments. Neuromuscular factors such as spasticity or low tone, coordination, involuntary movements, and the presence of tremors, should also be considered (Montgomery & Connolly, 1991). The assessment of each of these areas is provided in greater detail in chapters 5 (strength) and 7 (coordination).

Sensory Assessment

Vestibular function, vision, and somatosensation are the key areas associated with maintenance of balance, or posture (Nashner, 1996). For this reason, sensory testing should include assessment of the vestibular system, vision, and dorsal column–medial lemniscus system.

Vestibular.   Integrity of the vestibular system can be assessed clinically with a variety of tests that examine the interaction between the patient's visual and vestibular systems (Borello-France, Whitney, & Herdman, 1994). These tests include smooth pursuits, saccadic eye movements, vestibular ocular reflex (VOR), head thrust, rapid head shaking, and the Hallpike maneuver (a positional test) (Denham, 1996). Vestibular abnormalities may also be indicated through changes in functional positions as is seen with the Hallpike maneuver. Patient complaints of vertigo, nausea, or the presence of nystagmus when moving from one position to the next may indicate vestibular dysfunction. Other tests that can be performed, such as caloric tests and rotational tests, are discussed in the section on laboratory tests.

Smooth pursuits are assessed by instructing the patient to track an object with the eyes while the head remains stationary. The examiner should observe for involuntary horizontal as well as vertical movements of the eyes. These involuntary movements are often seen at the end range of the eye movement. For example, after tracking an object to the left, added beats, or movements of the eyes are noted as the eyes are fixed at the object within the left peripheral field. The appearance of nystagmus or a change in the quality of eye movements suggests an abnormality (Borello-France et al., 1994; Denham, 1996).

Saccadic eye movements are assessed by instructing the patient to look back and forth between two objects placed in a horizontal or vertical range. The presence of nystagmus or frequent overcorrection of eye movements to focus on the targets may indicate an abnormality (Borello-France et al., 1994; Denham, 1996).

The **vestibular ocular reflex (VOR)** is assessed when the patient focuses on a stationary object while actively moving the head from side-to-side or up and down. The ability to remain focused on the target is assessed as well as the presence of corrective saccades, which may indicate a vestibular deficit (Borello-France et al., 1994).

Head thrusts are performed by the therapist with a gentle but quick passive movement of the head to neutral, or center position, from a starting position of 30° off center. Evidence of nystagmus is observed by the therapist immediately after the movement (Denham, 1996). *Head shaking* is performed actively by the patient and consists of quick movements of the head back and forth 10 times. The therapist should observe the patient's eyes immediately after movement to determine the ability to fixate the eyes without hypoactive movements or the presence of nystagmus (Denham, 1996; Sharpe, 1994).

The *Hallpike maneuver* is a paroxysmal positional nystagmus test. To perform this test, the patient is in a long-sitting position on a treatment table and is instructed to move into a supine position (Fig. 8-4). During this movement the therapist guides the head into an extended and rotated position off the end of the table, to provide extension and rotation of the cervical spine (Denham, 1996). The head is rotated approximately 45° to one side (Oates, 1992). The examiner supports the head by placing his or her hands on either side of the patient's head. On reaching supine with the head extended and rotated, the therapist observes for the presence of nystagmus and asks how the patient feels.

Repeat the test, again starting from a long-sitting position, and rotate the head to the opposite side once the supine position is achieved. For example, if the head was rotated and flexed to the right in the first test, repeat the test, rotating and flexing the head to the left. This positional test activates the semicircular canals of the vestibular system. Complaints of vertigo, nausea, and the presence of nystagmus are indicative of vestibular dysfunction (Oates, 1992).

The assessment and treatment of vestibular abnormalities are advanced skills, both of which require additional training beyond most entry-level educational programs. However, entry-level therapists should be able to assess smooth pursuits, saccadic eye movements, and the VOR to determine if a vestibular impairment exists, which may require referral to a therapist trained in vestibular rehabilitation.

Vision. Visual system testing should include testing the patient's ability to see both far and near, within the peripheral field of vision. The presence of double vision as reported by the patient should also be tested, as should the presence of nystagmus in smooth pursuits or saccadic eye movements. Determining the patient's ability to see far can be accomplished by asking the patient to look down a hallway or across a room to identify markings, a sign, or a poster on a wall. Ask the patient to read a paper or magazine to assess close vision. While performing these tasks, ask if the patient experiences double vision when looking near or far.

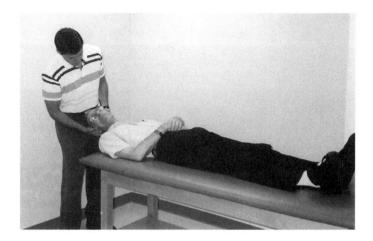

FIGURE 8-4. The Hallpike maneuver.

Test the peripheral visual fields by sitting in front of the patient and moving your hands forward, from behind both sides of the patient's head. Patients must keep their eyes focused on you. Initially place your hands back behind the patient's ears so that your hands are not within the patient's peripheral field of vision. Slowly bring your hands forward and instruct patients to report when they first see the hands within their visual field (Fig. 8-5).

As soon as the patient sees your hands, stop advancing them forward. With the hands stationary, wiggle the fingers on one hand, one at a time. Instruct the patient to point to the hand that is moving. This confirms the patient's ability to see both sides of the visual field. Continue to slowly move your hands through the peripheral field, occasionally stopping and wiggling the fingers to identify any blind spots.

See the section on the vestibular system for a description of techniques used to assess smooth pursuits and saccadic eye movements.

Somatosensation. Assessing the integrity of the dorsal column–medial lemniscus can be accomplished by testing for the ability to localize touch. Ask patients to close their eyes and identify various areas of their extremities that you touch. Success with this test indicates the dorsal columns, thalamocortical tract, and parietal cortex are functioning.

Testing proprioception and kinesthesia provides another indication of the integrity of the dorsal columns and may play a more important role in the patient's ability to maintain posture. Instruct patients to close their eyes, while one extremity is placed in various positions. Patients are instructed to match these positions with the opposite extremity. To test kinesthesia, continually move one extremity while the patient actively moves the opposite extremity in the same movement patterns.

Another test for assessing dorsal columns is the *Romberg* test (Cohen, 1993). Historically, this was the first test to assess balance. It was reported by Romberg in 1853 as a means to assess the integrity of kinesthetic pathways, specifically to assist in the diagnosis of tabes dorsalis.

Romberg's test includes both a time factor and the amount of body sway. These two components remain the primary emphasis of all balance testing performed today. To perform the Romberg test, patients stand with their eyes closed, their medial malleoli touching, and their arms folded across their chest. If they maintain this position for 30 seconds, the test is normal. The response is not normal if they open their eyes or unfold their arms before 30 seconds has passed (Fig. 8-6).

Assessing sway can be difficult, so videotaping is recommended (Begdie, 1968; Newton, 1989). The Romberg test was designed to examine the effects of posterior column disease on upright stance (Cohen, 1993).

Case Study

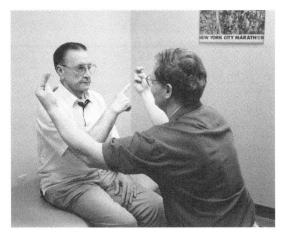

FIGURE 8-5. Assessing the patient's peripheral field of vision.

Mrs. Jackson's disability was assessed previously, with disabilities noted in:

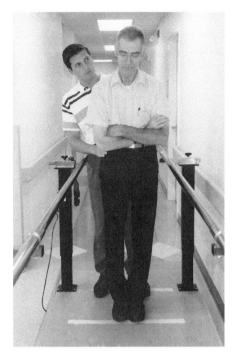

FIGURE 8-6. Patient performs the Romberg test.

- Sitting-to-standing—slow and deliberate movements to assume weight-bearing on both lower extremities; needed two-hand support on a walker placed in front of her.
- Standing—able to stand statically with two-hand support on the walker for 30 seconds with a symmetrical posture; dynamic standing was not assessed because patient was unable to statically stand without hand support.
- Ambulation—with the use of a walker for 50 feet with contact guard of the therapist; gait pattern slow; added use of vision to watch feet; did not pick each foot off the floor; slid each foot forward for the 50 feet.
- Climbing stairs—required vision to watch placement of feet and some as-

sistance of the therapist in stabilizing patient during single-limb support.

Because difficulty was noted in activities of functional mobility, assessment to identify impairments is performed.

Assessing the Impairment

Independent bed mobility, supine-to-sit activities, sitting statically, and moving in a sitting posture indicate adequate trunk strength and balance in sitting. Absence of vertigo, nausea, or nystagmus in functional movement requiring changes in head position and a negative VOR would rule out vestibular dysfunction. Difficulty moving to an upright bipedal posture and maintaining that posture, or dynamic movement in standing, suggest weakness or somatosensory loss in the lower extremities.

Assess lower extremity strength with manual muscle testing. To assess strength functionally, provide Mrs. Jackson with a stabilizing posture (eg, standing with a walker or in parallel bars) to determine strength of the extensor muscles used in the sit-to-stand maneuver. Can she perform this task symmetrically by pushing up off of both lower limbs and using her upper extremities for balance alone? Extensor muscles are important to test because they are active during the stance phase of single-limb support.

To assess balance, perform the Romberg test to rule out or confirm somatosensory dysfunction. If the Romberg test is positive, test the dorsal column–medial lemniscus system to assess proprioception and kinesthesia. A positive test for proprioception loss in the lower extremities indicates somatosensory loss as a potential cause of the difficulty with balance in standing and during gait.

Results of Impairment Testing

- Manual muscle testing reveals good (4/5) strength in muscles of the hip, knee, and ankle. Upper extremity strength is normal (5/5).
- Standing with a walker, the patient repeatedly moves from a sitting posture to standing five times without fatigue or asymmetrical movement.
- The Romberg test is positive with eyes closed; patient is unable to maintain narrow base of support and loses balance as soon as she closes her eyes.
- Proprioceptive testing of the lower extremities is inaccurate 8 of 10 trials.

GENERAL BALANCE TESTS

This section describes a variety of balance tests that can be performed to assess and quantify an individual's ability to maintain balance. Tests are noted to be for static or dynamic balance, or both.

With the exception of the Romberg, Fregly Graybiel, and Clinical Tests for Sensory Interaction for Balance, most of these tests are functionally based. The Romberg test and Clinical Tests for Sensory Interaction for Balance can be used to identify impairments. The remaining tests can be used to quantify the patient's ability to maintain static and dynamic postures and perform the movements required for daily activities.

Many of the tests described below require scoring on several activities, which, as suggested by their authors, can be totaled to determine some measure of balance. Because data collected in the majority of these tests consist of

ordinal data (ie, a ranking, such as normal, good, fair, poor, trace, zero) (Bork, 1993), the summation of test items is not reflective of the patient's ability to balance. Adding up various items on a test that uses ordinal scales will not provide a measurement reflective of the patient's ability to balance. The summation of item scores on an ordinal test cannot be compared to normative data of a population or to other patients because the total value is meaningless. Comparing items within the test can be useful in demonstrating the patient's progress, but should not be used as an aggregate score for balance. Clinical tests that use ordinal data are noted.

Romberg Test (Static)

Test positions, described above, are repeated here for convenience. Patients stand with their medial malleoli touching and arms folded across their chest and eyes closed. If they maintain this position for 30 seconds, the test is normal. The response is not normal if patients open their eyes or unfold their arms before 30 seconds has passed (see Fig. 8-6). Assessing sway can be difficult, so videotaping is recommended (Begdie, 1968; Newton, 1989).

The inability to achieve positions with eyes open suggests a cerebellar lesion; the inability to achieve positions with eyes closed suggests a somatosensory lesion. The Romberg test is a good example of the interrelatedness of the systems. Eyes open enables balance to be maintained (in the absence of a cerebellar lesion), with feedback processed from the visual field and somatosensory system. Closing the eyes forces the patient to rely only on the somatosensory system and may result in a positive test if this system is deficient. Therefore, if the Romberg test suggests a somatosensory lesion, further testing of somatosensory pathways (eg, position sense) is indicated.

Clinical Test for Sensory Interaction in Balance (Static)

This test (Shumway-Cook & Bahling-Horak, 1986) uses a progressive sequence of standing on a firm surface with the eyes open and closed; the eyes are open for the last sequence, but the visual input is distorted. The same progression is repeated while the patient stands on a foam surface, which distorts somatosensation during the three testing procedures. The visual conflict dome can be any type of dome—such as a Japanese lantern—that covers the head, to distort the visual input with movement of the body (Allison, 1995). Body sway is used to test sensory components of the postural control system (Shumway-Cook & Bahling-Horak, 1986) and was used by Romberg as a measurement of balance in his test.

Assessing sensory components requires that patients maintain standing for 30 seconds under the six different conditions (Fig. 8-7). Each square in Figure 8-7 is referred to as a cell (Nashner, 1996), and the impairment tested in a cell is described below. These six conditions alter somatosensory information entering the CNS. In all six testing procedures patients stand with feet either together or in tandem, with arms folded across the chest:

On firm surface
   Cell 1—eyes open; all three sensory systems assessed
   Cell 2—eyes closed; somatosensation assessed (Romberg test)
   Cell 3—visual conflict dome; visual integration of distorted information assessed

On foam surface
   Cell 4—eyes open; assesses distorted somatosensory
   Cell 5—eyes closed, referred to as the classical test for vestibular since eyes are closed and somatosensation is distorted

   Cell 6—eyes closed; distorted somatosensation and vision (Denham, 1996)

Each condition alters the availability and accuracy of visual and somatosensory information for postural orientation (Montgomery & Connolly, 1991). Amounts of body sway in the six different conditions are recorded (Shumway-Cook, & Bahling-Horak, 1986; Shumway-Cook & Horak, 1990).

A scale to quantify amounts of sway may include:

- Subjective assessment based on a numerical ranking system (eg, 1 = minimal sway, 2 = mild sway, 3 = moderate sway, and 4 = fall)
- Time standing erect in each position and condition, or
- Use of grids and plumb lines to record body displacement (Shumway-Cook & Bahling-Horak, 1986).

Any report by patients of nausea or dizziness should be recorded, as well as movement strategies used to maintain stability (Shumway-Cook & Bahling-Horak, 1986).

Fregly and Graybiel Quantitative Ataxia Test Battery (Static and Dynamic)

Components of the Fregly and Graybiel test are the most commonly used balance tests in the clinic today. However, test positions are not necessarily functional. The battery consists of six test conditions. Only two measurements are recorded: (1) the time standing in the test position, and (2) the number of steps taken without falling. Body sway was not indicated by Fregly and Graybiel as a factor to be assessed in these testing conditions (Begdie, 1968; Duncan, Weiner, Chandler, & Studenski, 1990; Fregly,

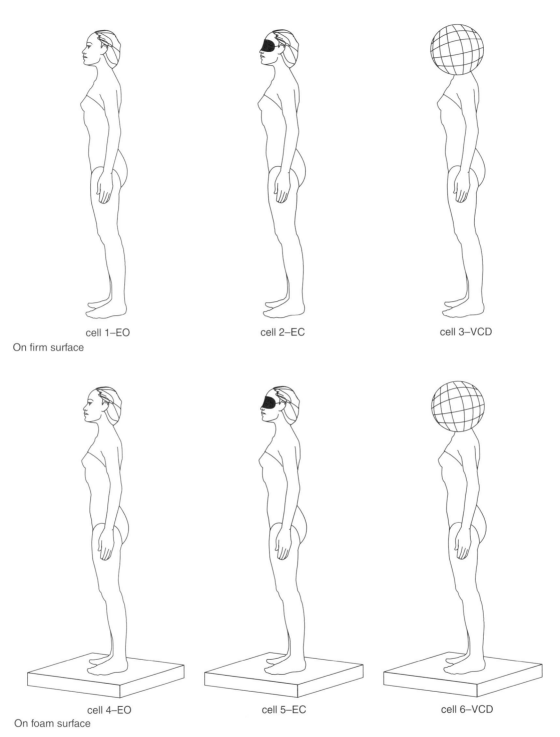

cell 1–EO   cell 2–EC   cell 3–VCD

On firm surface

cell 4–EO   cell 5–EC   cell 6–VCD

On foam surface

FIGURE 8-7. Clinical test for sensory interaction in balance. Key: EO = eyes open; EC = eyes closed; VED = visual conflict dome.

Graybiel, & Smith; 1972; Fregly, Smith & Graybiel, 1972; Newton, 1989).

1. *Sharpened Romberg.* Patients stand in tandem (heel-to-toe position) with their
   arms folded across their chest and eyes
   open for 60 seconds. Four trials are performed with the time of each trial recorded. Maximum score is 240 seconds
   (60 seconds × 4 trials).
2. *Walk on balance beam, eyes open.* Patients
   walk heel-to-toe on the balance beam
   with their eyes open and arms folded
   across their chest. They are allowed two
   steps for positioning and then continue
   for an additional five steps (Fig. 8-8).
   This sequence is repeated three times
   for a total of 15 steps. The original test
   described by Fregly was performed on

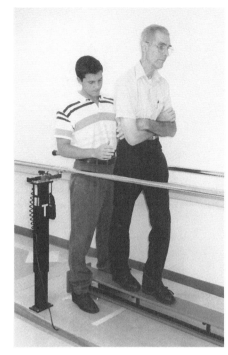

FIGURE 8-9. Patient standing on a balance beam in
tandem with the therapist.

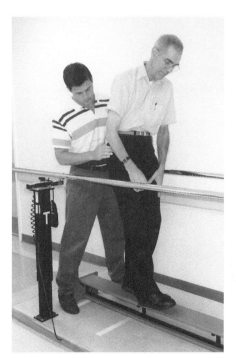

FIGURE 8-8. Patient walks on the balance beam with
his eyes open.

balance beams of varying widths, the
narrowest of which was 0.75 inches.
3. *Stand with eyes open.* The test is similar to
   the sharpened Romberg with the exception that the patient stands in tandem
   (heel-to-toe) position on a balance
   beam. The patient maintains this position with arms folded across his or her
   chest for 60 seconds (Fig. 8-9). Three
   trials are performed with a maximum
   score of 180 seconds. This test was originally performed on a 0.75 inch balance
   beam.
4. *Stand with eyes closed.* Patients now stand
   on a 2.25-inch balance beam with arms
   folded across the chest. Time standing
   on the balance beam with eyes closed is
   recorded for a maximum of 60 seconds
   for each of three trials.

5. *Stand on one leg, eyes closed.* Patients stand on a firm surface on one lower extremity, with arms folded across the chest for 30 seconds. They are allowed to choose which lower extremity they stand on and complete five trials of this activity. The maximum amount of time is 150 seconds for the five trials. This test was later revised to include standing on each lower extremity (Fregly, Smith, & Graybiel, 1972).

6. *Walk on floor with eyes closed.* Patients walk at a normal speed in tandem for 10 steps with eyes closed. Three trials are given for a maximum of 30 steps (Fig. 8-10).

Clinicians have used one or more of the testing positions described by Fregly and Graybiel to assess balance or treat balance dysfunctions (Bohannon, Larkin, Cook, Gear, & Singer, 1984; Duncan, Chandler, Studenski, Hughes, & Prescott, 1993; Gehlsen & Whaley, 1990; Horak, Jones-Rycewicz, Black, & Shumway-Cook, 1992; Judge, Lindsey, Underwook, & Winsemius, 1993; Lee, Deming, & Sahgal, 1988). However, the reader should now appreciate that the patient's performance in any of these testing positions does not assist the clinician in determining the cause of the balance dysfunction.

Berg Balance Scale (Static and Dynamic)

This ordinal scale evaluates patient performance on 14 tasks commonly performed in everyday life (Berg, Maki, Williams, Holliday, & Wood-Dauphinee, 1992; Berg, Wood-

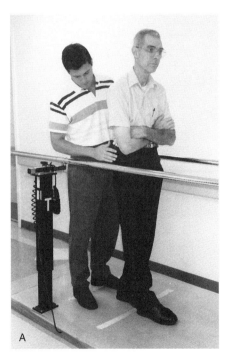
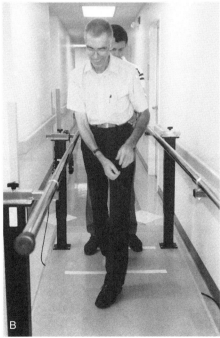

FIGURE 8-10.   *(A,B)* Patient walks in tandem with the therapist. The patient's eyes should be closed for this test.

Dauphinee, Williams, & Gayton, 1989; Ratliffe, Alba, Hallum, & Jewell, 1987). Each task is scored from 0 to 4, with 0 = unable to perform, and 4 = able to perform the task safely and independently. Inability to perform all of these movements may be an indicator that patients are at risk for falls.

Items tested on the scale include:

- Sitting to standing
- Standing unsupported
- Sitting unsupported
- Standing to sitting
- Transferring
- Standing with eyes closed
- Standing with feet together
- Reaching forward with outstretched arm
- Retrieving object from floor
- Turning to look behind
- Turning 360°
- Placing alternate foot on stool
- Standing with one foot in front
- Standing on one foot

"Get Up and Go" Test (Static and Dynamic)

This test evaluates the patient's ability to rise from a chair, walk, and return to sitting (Mathlas, Mayak, & Isaacs, 1986). The starting position is in a high-back chair with armrests. Patients rise from the chair, stand still momentarily, walk toward a wall, turn without touching the wall, walk back to the chair, turn around, and then sit down. Examiners observe this activity and score patient balance using a 5-point scale:

1 = normal
2 = very slightly abnormal
3 = mildly abnormal
4 = moderately abnormal
5 = severely abnormal

To be assigned a score of "normal," patients must not display any risk of falling (ie, no postural sway or excessive movement to maintain balance). Patients who appear at risk of falling during testing procedures receive a 5 (severely abnormal) (Mathlas et al., 1986).

Timed "Up and Go" Test (Dynamic)

This is a modified version of the "Get Up and Go" test. In this test, patients walk to a line placed 10 feet away from a chair, turn, walk back to the chair, and sit down. Patients are timed in this test. The score assigned is the time required (in seconds) to complete the test. Time starts at the examiner's command of "go" and ends when patients sit back in the chair (Posiadlo & Richardson, 1991).

Clinical Balance Assessment (Static)

This assessment is based on five items, one of which is self-report by patients (Lee et al., 1988). Items and criteria for scoring the balance test are:

1. Number of falls in the past 2 weeks

0 = more than two
1 = one to two
2 = none

2. Stance tests: standard—eyes open and closed; tandem—eyes open and closed

0 = unable to maintain for 5 seconds
1 = presence of unsteadiness, swaying, or deviation even if position is maintained for 5 seconds or more
2 = maintains steady position for more than 5 seconds

3. Standing without support

0 = cannot stand without support
1 = can stand erect for less than 1 minute, or can stand for a longer time but sways somewhat
2 = good standing balance, can maintain balance for more than 1 minute without insecurity

4. Standing on one lower extremity

0 = position cannot be maintained for more than a few unstable seconds
1 = can stand in balanced position between 4 to 9 seconds
2 = can maintain balanced position for more than 10 seconds

5. Tilting reactions in standing. Tilting reactions are defined as either lateral trunk and neck flexion toward the side being pushed, rotation of trunk and neck toward the side being pushed, or abduction of the arm and leg on the side being pushed. Ordinal data are used throughout this test.

0 = no reaction observed
1 = delayed or incomplete reactions
2 = normal reactions

Functional Reach (Dynamic)

This test uses a leveled yardstick mounted onto a wall at the height of the patient's acromion process. The patient stands without shoes and socks in a normal, relaxed stance beside the wall where the yardstick is mounted (foot tracings are made to reproduce standing position). The patient then extends one arm, with the hand made into a fist. Placement of the third metacarpal along the yardstick is recorded. The patient then reaches forward as far as possible without losing balance or taking a step forward. Placement of the third metacarpal is again re-

corded (Fig. 8-11). The upper extremity is not allowed to touch the wall during the procedure. The measurement at rest is subtracted from the measurement at the farthest point of reach to obtain the value.

Three trials of the functional reach are performed, with an average of the three measurements reported (Duncan et al., 1990; Weiner, Duncan, Chandler, & Studenski, 1992). Age-related changes in functional reach have been reported (Duncan et al., 1990):

> In the 20- to 40-year-old range, reach was 16.73 inches for men and 14.64 for women.
> In the 41- to 69-year-old range, reach was 14.98 inches for men and 13.81 for women.
> For those aged 70 to 87, reach was 13.16 inches for men and 10.47 for women.

Tinnetti Tests (Static and Dynamic)

Mary Tinnetti is a physician who has explored problems associated with falling, and measures that can be used to identify individuals at risk of falling. She has emphasized the need for balance instruments that (1) require no equipment and little experience so they can be used clinically; (2) are reliable yet sensitive to significant changes; and (3) reflect position changes and gait maneuvers used during normal daily activities (Tinnetti, 1986; Tinnetti, Williams, Franklin, & Mayewski, 1986; Topper, Maki, & Holliday, 1993).

The following activities are components of the Tinnetti test for balance, which are used to identify patients at risk for falling:

• Rising from and sitting in a chair
• Standing with eyes open and closed
• Withstanding a nudge on the sternum
• Turning the neck
• Turning in place
• Back extension

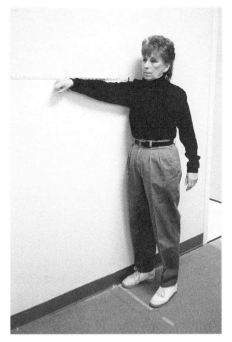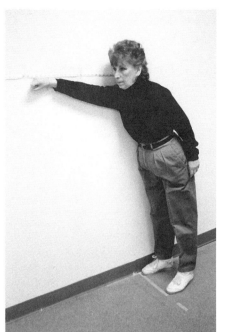
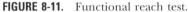

FIGURE 8-11. Functional reach test.

- Standing on one leg
- Reaching up and bending over

Each of these activities is scored using a 3-point scale, with 0 representing inability to do the task; 1 requiring some assistance; and 2 able to perform the task without support or assistance.

Tinnetti also developed an assessment for gait, which uses a similar scale for scoring. The gait assessment includes:

- Initiation of gait
- Step length, height, symmetry, and continuity
- Path deviation
- Trunk sway
- Walking stance
- Turning while walking
- Ability to walk faster (Tinnetti, 1986)

Fukuda Stepping Test (Dynamic)

Patients step into centers of two concentric circles with diameters of 1 and 2 meters. Circles are marked in 30° increments, increasing from 0° to 180°.

Patients are blindfolded and, from the center of the circle, take high marching steps up to a maximum of 100 steps at normal walking speeds. Their arms are horizontal while they complete this excessive hip flexion stepping (Mewton, 1989). Examiners observe changes in postural sway, arm position, and displacement of feet from the starting position. Objective values can be obtained related to the distance traveled from the starting position and the amount of rotation that occurred within the circle from the starting point. Reliability has not been established for this test.

Postural Stress Test

Developed by Wolfson and his colleagues, this test is used to determine individual responses to backward displacement. This test can be performed in clinics using wall-mounted pulleys.

Patients stand with a pulley system attached to their waist; the other end of the contraption is attached to weights of 1.5%, 3%, and 4.5% of their body weight. Various weights are dropped and patient responses to the backward displacement is videotaped. Patients try to maintain their position without moving their feet. The videotape is analyzed to determine if patients lost their balance (score of 0) or were able to maintain their balance (score of 1). A major difference of this test is that displacement is applied to the pelvis rather than to the feet, which are used in other displacement tests (Leonard, 1990; Newton, 1989; Wolfson, Whipple, Amerman, & Kleinberg, 1986).

A similar test was performed by Lee and coworkers (1988) using digital displacement of hip and trunk movements. Displacement was recorded by computer as weights were applied for a maximum of 2 seconds.

• •

LABORATORY TESTS

The tests described in this section are those that require equipment not ordinarily found in physical therapy clinics, or tests not routinely performed by physical therapists (eg, caloric and rotational tests, which are performed by physicians). In physical therapy clinics that are located in centers for balance dysfunction, this testing would be performed by professionally trained personnel at the center.

Platform Perturbation Tests

These tests have been used in several studies to measure balance (Black, Wall, Conrad, Rockette, & Kitch, 1982; Diener, Dichgans, Bacher, & Gompe, 1984; Ekdahl, Jarnio, & Andersson, 1989; Leonard, 1990; Mauritz, Dichgans, & Hueschmidt, 1979; Topper et al., 1993). The platform perturbation tests require a multicomponent force measurement platform interfaced with a computer.

The purpose of the test is to measure patients' sway as they stand on a platform that contains a force transducer. The platform is connected to a computer that analyzes the forces produced as the patient is in standing position and experiences body sway. Patients assume various positions (eg, quiet standing with eyes open and closed; a comfortable stance width; narrow stance; and an in-tandem position with right and left feet leading alternately) (Black et al, 1982; Diener et al., 1984; Ekdahl et al., 1989; Leonard, 1990; Mauritz, 1979; Topper et al., 1993).

In one study (Lehman et al., 1990), subjects were also exposed to distorted visual feedback from a visual conflict dome as they stood on a foam mat platform. Measurements of sway were recorded by the computer. Other studies had subjects shift their weight forward, backward, left, and right as far as possible. Tests of weight-shifting were done with feet apart in a comfortable stance and also with feet together (Murray, Sireg, & Sepic, 1975).

Ekdahl and coworkers (1989) also examined platform perturbation tests in healthy women and men, 20 to 64 years of age. They concluded that "Force platform results correlated significantly with the results of the functional tests. The findings suggest the functional balance tests, with the possible exception of the coordination test, to be of value in clinical practice" (Ekdahl et al., 1989, p. 193).

The functional tests performed in this study included standing on one leg with the other slightly flexed, standing with the eyes open and then closed, and walking as fast as possible for 30 meters and taking only one turn made during that distance. The activities of standing on one leg, and with eyes open and closed, appear similar to the Fregly Graybiel tests described above. Neither of these tests are functional. However, walking 30 meters as fast as possible and making a turn is a functional activity. The coordination test examined concomitant flexion of one arm and the alternate leg as fast as possible for 30 seconds (Ekdahl et al., 1989).

Caloric Tests

The caloric test, usually performed by a physician, involves injecting water or air into the semicircular canals to alter the temperature of the inner ear (Fox & Cohen, 1993). The air or water produces a temperature gradient that results in nystagmus. This procedure tests each labyrinth separately to identify the location of a peripheral lesion (Fox & Cohen, 1993). With an intact vestibular system, warmth produces nystagmus toward the stimulated ear, and cold produces nystagmus away from the stimulated ear (Herdman, 1994).

Rotational Tests

The rotation tests examine the horizontal semicircular canals. Like the caloric tests, they too are used to identify vestibular lesions. Patients are rotated in a chair, and throughout the rotation, they are questioned to maintain mental alertness. After a predetermined time, rotation is stopped and the patient's visual responses are observed for both timing of movements and magnitude. Both of these variables are calculated with an equation to determine the presence of a lesion (Herdman, 1994).

TREATMENT OF BALANCE DYSFUNCTION

Determining origins of balance dysfunctions greatly assists in development of treatment plans. Difficulty maintaining balance may result from muscle weakness, vestibular disorders, visual deficits, or loss of somatosensory input.

Weakness can be addressed with many of the exercises described in Chapter 5, or in the general balance program which appears later in this chapter. If patients are able to maintain static postures, emphasis should be on dynamic exercises. Recommendations for treating somatosensory loss are presented in this section, as are treatments for vestibular–ocular dysfunction. It has been demonstrated that the neuroplasticity of the CNS enables recovery of balance for vestibular patients (Shumway-Cook & Horak, 1990). The loss of visual feedback experienced by many patients is most often compensated for by enhanced feedback of other senses.

In the event that a specific etiology cannot be identified, referral to a physical therapist trained in vestibular rehabilitation, or physicians trained in otolaryngology or neurology, may be of some assistance. Lacking a specific diagnosis, physical therapists should identify functional postures and activities that challenge the patient's balance, and design treatment programs around those activities. The general balance section described later provides several ideas for activities to be performed to improve patient balance.

It is important to address education related to safety issues with patients and their families. It may be necessary to modify the home to prevent falls. You may need to instruct the patient's family to leave lights on at night and remove any unnecessary clutter from hallways or walkways. In addition, patients should avoid working in any environment that places them at great heights (Shumway-Cook & Horak, 1990).

Weakness

Strengthening weak muscles that contribute to postural instability can be accomplished with a variety of exercises or functional activities. Chapter 5 describes several functional tasks that can be used to increase stability and dynamic movement, as well as exercises to increase individual muscle strength. However, whenever possible, standing and dynamic functional activities should be incorporated to enhance strength and to challenge the CNS in the maintenance of balance. Activities suggested under the general balance program are also appropriate for use with patients who have weakness that results in postural instability.

Patients who display weakness in specific movement strategies (eg, ankle strategy) needed to maintain balance should be placed in positions where those movement strategies are needed to facilitate the activation of weak muscles. To strengthen those muscles, have patients start with small sways in various ranges (keeping knees and hips straight and body in midline) (Lehmann et al., 1990; Montgomery & Connolly, 1991).

For example, have patients with weak dorsiflexors stand in parallel bars and practice leaning posteriorly within a small range of movement. As they lean posteriorly, dorsiflexors become activated as part of the equilibrium response. The patient in Figure 8-1, shown earlier, demonstrates the activity on his noninvolved leg; he does not have the response on his involved leg. Strengthening dorsiflexors in this patient may require sitting activities on a therapeutic ball with the same stimulus, rolling the ball posteriorly. When sitting, hips and knees are also in flexion, which may increase activation of the anterior tibialis.

Vestibular Dysfunction

Patients with vestibular dysfunction experience problems of vertigo and nausea, in addition to a disturbance in balance. The symptoms experienced should be considered when treating patients with vestibular dysfunctions. Treatment for these patients most often emphasizes movement and positioning to reproduce symptoms in order to train the CNS to compensate for the vestibular dysfunction.

According to Shumway-Cook and Bahling-Horak (1986), "Sensorimotor activity is thought to enable the physiologic mechanisms underlying vestibular compensation to act. These mechanisms include central sensory substitution, rebalancing tonic activation in central vestibular pathways, and vestibular habituation" (p. 175). The ability of the CNS to compensate for vestibular problems appears to be the result of neuroplasticity (Shumway-Cook & Horak, 1990), which may entail substitution of other sensory feedback and reprogramming information transmitted by the vestibulospinal tracts.

Habituation exercises (repeatedly positioning the patient in positions that elicit symptoms) consist of repetitive movements and positions that reproduce vertigo. Movements and positions vary and should be specific to the patient's position of complaint. The patient in Figure 8-12 is gradually being positioned from supine into upright sitting. Wedges and pillows are used to support him through varying degrees of elevation of his head from the bed.

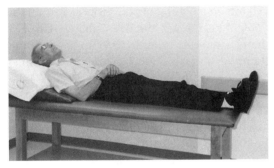

FIGURE 8-12. The patient moves from this posture to full upright sitting. The goal is for the patient to move from lying directly on the table up into sitting without vertigo.

With each change in position toward upright, symptoms of vertigo and nystagmus may reappear. Positions are maintained until the symptoms disappear. Once symptoms are gone, the head is again moved into more upright postures. Patients may also be moved through the full range (ie, from supine to full upright sitting posture) if they can tolerate the intensity of the symptoms. Moving through the full range without symptoms is the ultimate goal of treatment.

During the first week of therapy, only two movements or positions that elicit symptoms should be addressed. Gradually, other movements and positions that elicit vertigo can be added, until all symptoms diminish and patients are free of vertigo. Patients should perform movements and positioning activities 5 to 10 times, and repeat them at least 3 times a day (Shumway-Cook & Horak, 1990). Functional movements, such as reaching up into cabinets, bending down and reaching into low cabinets, vacuuming, and climbing the stairs, should be included in treatment programs. Performance of these functional activities assists the CNS in compensating for vestibular dysfunction in all functional movement patterns.

Treatment for lesions of the peripheral vestibular system may include rapid repositioning of the head if the problem is one of displaced **otoconia** (calcium carbonate crystals that provide the membrane overlying the hair cells in the inner ear receptors [saccule] with a specific gravity) onto the **cupula** (a gelatinous cap in which the hair cells are embedded) of the posterior semicircular canal. Rapid repositioning may assist in dislodging the displaced otoconia. Sitting and bouncing on a therapy ball or the patient's bed is another technique to reposition the displaced otoconia. Repetitive performance of the habituation exercises that involve movement can also help the CNS compensate for vestibular dysfunction (eg, moving from a modified Hallpike position quickly into sitting) (Shumway-Cook & Horak, 1990).

Patients who have vestibular dysfunction often have concomitant muscle imbalance that develops from strategies to minimize head and trunk movement that may cause vertigo. Muscle imbalances (eg, tight sternocleidomastoid) should be addressed before, or in addition to, vestibular treatments.

The vestibular–ocular reflex may be impaired in patients with vestibular dysfunction. The following exercises may increase the VOR:

- In sitting position: visual tracking exercises of any moving object while keeping the head still. Instruct the patient to move a pencil back and forth in front of the face. This activity may have to be started with small ranges of eye movements if the patient complains of nystagmus, nausea, or vertigo. The progression of the exercise should be to a wider range of horizontal or vertical movements, and to a position of standing. As a further challenge, have the patient practice visual tracking while walking or ascending and descending stairs. (Note: Provide appropriate guarding during these two activities.) (Denham, 1996)

• In sitting position: eyes fixed while the head is moved passively by the therapist. First perform slowly, then with increasing speed, progressing to active movements. Once patients can perform active movements, have them progress to a position of standing, walking, and walking while reading a magazine and performing the VOR (Denham, 1996).

These exercises should be performed first in sitting, progressing to standing, to walking on a firm surface, and to walking on varying surfaces (Shumway-Cook & Horak, 1990). These exercises can also be added to any of the dynamic balance activities listed at the end of this chapter.

Rehabilitation of vestibular disorders has grown tremendously over the past several years. Treatment approaches addressing vestibular dysfunction have been designed by Cawthorne-Cooksey, Norré, Brandt & Daroff, and others (Herdman, 1994). Vestibular assessment and rehabilitation are recognized by the authors of this text as an advanced skill of the physical therapist. Readers who are interested in this area of neurorehabilitation are referred to *Vestibular Rehabilitation* by Susan Herdman (see annotated references) or to any number of continuing education courses that provide training in this specific area of rehabilitation.

Somatosensory Loss

Treating patients with somatosensory loss may include use of the external environment or additional stimuli to increase their awareness of their extremities. Changing the external environment or stimulus may increase awareness or assist in retraining perception of the environment.

Patients who rely on hard, smooth surfaces for somatosensory feedback should practice walking on irregular or soft surfaces (Shumway-Cook & Horak, 1989). Walking barefoot changes surface stimuli used in ambulation. Standing on stable surfaces with distortion of visual cues (ie, looking through a prism) is helpful for patients who rely heavily on visual cues. This activity requires patients to use available somatosensory information rather than visual feedback (Shumway-Cook & Horak, 1990).

Use of a force plate for biofeedback with weight shift has been beneficial in patients with hemiparesis (Leonard, 1990; Ratliffe et al., 1987). In this activity, patients begin with static standing and equal weight distribution, then move from a standing position to sitting, and from a sitting position to standing. In both of these movements, equal weight distribution should be maintained through the lower extremities. Therapists may incorporate lateral weight shift from limb to limb, anteroposterior weight shift with the involved limb forward and then behind, and stepping in place (Leonard, 1990; Shumway-Cook, Anson, & Haller, 1988).

To increase somatosensory input for trunk alignment, position patients (in midline) with their backs against a chair or wall. The wall or back of a chair provides additional sensory information on trunk alignment. Therapists may use visual cues (mirror) as needed to maintain midline posture and then withdraw these visual cues and wall or chair stimuli. Patients need to maintain this upright posture without additional sensory cues (Fig. 8-13). Patients may stand without shoes or socks to increase input through their feet (Shumway-Cook & Horak, 1989).

Patients who display loss of somatosensory input may be treated with weights placed on their ankles or on assistive devices to increase sensory stimulation (Fig. 8-14). Wearing a weighted belt has also shown some benefit in decreasing postural sway in patients with intact

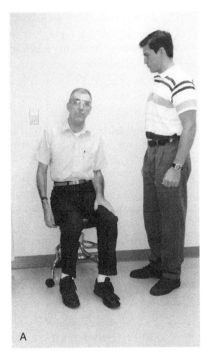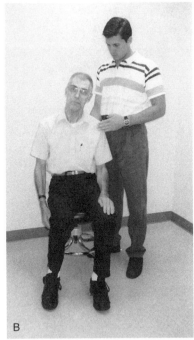

FIGURE 8-13. (*A*) The patient uses the wall for sensory feedback. (*B*) When the patient is moved away from the wall, no sensory cues can be perceived through the back.

somatosensation, by increasing somatosensory input (Ratliffe et al., 1987).

Overuse of visual compensation in sensory-deprived conditions should also be addressed in treatment programs. To decrease reliance on visual input, therapists may place blinders on patients, or blindfold them, and then assist them into positions where their static or dynamic balance will be challenged. This again forces patients to use whatever somatosensory feedback is available.

Conversely, for patients who are unable to use somatosensory processing, mirrors may be used to integrate visual input to achieve midline sitting or stance. Mirrors should be withdrawn as soon as patients develop appropriate CNS compensation to maintain midline without visual feedback.

General Balance Program

In the event that specific etiologies for balance dysfunctions are unknown, a general balance program can be used to address patient disabilities. The general balance program can also be used as an adjunct to other specific treatment directed toward a known balance impairment.

For example, patients with diminished somatosensation or vestibulo–ocular deficits can perform general balance exercises as a way to improve their functional movement, and can practice the activities to address their impairment. Activities used in a general balance program are based on functional needs experienced by the patient (eg, patients unable to sit or stand should first work on static activities in one of these positions). Many of the exercise

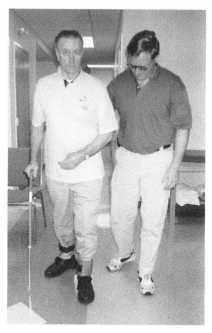

FIGURE 8-14. Patient walks with weights on his ankles.

activities described in this section will also improve strength and posture, thereby enabling patients experiencing weakness to benefit from these activities.

Verbal cues can be used with these activities to assist in maintaining balance. Manual support should be provided only as needed (Carr & Shepherd, 1987). Patients should experience a loss of balance (in a guarded environment) to learn how to move to regain their balance. Activities should be progressed to continually challenge the patient's ability to maintain balance. Activities listed below progress from static to dynamic, and from lower level to higher level activities.

Static

Patients begin by sitting unsupported. If they are unable to sit unsupported, then start with two-handed support and progress to one-

handed support, then to sitting unsupported. Vary the surfaces (hard to soft) that patients sit on, and the height of the surface, when working on static sit techniques.

Patients progress to standing in parallel bars with both hands on the bars. Patients should practice removing one hand at a time, progressing to unsupported standing. If they have difficulty standing without hand support, try widening their base of support. Once they have accomplished standing unsupported on hard, smooth surfaces, challenge their balance by putting them on uneven surfaces. Different surfaces may be rugs, floor mats, or pieces of foam. The patient's eyes may be open and closed while working on this technique.

From standing unsupported, have the patient progress to a narrow base of support, and eventually to the Romberg stance. When patients achieve the Romberg stance satisfactorily, they should then attempt it again with their eyes closed.

Starting with a comfortable base of support and both hands on parallel bars, patients should stand on one leg or in tandem. Once they are in this position, direct them to slowly remove their hand support and practice maintaining their balance in a single-leg stand or in tandem stand (see Fig. 8-10). Alternate between each leg in the single-leg stance and the front leg in the tandem stance.

Dynamic

When the patient is performing dynamic activities, the therapist should be positioned to guard the patient and provide assistance in maintaining balance if needed. Therapists should allow patients to move off balance to "feel" what it is like to lose their balance, but the therapist should be ready to assist in the event of a total loss of balance. Enabling patients to move off balance will facilitate their ability to learn how to respond to external forces and regain their balance. However, patients should never be placed in positions where they are at risk for falling.

The lowest level dynamic activity is moving from a position of supine to sitting at the edge of the bed or mat. Therapists should provide assistance as needed to enable patients to accomplish tasks, but as soon as possible, decrease or eliminate manual assistance.

Once the patient has assumed an unsupported static sit, ask the patient to look up and down, and from side to side. This head movement will activate the vestibular system, which should provide sensory feedback for this task. Progress from static sit unsupported to reaching activities to the same side (right arm to right side), to crossing midline (right arm to left side). Patients should reach for objects when performing this activity so that there is motivation to move within a specific range (Fig. 8-15). This same activity can be performed in static stand unsupported in parallel bars.

Have patients support themselves in the static sit posture by placing their hands on the mat or bed. Then ask them to stand up. During this movement, look for symmetry and bilateral support on both lower extremities. If patients are unsuccessful in moving symmetrically, place a mirror in front of them to increase the visual input and to emphasize symmetrical movements. If patients are bearing weight only on the noninvolved lower extremities, place the noninvolved hand on the involved knee and direct them to push off the involved knee with the noninvolved hand. This will encourage weight-bearing through the involved lower extremities (Carr & Shepherd, 1987).

As patients are able to accomplish this task with the support of two hands, progress them to one-hand support and then unsupported. Again emphasize symmetry and equal weight-bearing through both lower extremities. To make this task easier or harder, change seat heights (Fig. 8-16).

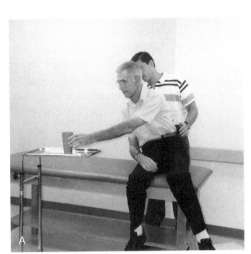
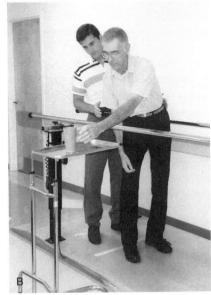

FIGURE 8-15. The patient reaches for an object while sitting (*A*) and standing (*B*).

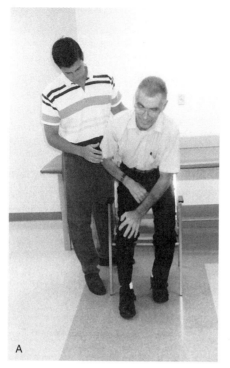 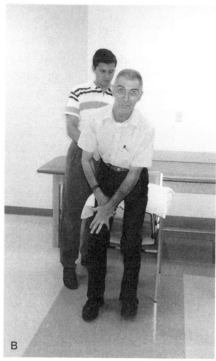

FIGURE 8-16. (*A,B*) Patient moves from sitting to a symmetrical stance from seats of different heights.

Patients can practice taking one step forward and one step back while standing in parallel bars with one- or two-hand support (Fig. 8-17). Alternate the leg performing the stepping motion to increase weight-bearing on the involved limbs. The nonmoving limb provides the stabilization needed for balance. Progress the patient to standing unsupported and stepping forward and back.

Have the patient assume the supine position from standing on a floor mat. From the supine position, the patient can move back to standing. You can alter the movement patterns by asking the patient to move to prone positions on the floor mats. Each technique activates the vestibular system in addition to challenging the patient's dynamic balance. Provide careful guarding as patients move through these sequences.

Trunk strength and dynamic balance can be addressed by throwing and catching large therapy balls with patients in a variety of positions: kneeling, half-kneeling, sitting, and standing (Fig. 8-18). Throwing the ball directly at patients will cause head and upper extremity movement. Progress to throwing the ball to either side of the patient. To catch the ball, the patient will have to rotate, flex and/or extend the trunk.

Ambulation is the most common dynamic functional activity. In gait training, therapists often start patients with assistive devices to stabilize their balance. However, to improve patient balance the CNS must be challenged continually to respond to unstable environments.

To emphasize balance training, progress to less stabilizing devices (eg, from a walker to a

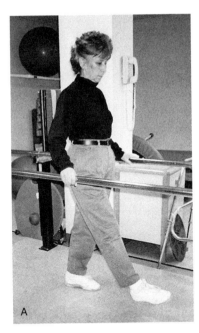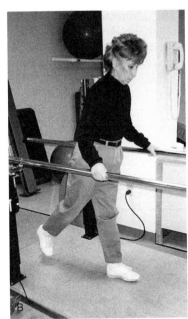

FIGURE 8-17. Patient standing between parallel bars steps forward (*A*) and then back (*B*). This should be progressed to no hand support.

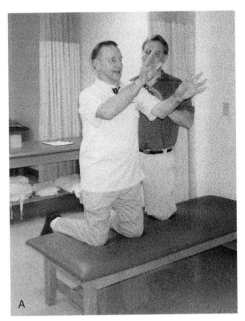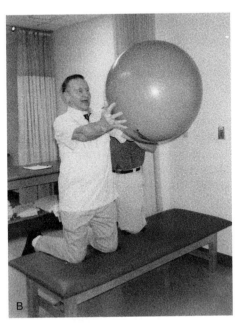

FIGURE 8-18. (*A,B*) Patient catches a therapy ball while kneeling.

cane); gradually move toward having the patient ambulate with no device at all, if possible. Walking speed should also be varied to challenge the motor and sensory systems to function in maintaining balance.

Terrain that patients walk on may be altered as well to challenge their ability to balance. A rug or floor mat can be used for irregular surfaces in institutional settings (Fig. 8-19). Ambulation outdoors should emphasize walking on grass, gravel, or sand. During ambulation activities the therapist should maintain close guarding, but keep his or her hands off patients to enable them to use movement strategies to maintain balance.

The patient's base of support for walking can be altered from a wide base, to a narrow base, to tandem walking on a line. When decreasing the base of support, have the patient practice walking backward to improve balance responses. This eliminates visual input in place-

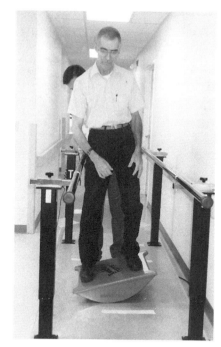

FIGURE 8-20.   Patient shifts weight on an equilibrium board while standing between parallel bars.

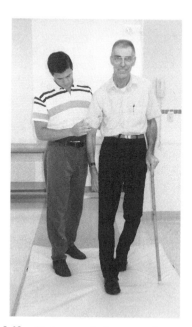

FIGURE 8-19.   Patient ambulates on floor mat with the assistance of a cane.

ment of the feet in the narrow base or tandem walk.

Additional gait activities to be practiced include side-stepping, walking forward crossing legs, walking backward crossing legs, and high stepping. All of these should emphasize symmetry of movement, equal weight-shifting between each leg, and the elimination of upper extremity support for balance.

Balancing on an equilibrium board, or wobble board, placed between parallel bars will emphasize weight-shifting from side to side or forward and back (depending on how patients are positioned on the board). When beginning this activity, allow patients to use two-hand support on parallel bars, progressing to one-hand support, and eventually to using no support at all (Fig. 8-20). Mirrors can be added to allow the patient to process more visual cues to assist in maintaining balance. To make this activity even more difficult, have patients close their eyes while shifting weight on the board.

Next, patients may practice kicking a ball placed in front of their feet while standing in parallel bars or in a guarded environment (Fig. 8-21). Progress patients to kicking a ball that is rolled to them. To increase the difficulty of the task, change the speed at which, and the direction in which (ie, to either side of the patient), the ball is rolled. Emphasize kicking with alternate legs to work on the stability and balance of each leg, with dynamic movement of the opposite leg.

Additional progressions of this activity may include performing it without using parallel bars, and using smaller balls. Another progression may include having the patient kick the ball against a wall. Have the patient stand 5 feet from a wall and kick the ball into the wall. The patient must be prepared to stop the ball as it returns before the next kick.

Patients can practice dribbling a ball with either their hands or feet. In either instance, their balance is challenged as they attempt to maintain control over the ball. Again vary the speed and direction that patients walk (eg, turn while dribbling or dribble in a large circle) to increase the difficulty of the task.

Walking through an obstacle course that requires navigation around and over objects is another challenge for patients with balance dysfunctions. Time to complete the obstacle course can be recorded, as well the number of objects patients hit with their feet, and whether or not they lost their balance. Progression for this activity may include speed and dribbling a ball through the obstacle course (Fig. 8-22).

Having patients ambulate in crowded hallways with irregular surfaces is a more functional way to address high level balance control.

T'ai chi exercises have been recommended for balance dysfunction because they involve slow, controlled movements, while emphasizing good postural control and single-leg stance (Judge et al., 1993).

General Strengthening and Aerobic Exercise

Patients who have balance dysfunction frequently become deconditioned because of self-imposed immobility arising from fear related to loss of balance or falling. Introduce conditioning exercises as the patient is able to maintain a center of gravity over static and dynamic bases of support.

General strengthening or conditioning exercises should be added gradually to existing balance exercises to enhance the patient's general conditioning. Care should be taken with the type of conditioning exercises used to prevent activities that could lead to loss of balance. For example, if marching in place on a mini-

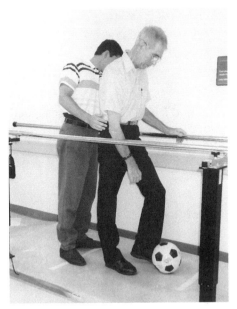

FIGURE 8-21. Patient practices kicking a soccer ball while using parallel bars for support.

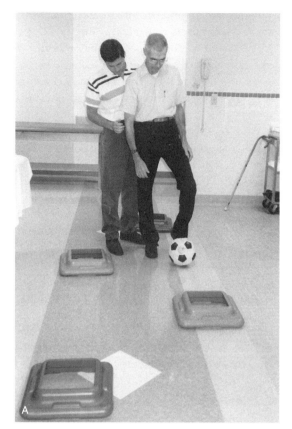 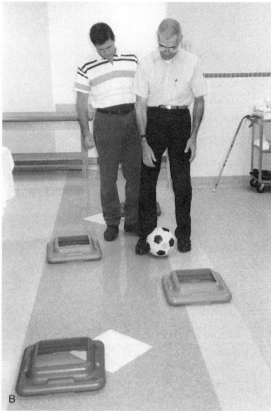

FIGURE 8-22. *(A,B)* Patient dribbles a soccer ball through an obstacle course.

trampoline is used, allow patients to use two-hand support on parallel bars when initiating this activity. As balance improves, the hand support can be reduced to one-hand support, and eventually to unsupported. Examples of general strengthening or aerobic exercise include:

- Stationary bike
- Repeated step-ups on training stairs or step-up
- Kinetron or Stairmaster
- Light weights on extremities; active ROM performed sitting or preferably standing
- Walking or jogging

- Modified aerobic exercise class based on patient's balance abilities
- Mini-trampoline
- Rowing

Case Study

Mrs. Jackson's impairment and disability have been assessed. Functional mobility was limited in moving from sitting-to-standing, standing, ambulation, and stair climbing. Impairments were identified as weakness (4/5 strength) and diminished somatosensation in the lower extremities.

Functional assessment of balance was performed with the Functional Reach Test. Mrs. Jackson, who is 42 years old, was able to reach 6.2 inches (normal value for this age and gender is 13.8).

Treatment of Mrs. Jackson

Treatment should focus on increasing somatosensory feedback from the lower extremities. This can be accomplished by applying weights to Mrs. Jackson's lower extremities, having her ambulate without shoes or on uneven surfaces, and adding visual feedback from a mirror.

Somatosensory feedback should be provided initially during all functional activities. Make the patient aware of her own internal biofeedback system (eg, watching muscles contract, seeing joints move) to increase her awareness of her lower limbs. To increase control of movements (in the absence of diminished feedback), perform functional movements within a shortened range and at a slow rate. Progress this to an increased range and faster movement.

Limitations in functional mobility were identified as moving from sitting-to-standing, standing, and ambulation. Functional reach was limited by 50%. All of these tasks, including functional reach, should be practiced during treatment sessions. All of the activities to address the diminished sensation will also be effective in increasing strength in the lower extremities. Climbing stairs should be used as an activity to increase somatosensation and strength. See Chapters 6 and 7 on coordination and sensory dysfunction for additional treatment ideas.

SUMMARY

- Balance was defined as the integration of vestibular, visual, and somatosensory information with an intact musculoskeletal system, to maintain the body's center of gravity over its base of support.
- Maintaining balance requires the complex interaction of the neuromuscular and musculoskeletal systems.
- A disruption of any component of these two systems (vestibular, visual, somatosensory, or strength and ROM) can result in a disability.
- Specific testing should be performed to identify the cause of the balance dysfunction, to enable the development of an appropriate treatment program.
- Standardized instruments are available to quantify an individual's ability to maintain balance. The majority of the tests described are functionally based, with the exception of the Romberg, Fregly Graybiel, and Clinical Tests for Sensory Interaction for Balance.
- Treatments should be designed for specific impairments, such as vestibular, visual, somatosensory deficits, or weakness. Progression of treatment should include retraining for functional mobility at the highest level attainable.

REFERENCES

Allison, L. (1995). Balance disorders. In D. Umphred (Ed.). *Neurological rehabilitation*. St. Louis: Mosby-Year Book.

Begdie, GH. (1968). The assessment of imbalance. *Physiotherapy, 55,* 411–414.

Berg, K, Wood-Dauphinee, S, Williams, JI, & Gayton, D. (1989). Measuring balance in the elderly: Preliminary development of an instrument. *Physiotherapy Canada, 41*(6), 304–311.

Berg, KQ, Maki, BE, Williams, JI, Holliday, PJ, & Wood-Dauphinee, SL. (1992). Clinical and laboratory measures of postural balance in an elderly population. *Archives of Physical Medicine and Rehabilitation, 73,* 1073–1080.

Black, FO, Wall, C, Conrad, C, Rockette, HE, & Kitch, R. (1982). Normal subject postural sway during the Romberg test. *American Journal of Otolaryngology, 3,* 309–318.

Bohannon, RW, Larkin, PA, Cook, AC, Gear, J, & Singer, J. (1984). Decrease in timed balance test scores with aging. *Physical Therapy, 64,* 1066–1070.

Borello-France, D. (1996). Central vestibular disorders. *Neurology Report, 20*(3), 54–60.

Borello-France, D, Whitney, S, & Herdman, SJ. (1994). Assessment of vestibular hypofunction. In SJ. Herdman (Ed.). *Vestibular rehabilitation.* Philadelphia: Davis.

Bork, CE. (1993). *Research in physical therapy.* Philadelphia: Lippincott.

Carr, JH, & Shepherd, RB. (1987). *Movement science, foundations for physical therapy in rehabilitation.* Rockville, MD: Aspen.

Cohen, H. (1993). *Neuroscience for rehabilitation.* Philadelphia: Lippincott.

Cooke, D. (1996). Central vestibular disorders. *Neurology Report, 20*(3), 22–29.

Denham, T. (1996). *Physical therapy evaluation of the dizzy patient.* Presented at New York University Medical Center Conference, Evaluation and Management of the Patient with Dizziness: New Perspectives on Diagnosis and Rehabilitation.

Diener, HC, Dichgans, J, Bacher, M, & Gompe, B. (1984). Quantification of postural sway in normals and patients with cerebellar diseases. *Electroencephalography and Clinical Neurophysiology, 57,* 134–142.

Duncan, PW, Chandler, J, Studenski, S, Hughes, M, Prescott, B. (1993). How do physiological components of balance affect mobility in elderly men? *Archives of Physical Medicine and Rehabilitation, 74,* 1343–1349.

Duncan, PW, Weiner, DK, Chandler, J, & Studenski, S. (1990). Functional reach: A new clinical measure of balance. *Journal of Gerontology, 45*(6), M192–197.

Ekdahl, C, Jarnio, GB, & Andersson, SI. (1989). Standing balance in healthy subjects. *Scandinavian Journal of Rehabilitation Medicine, 21,* 187–195.

Fox, CR, & Cohen H. (1993). The visual and vestibular systems. In H. Cohen (Ed.). *Neuroscience for rehabilitation* (pp. 97–125). Philadelphia: Lippincott.

Fregly, AR, Graybiel, A, & Smith, MJ. (1972). Walk on floor eyes closed (wofec): A new addition to an ataxia test battery. *Aerospace Medicine, 43*(4), 395–399.

Fregly, AR, Smith, MJ, & Graybiel, A. (1972). Revised normative standards of performance of men on a quantitative ataxia test battery. *Acta Otolaryngology, 75,* 10–16.

Gehlsen, GM, & Whaley, MH. (1990). Falls in the elderly: Part II, balance, strength, and flexibility. *Archives of Physical Medicine and Rehabilitation, 71,* 739–741.

Herdman, SJ. (Ed.). (1994). *Vestibular rehabilitation.* Philadelphia: Davis.

Horak, FB. (1987). Clinical measurement of postural control in adults. *Physical Therapy, 67*(12), 1881–1885.

Horak, FB, Jones-Rycewicz, C, Black, FO, & Shumway-Cook, A. (1992). Effects of vestibular rehabilitation on dizziness and imbalance. *Otolaryngology—Head and Neck Surgery, 106*(2), 175–180.

Judge, JO, Lindsey, C, Underwook, M, & Winsemius, D. (1993). Balance improvements in older women: Effects of exercise training. *Physical Therapy, 73*(4), 254–265.

Kandell, ER, Schwartz, JH, & Jessel, TM. (1991). *Principles of neuroscience* (3rd ed.). East Norwalk, CT: Appleton & Lange.

Lee, WA, Deming, L, & Sahgal, V. (1988). Quantitative and clinical measures of static standing balance in hemiparetic and normal subjects. *Physical Therapy, 68,* 970–976.

Lehmann, JF, Boswell, S, Price, R, Burleigh, A, deLateur, BJ, Jaffe, KM, & Hertling, D. (1990). Quantitative evaluation of sway as an indicator of functional balance in post-traumatic brain injury. *Archives of Physical Medicine and Rehabilitation, 71,* 955–962.

Leonard, E. (1990). Balance tests and balance responses: Performances changes following a CVA. A review of the literature. *Physiotherapy Canada, 42*(2), 68–72.

Mathlas, S, Mayak, USL, Isaacs, B. (1986). Balance in elderly patients: The ''get-up and go'' test. *Archives of Physical Medicine and Rehabilitation, 67,* 387–389.

Mauritz, KH, Dichgans, J, & Hueschmidt, A. (1979). Quantitative analysis of stance in late cortical cerebellar atrophy of the anterior lobe and other forms of cerebellar ataxia. *Brain, 102,* 461–482.

Montgomery, PC, & Connolly, BH. (1991). *Motor control and physical therapy. Theoretical framework practical application.* Hixson, TN: Chattanooga Group Inc.

Murray, MP, Seireg, AA, & Sepic, SB. (1975). Normal postural stability and steadiness: Quantitative assessment. *Journal of Bone and Joint Surgery, 57A*(4), 510–516.

Nashner, LM. (1996). *A global perspective of the balance system.* Presented at New York University Medical Center Conference, Evaluation and Management of the Patient with Dizziness: New Perspectives on Diagnosis and Rehabilitation.

Newton, R. (1989). Review of tests of standing balance abilities. *Brain Injury, 3*(4), 335–343.

Oates, J. (1992). Post-concussive balance dysfunction: A physical therapy assessment. *Neurology Report, 16*(2), 16–21.

Posiadlo, D, & Richardson, S. (1991). The timed ''up & go'': A test of basic functional mobility for frail elderly persons. *Journal of the American Geriatrics Society, 39,* 142–148.

Ratliffe, KT, Alba, BM, Hallum, A, & Jewell, M. (1987). Effects of approximation on postural sway in healthy subjects. *Physical Therapy, 67*(4), 502–506.

Sharpe, JA. (1994). Assessment and management of central vestibular disorders. In SJ. Herdman (Ed.). *Vestibular rehabilitation.* Philadelphia: iDavis.

Shumway-Cook, A, Anson, D, & Haller, S. (1988). Postural sway biofeedback: Its effect on reestablishing stance stability in hemiplegic patients. *Archives of Physical Medicine and Rehabilitation, 69,* 395–400.

Shumway-Cook, A, & Bahling-Horak, F. (1986). Assessing the influence of sensory interaction on balance. *Physical Therapy, 66,* 1548–1550.

Shumway-Cook, A, & Horak, F. (1989). Vestibular rehabilitation: An exercise approach to managing symptoms of vestibular dysfunction. *Seminars in Hearing, 10*(2) 196–208.

Shumway-Cook, A, & Horak, FB. (1990). Rehabilitation strategies for patients with vestibular deficits. *Neurologic Clinics, 8*(2), 441–456.

Shumway-Cook, A, & Woollacott, M. (1995). *Motor control–theory and practical applications.* Baltimore: Williams & Wilkins.

Stones, MJ, & Kozma, A. (1987). Balance and Age in the Sighted and Blind. *Archives of Physical Medicine and Rehabilitation, 68,* 85–89.

Tinnetti, ME. (1986). Performance-oriented assessment of mobility problems in elderly patients. *Journal of the American Geriatrics Society, 34,* 119–126.

Tinnetti, ME, Williams, T, Franklin, B, & Mayewski, R. (1986). Fall risk index for elderly patients based on number of chronic disabilities. *American Journal of Medicine, 80,* 429–434.

Topper, AK, Maki, BE, & Holliday, PJ. (1993). Are activity-based assessments of balance and gait in the elderly predictive of risk of falling and/or type of fall? *Journal of the American Geriatrics Society, 41*(5), 479–487.

Umphred, DA. (1990). *Neurological rehabilitation* (2nd. ed.). St. Louis: Mosby-Year Book.

Weiner, DK, Duncan, PW, Chandler, J, & Studenski, SA. (1992). Functional reach: A marker of physical frailty. *Journal of the American Geriatrics Society, 40*(5), 203–207.

Whitney, SL, & Borello-France, B. (1993). Objective measures of balance: What's new. Department of Physical Therapy, University of Pittsburgh.

Winstein, C, & Mitz, AR. (1993). The motor system II: Higher centers. In H. Cohen (Ed.). *Neuroscience for rehabilitation* (pp. 176–217). Philadelphia: Lippincott.

Wolfson, LL, Whipple, R, Amerman, P, & Kleinberg, A. (1986). Stressing the postural response. A quantitative method for testing balance. *Journal of the American Geriatrics Society, 34,* 845–850.

Woollacott, MH, & Shumway-Cook, A. (1990). Changes in posture control across the life span–a systems approach. *Physical Therapy, 70*(12), 799–807.

● ●

SUGGESTED READINGS

Allison, L. (1995). Balance disorders. In D. Umphred (Ed.). *Neurological rehabilitation.* St. Louis: Mosby Year Book.

> This chapter reviews the systems approach to balance, clinical assessment of balance, problem identification, goal setting, and treatment planning for balance disorders, balance retraining techniques, and two case studies.

American Physical Therapy Association. (1996, September). Vestibular rehabilitation. A special issue of *Neurology Report, 20,* published by Neurology Section, American Physical Therapy Association.

This collection of articles examines unilateral peripheral vestibular lesions, computerized dynamic posturography in balance disorders, central vestibular disorders, acoustic neuromas leading to unilateral vestibular lesions, bilateral vestibular disease, treatment of benign paroxysmal positional vertigo, and physical therapy management of bilateral peripheral vestibular loss.

Cohen, H. (1993). *Neuroscience for rehabilitation.* Philadelphia: Lippincott.

Several chapters in this text provide an excellent foundation of the anatomy and physiology of the sensory systems involved in balance. Chapters include The Somatosensory Systems, The Visual and Vestibular Systems, and The Motor System II: Higher Centers.

Herdman, SJ. (Ed.). (1994). *Vestibular rehabilitation.* Philadelphia: Davis.

This comprehensive text addresses the anatomy and physiology of the normal vestibular system, the role of this system in postural control and abnormalities of posture, the medical assessment and management of vestibular dysfunction, and rehabilitation assessment and management.

Standardized Measures of Disability

This text has emphasized the assessment of functional mobility in patients with neurological dysfunction. The analysis of their movement is based on an understanding of what is normal, as well as on the observation of abnormal movement, or the alternative strategies, used to accomplish a given functional task. The analysis considers both the quality and quantity of movement, although quality is difficult to measure. Functional movement is measured in terms of the level of independence with which the patient is able to accomplish it. Symmetry, or lack thereof, may be used to provide a limited measure of the quality of movement.

Incorporating standardized functional assessment scales into the analysis of functional movement allows for the use of objective measurement values. The Functional Independence Measure (FIM) is a basic indicator of the severity of disability and the burden of care. The FIM consists of a 7-point scale to designate major changes in functional behavior from dependence to independence. With the FIM and other standardized functional assessment tools, the therapist is able to:

- Make objective measures of functional mobility
- Enhance communication of a patient's status and progress within and across disciplines
- Provide uniformity of documented outcomes
- Measure treatment efficacy

The responsible parties in rehabilitation (physicians, physicians' assistants, nurses, nurse practitioners, physical therapists, occupational therapists, and speech therapists) should be involved in the selection of assessment tools suitable to their patient populations. A functional assessment tool that incorporates all disciplines will enhance the level of communication and treatment provided to the patient.

The following scales are presented in this appendix:

- Barthel
- FIM
- Rivermead Mobility Index
- SF-36
- 12-Item Health Status Questionnaire (HSQ-12)

Barthel Index. The Barthel index measures the degree of assistance required by an individual to perform 10 items of mobility and self-care. The scale is based on a total score of 20 points, which reflects independence in all 10 activities. The range of scoring for each item varies from 0 to 1 or 0 to 4. In grooming and bathing the range of scores is 0 to 1, with 1 representing independence. In bowel, bladder, toilet use, feeding, dressing, or climbing stairs, the range of scores is 0 to 2, with 1 representing a level of dependence and 2 representing independence. Transfers and mobility are scored from 0 to 3, with 1 and 2 representing a level of

(*Text continues on page 230*)

Bowels

0 = incontinent (or needs to be given enema)
1 = occasional accident (once a week)
2 = continent

Bladder

0 = incontinent, or catheterized and unable to manage alone
1 = occasional accident (maximum once per 24 hours)
2 = continent

Grooming

0 = needs help with personal care
1 = independent face/hair/teeth/shaving (implements provided)

Toilet Use

0 = dependent
1 = needs some help, but can do something alone
2 = independent (on and off, dressing, wiping)

Feeding

0 = unable
1 = needs help cutting, spreading butter, etc.
2 = independent

Transfer (bed to chair and back)

0 = unable, no sitting balance
1 = major help (one or two people, physical), can sit
2 = minor help (verbal or physical)
3 = independent

Mobility

0 = immobile
1 = wheelchair independent, including corners
2 = walks with help of one person (verbal or physical)
3 = independent (but may use any aid; for example, cane)

Dressing

0 = dependent
1 = needs help but can do about half unaided
2 = independent (including buttons, zips, laces, etc.)

Stairs

0 = unable
1 = needs help (verbal, physical, carrying aid)
2 = independent

Bathing

0 = dependent
1 = independent (or in shower)

Total 0–20

LEVELS		
	7 Complete Independence (Timely, Safely) 6 Modified Independence (Device)	NO HELPER
	Modified Dependence 5 Supervision 4 Minimal Assist (Subject = 75% +) 3 Moderate Assist (Subject = 50% +) Complete Dependence 2 Maximal Assist (Subject = 25% +) 1 Total Assist (Subject = 0% +)	HELPER

	ADMIT	DISCHG	FOL-UP
Self-Care			
A. Eating			
B. Grooming			
C. Bathing			
D. Dressing - Upper Body			
E. Dressing - Lower Body			
F. Toileting			
Sphincter Control			
G. Bladder Management			
H. Bowel Management			
Transfers			
I. Bed, Chair, Wheelchair			
J. Toilet			
K. Tub, Shower			
Locomotion			
L. Walk/wheelchair	Walk / Wheelchair / Both	Walk / Wheelchair / Both	Walk / Wheelchair / Both
M. Stairs			
Motor Subtotal Score			
Communication			
N. Comprehension	Auditory / Visual / Both	Auditory / Visual / Both	Auditory / Visual / Both
O. Expression	Vocal / Non–vocal / Both	Vocal / Non–vocal / Both	Vocal / Non–vocal / Both
Social Cognition			
P. Social Interaction			
Q. Problem Solving			
R. Memory			
Cognitive Subtotal Score			
Total FIM			

NOTE: Leave no blanks; enter 1 if patient not testable due to risk

FIGURE A-1. Functional Independence Measure (Adult FIM™).

DISPLAY A-2
Rivermead Motor Assessment

Section
   Item   **Score**

Gross function

1. Sit unsupported
   Without holding on, on edge of bed, feet unsupported.   _____

2. Lying to sitting on side of bed
   Using any method.   _____

3. Sitting to standing
   May use hands to push up. Must stand up in 15 sec and stand   _____
   for 15 sec, with an aid if necessary.

4. Transfer from wheelchair to chair towards unaffected side   _____
   May use hands.

5. Transfer from wheelchair to chair towards affected side   _____
   May use hands.

6. Walk 10 m indoors with an aid   _____
   Any walking aid. No stand-by help.

7. Climb stairs independently   _____
   Any method. May use bannister and aid—must be a full flight
   of stairs.

8. Walk 10 m indoors without an aid   _____
   No stand-by help. No caliper, splint or walking aid.

9. Walk 10 m, pick up bean bag from floor, turn and carry back   _____
   Bend down any way, may use aid to walk if necessary. No
   stand-by help. May use either hand to pick up bean bag.

10. Walk outside 40 m   _____
    May use walking aid, caliper or splint. No stand-by help.

11. Walk up and down four steps   _____
    Patient may use an aid if he would normally use one, but may
    not hold on to rail. This is included to test ability to negotiate
    curb or stairs without a rail.

12. Run 10 m   _____
    Must be symmetrical.

13. Hop on affected leg five times on the spot   _____
    Must hop on ball of foot without stopping to regain balance.
    No help with arms.

Gross function total   _____

INSTRUCTIONS: This survey asks for your views about your health. This information will help keep track of how you feel and how well you are able to do your usual activities.

Answer every question by marking the appropriate oval. If you are unsure about how to answer a question, please give the best answer you can.

MARKING INSTRUCTIONS

- Use a No. 2 Pencil ONLY.
- Make dark heavy marks that fill the oval completely.
- Erase unwanted marks cleanly.
- Make no stray marks on this answer sheet.

PROPER MARK ⬭ ⬬ ⬭ IMPROPER MARKS

Before beginning this questionnaire...
Please print your ID number in the boxes to the right and then fill in the appropriate oval next to each number.
If you don't know your number, please ask the person who gave you this questionnaire.

ID NUMBER

	0	1	2	3	4	5	6	7	8	9
	0	1	2	3	4	5	6	7	8	9
	0	1	2	3	4	5	6	7	8	9
	0	1	2	3	4	5	6	7	8	9
	0	1	2	3	4	5	6	7	8	9
	0	1	2	3	4	5	6	7	8	9
	0	1	2	3	4	5	6	7	8	9
	0	1	2	3	4	5	6	7	8	9
	0	1	2	3	4	5	6	7	8	9
	0	1	2	3	4	5	6	7	8	9
	0	1	2	3	4	5	6	7	8	9

Now begin with the questions below.

1. In general, would you say your health is: (Mark only one.)
   1 ① **Excellent**
   ② **Very good**
   ③ **Good**
   ④ **Fair**
   ⑤ **Poor**

2. **Compared to one year ago**, how would you rate your health in general now? (Mark only one.)
   2 ① **Much better now than 1 year ago**
   ② **Somewhat better now than 1 year ago**
   ③ **About the same as 1 year ago**
   ④ **Somewhat worse now than 1 year ago**
   ⑤ **Much worse now than 1 year ago**

FIGURE A-2. Health Status Profile—SF-36.™ (© 1994 Response Technologies, Inc. East Greenwich, R.I. 02816. Used with permission.)

(continued)

The following items are about activities you might do during a typical day. Does **your health now limit you** in these activities? If so, how much? (Mark one oval on each line.)

	Yes, Limited A Lot	Yes, Limited A Little	No, Not Limited At All
3. **Vigorous activities,** such as running, lifting heavy objects, participating in strenuous sports	①	②	③
4. **Moderate activities,** such as moving a table, pushing a vacuum cleaner, bowling, or playing golf	①	②	③
5. Lifting or carrying groceries	①	②	③
6. Climbing **several** flights of stairs	①	②	③
7. Climbing **one** flight of stairs	①	②	③
8. Bending, kneeling, or stooping	①	②	③
9. Walking **more than a mile**	①	②	③
10. Walking **several blocks**	①	②	③
11. Walking **one block**	①	②	③
12. Bathing or dressing yourself	①	②	③

During the **past 4 weeks,** have you had any of the following problems with your work or other regular daily activities **as a result of your physical health?** (Mark one oval on each line.)

	Yes	No
13. Cut down the **amount of time** you spent on work or other activities	①	②
14. **Accomplished less** than you would like	①	②
15. Were limited in the **kind** of work or other activities	①	②
16. Had **difficulty** performing the work or other activities (for example, it took extra effort)	①	②

PLEASE TURN CARD OVER TO COMPLETE QUESTIONNAIRE

FIGURE A-2. (*Continued*)

This is Side 2 of the Questionnaire.
Make sure you complete the OTHER side first.

During the **past 4 weeks**, have you had any of the following problems with your work or the other regular daily activities **as a result of any emotional problems** (such as feeling depressed or anxious)? (Mark one oval on each line.)

17. Cut down on the **amount of time** you spent on work or other activities	① Yes	② No
18. **Accomplished less** than you would like	① Yes	② No
19. Didn't do work or other activities as **carefully** as usual	① Yes	② No

20. During the **past 4 weeks**, to what extent has your physical health or emotional problems interfered with your normal social activities with family, friends, neighbors, or groups? (Mark one oval.)

① Not at all ② Slightly ③ Moderately ④ Quite a bit ⑤ Extremely

21. How much **bodily** pain have you had during the **past 4 weeks**? (Mark one oval.)

① None ② Very mild ③ Mild ④ Moderate ⑤ Severe ⑥ Very severe

22. During the **past 4 weeks**, how much did **pain** interfere with your normal work (including both work outside the home and housework)? (Mark one oval.)

① Not at all ② A little bit ③ Moderately ④ Quite a bit ⑤ Extremely

These questions are about how you feel and how things have been with you **during the past 4 weeks**. For each question, please give the one answer that comes closest to the way you have been feeling. How much of the time during the **past 4 weeks**... (Mark one oval on each line.)

	All of the Time	Most of the Time	A Good Bit of the Time	Some of the Time	A Little of the Time	None of the Time
23. Did you feel full of pep?	①	②	③	④	⑤	⑥
24. Have you been a very nervous person?	①	②	③	④	⑤	⑥
25. Have you felt so down in the dumps that nothing could cheer you up?	①	②	③	④	⑤	⑥
26. Have you felt calm and peaceful?	①	②	③	④	⑤	⑥
27. Did you have a lot of energy?	①	②	③	④	⑤	⑥
28. Have you felt downhearted and blue?	①	②	③	④	⑤	⑥
29. Did you feel worn out?	①	②	③	④	⑤	⑥
30. Have you been a happy person?	①	②	③	④	⑤	⑥
31. Did you feel tired?	①	②	③	④	⑤	⑥

FIGURE A-2. (*Continued*)

32. During the **past 4 weeks,** how much of the time has your **physical health or emotional problems** interfered with your social activities (like visiting with friends, relatives, etc.)? (Mark one oval.) — 32

① **All of the time** ② **Most of the time** ③ **Some of the time** ④ **A little of the time** ⑤ **None of the time**

How **true** or **false** is **each** of the following statements for you?		Definitely True	Mostly True	Don't Know	Mostly False	Definitely False
33. I seem to get sick a little easier than other people	33	①	②	③	④	⑤
34. I am as healthy as anybody I know	34	①	②	③	④	⑤
35. I expect my health to get worse	35	①	②	③	④	⑤
36. My health is excellent	36	①	②	③	④	⑤

37. Are you male or female — 37 ① **Male** ② **Female**

38. How old were you on your last birthday? — 38

① **less than 18** ② **18-24** ③ **25-34** ④ **35-44** ⑤ **45-54** ⑥ **55-64** ⑦ **65-74** ⑧ **75+**

DO NOT WRITE IN THIS SPACE

THANK YOU FOR YOUR TIME

FOR OFFICE USE ONLY Ⓐ Ⓑ Ⓒ Ⓓ Ⓔ

FIGURE A-2. *(Continued)*

1. In general, would you say your health is (*circle one number*):

Excellent	1	Fair	4
Very Good	2	Poor	5
Good	3		

The following items are about activities you might do during a typical day. Does your health now limit you in these activities? If so, how much?

	(*circle one number on each line*)		
	Yes, limited a lot	Yes, limited a little	No, not limited at all
2. Lifting or carrying groceries	1	2	3
3. Climbing **several** flights of stairs	1	2	3
4. Walking **several** blocks	1	2	3

5. During the **past 4 weeks,** how much difficulty did you have doing your work or other regular daily activities **as a result of your physical health?** (*circle one number*)

None at all	1	Quite a bit	4
A little bit	2	Could not do daily work	5
Some	3		

6. During the **past 4 weeks,** to what extent have you accomplished less than you would like in your work or other daily activities **as a result of emotional problems** (such as feeling depressed or anxious)? (*circle one number*)

Not at all	1	Quite a bit	4
Slightly	2	Extremely	5
Moderately	3		

7. During the **past 4 weeks,** to what extent has your physical health or emotional problems interfered with your normal social activities with family, friends, neighbors, or groups? (*circle one number*)

Not at all	1	Quite a bit	4
Slightly	2	Extremely	5
Moderately	3		

8. How much bodily pain have you had during the **past 4 weeks?** (*circle one number*)

None	1	Moderate	4
Very mild	2	Severe	5
Mild	3	Very severe	6

These questions are about how you feel and how things have been with you during the **past 4 weeks.** For each question, please give the one answer that comes closest to the way you have been feeling.

How much of the time during the **past 4 weeks** . . .

	(*circle one number on each line*)					
	All of the time	Most of the time	A good bit of the time	Some of the time	A little of the time	None of the time
9. Have you felt calm and peaceful?	1	2	3	4	5	6
10. Did you have a lot of energy?	1	2	3	4	5	6
11. Have you felt downhearted and blue?	1	2	3	4	5	6
12. Have you been a happy person?	1	2	3	4	5	6

FIGURE A-3. The 12-item Health Status Questionnaire (HSQ-12). (Copyright © 1995 by Health Outcomes Institute.)

dependence and 3 representing independence. The 10 items and scoring are depicted in Display A-1.

Functional Independence Measure. The FIM was designed to include only a minimum number of items. It measures disability, not impairment, and is based on observed performance of the patient initiating and/or completing the functional tasks. A 7-point scale is used to denote the level of independence (scores of 6 or 7) or dependence (scores of 1–5) in the performance of 18 different items. The total score of the FIM can be reported, but more often subscores for motor and cognitive performance are used. (See Fig. A-1.)

Rivermead Mobility Index. The Rivermead Mobility Index was originally designed as the Rivermead Motor Assessment to measure impairment as well as functional mobility. Most recently it has been used primarily as an index of mobility because these items are easy and quick to perform. The scoring is either a 1 if patients can perform the activity, or a 0 if they cannot. The total number of items on the mobility index is 13. (See Display A-2.)

SF-36. This quality-of-life questionnaire is the same as the MOS 36-Item Short-Form Health Survey. The questionnaire was originally developed from the Rand 36-item questionnaire. The SF-36 assesses eight health attributes: physical function, role limitations due to physical health, role limitations due to emotional problems, energy and fatigue, emotional well-being, social functioning, pain, and general health. The questionnaire is completed by patients based on how they are feeling or functioning. This tool assesses patients' quality of life in addition to their functional abilities. (See Fig. A-2.)

12-Item Health Status Questionnaire (HSQ-12). The HSQ-12 is similar to, albeit a shortened version of, the 36-Item Health Status Questionnaire. The HSQ-12 was recently published by the Health Outcomes Institute (2001 Killebrew Dr., Suite 122, Bloomington, MN 55425). Like the SF-36, the HSQ-12 measures eight health attributes: physical functioning, role limitations due to physical factors, bodily pain, health perception, energy and fatigue, social functioning, role limitations due to mental factors, and mental health. (See Fig. A-3.)

Validity and Reliability of Standardized Instruments

This appendix identifies references for the validity and reliability of the standardized tests described in this textbook. The tables include:

- Instruments to Measure Mobility and Disability
- Instruments to Measure Quality of Life

- Instruments to Measure Weakness/ Motor Loss
- Instruments to Measure Balance Dysfunction
- Instruments to Measure Incoordination
- Instruments to Measure Sensory/ Perceptual Dysfunction

TABLE B-1. Instruments to Measure Mobility and Disability

Instrument	Chapter in Text	References
Mobility		
Rivermead Mobility Index	Chap. 1 Chap. 3 Appendix A	Wade, Collen, Robb, & Warlow (1992) Collen, Wade, Robb, & Bradshaw (1991)
Disability		
Barthel Index	Chap. 1 Chap. 3 Appendix A	Gresham, Phillips, & Labi, (1980) Wade & Hewer (1987) Hertanu, Demopoulus, Yang, Calhoun, & Fenigstein (1984) Duncan (1992) Wade & Collen, (1988) Shinar, Gross, Bronstein, et al. (1987)
Functional Independence Measure (FIM)	Chap. 1 Chap. 3 Appendix A	Hamilton, Granger, Sherwin, Zielezny, & Tashman (1987) Granger & Hamilton (1990) Hamilton, Laughlin, Granger, & Kayton (1991)

TABLE B-2.   Instruments to Measure Quality of Life

Name of Test	Chapter in Text	References
SF-36, Medical Outcomes Study (MOS), 36-Item Short Form Health Survey	Chap. 1 Appendix A	Ware & Sherbourne (1992)
Health Status Questionnaire (HSQ-12)	Chap. 1 Appendix A	Health Outcomes Institute

TABLE B-3.   Instruments to Measure Weakness/Motor Loss

Name of Test	Chapter in Text	References for Validity and Reliability
Manual Muscle Test	Chap. 5	Iddings, Smith, & Spencer (1961)
Hand-held dynamometer	Chap. 5	Bohannon & Andrews (1987)
Isokinetic dynamometer	Chap. 5	Hasu, Masatoshi & Kikuchi (1980) Mayer, Smith, Kondraske, Gatchell, Suzuki, & Enclo

TABLE B-4.   Instruments to Measure Balance Dysfunction

Name of Test	Chapter in Text	References for Validity and Reliability
Berg Balance Scale	Chap. 8	Berg, Maki, Williams, Holliday, & Wood-Daphnee (1992) Berg, Wood-Daphnee, Williams, & Gayton (1989)
Timed "Up and Go"	Chap. 8	Posiadlo & Richardson (1991) Mathlas, Nayak, & Isaacs (1986)
Functional Reach	Chap. 8	Duncan, Weiner, Chadler, & Studenski (1990) Weiner, Duncan, Chadler, & Studenski (1992)

TABLE B-5. Instruments to Measure Incoordination

Name of Test	Chapter in Text	References for Validity and Reliability
Rivermead Motor Assessment	Chap. 1 Chap. 3 Appendix A Chap. 7	Collen, Wade, & Bradshaw (1990) Collen, Wade, Robb, & Bradshaw (1991)
Box & Block Test	Chap. 7	Mathiowetz, Volland, Kashman, & Weber (1985) Desrosiers, Bravog, Hebert, Dutil, & Mercier (1994)
Jebsen Hand Function	Chap. 7	Jebsen, Taylor, Trieschmann, Trotter, & Howard (1969)
Fitts' Tapping Test	Chap. 7	Williamson & Leiper (1993)
Frenchay Arm Test	Chap. 7	DeSouza, Langton Hewer, & Miller (1980) Berglund & Fugl-Meyer (1986)

TABLE B-6. Instruments to Measure Sensory/Perceptual Dysfunctions

Name of Test	Chapter in Text	References for Validity and Reliability*
Ayers Figure-Ground Test	Chap. 6	Ayers (1987)
The Space Visualization Test of the Sensory Integration and Praxis Test	Chap. 6	children only, Ayers (1987)
Right-Left Orientation Test	Chap. 6	
Schenkenberg Line Bisection Test	Chap. 6	
Goodglass & Kaplan Test of Apraxia	Chap. 6	

*The validity and reliability of the tests listed in this table is limited.

REFERENCES

Berglund, K, & Fugl-Meyer, AR. (1986). Upper extremity function in hemiplegia: A cross-validation study of two assessment methods. *Scandinavian Journal of Rehabilitation Medicine 18*(4), 155–157.

Bohannon, RW, & Andrews, AW. (1987). Interrater reliability of hand-held dynamometry. *Physical Therapy 67*(6), 931–940.

Collen, FM, Wade, DT, & Bradshaw, CM. (1990). Mobility after stroke: Reliability of measures of impairment and disability. *International Disability Studies 12,* 6–9.

Collen, FM, Wade, DT, Robb, GF, & Bradshaw, CM. (1991). The Rivermead Mobility Index: A further development of the Rivermead Motor Assessment. *International Disability Studies 13,* 50–54.

DeSouza, LH, Langton Hewer, R, & Miller, S. (1980). Assessment of recovery of arm control in hemiplegic stroke patients: Arm function test. *International Rehabilitation Medicine 2,* 3–9.

Duncan, PW. (1992). Contemporary management of motor control problems: Proceedings of the II Step Conference. In *Stroke: Physical therapy assessment and treatment.* Alexandria, VA: Foundation for Physical Therapy.

Granger, CV, & Hamilton, BB. (1990). Measurement of stroke rehabilitation outcome in the 1980s. *Stroke 21* (Suppl. 110), 1146–1147.

Gresham, GE, Phillips, TF, & Labi, ML. (1980). ADL status in stroke: Relative merits of three standard indexes. *Archives of Physical Medicine and Rehabilitation 61*(8), 355–358.

Hamilton, BB, Granger, CV, Sherwin, FS, Zielezny, M, & Tashman, JS. (1987). A uniform national data system for medical rehabilitation. In MJ. Fuhrer (Ed.). *Rehabilitation outcomes: Analysis and measurement.* Baltimore: Brookes.

Hamilton, BB, Laughlin, JA, Granger, CV, & Kayton, RM. (1991). Interrater agreement of the seven level functional independence measure (FIM). *Archives of Physical Medicine and Rehabilitation 72,* 790.

Hasu, M, Fujiwara, M, & Kikuchi, S. (1980). A new method of quantitative measurement of abdominal and back muscle strength. *Spine 5*(2), 143–148.

Hertanu, JS, Demopoulos, JT, Yang, WC, Calhoun, WF, & Fenigstein, HA. (1984). Stroke rehabilitation: Correlation and prognostic value of computerized tomography and sequential functional assessments. *Archives of Physical Medicine and Rehabilitation 65*(9), 505–508.

Iddings, DM, Smith, LK, & Spencer, WA. (1961). Muscle testing, Part 2: Reliability in clinical use. *Physical Therapy Review 41,* 249–256.

Mayer, TG, Vanharanba, H, Gatchel, RJ, Mooney, V, Barnes, D, Judge, L, Smith, S, & Terry, A. (1989). Comparison of CT scan muscle measurements and isokinetic trunk strength in postoperative patients. *Spine 14,* 33–36.

Shinar, D, Gross, CR, Bronstein, KS, et al. (1987). Reliability of the Activities of Daily Living Scale and its use in telephone interviews. *Archives of Physical Medicine and Rehabilitation 68,* 723–728.

Wade, DT, Collen, FM, Robb, GF, & Warlow, CP. (1992). Physiotherapy intervention late after stroke and mobility. *British Medical Journal 304*(6827), 609–613.

Wade, DT, & Collin, C. (1988). The Barthel ADL Index: A standard measure of physical disability? *International Disability Studies 10*(2), 64–67.

Wade, DT, & Hewer, RL. (1987). Functional abilities after stroke: Measurement, natural history and prognosis. *Journal of Neurology, Neurosurgery, and Psychiatry 50*(2), 177–182.

Ware, JE, & Sherbourne, CD. (1992). The MOS 36-item short-form health survey (SF-36): I. Conceptual framework and item selection. *Medical Care 30*(6), 473–483.

abnormal tone: Abnormal force with which a muscle resists being lengthened; abnormal stiffness

actin: A muscle protein found on the I band of the sarcomere

action potential: A transient electrical signal that results in a chemical synapse at a motor unit

active assistive exercise (AAE): Active exercises performed by a patient throughout a full or partial range of motion (ROM) with the assistance of a therapist in functional, gravity-eliminated planes

active resistive exercises (ARE): Those performed by a patient with resistance provided by a therapist or via other resistive equipment, such as free weights

afferent connections: Those that carry messages to the central nervous system (CNS)

agnosia: The inability to recognize objects

agonist: Muscles that are the prime movers. They contract, as opposed to *relax* during a given movement. (See *antagonist.*)

akinesia: Absence of movement, either complete or partial

alpha motor neurons: Located subcortically, neurons that conduct impulses from the CNS to the periphery to produce a motor response, such as movement

antagonist: Muscles that counteract the action of the prime movers

approximation: A physical therapy technique in which the bones of a joint are brought together

apraxia: Loss of the ability to perform movement in the absence of motor or sensory impairments
    constructional: Inability to produce designs in two or three dimensions by copying, drawing, or constructing

ideational: Inability to correlate purpose and accomplishment of tasks; believed to be caused by a disruption in the conceptual organization of movement

ideomotor: Inability to carry out purposeful movement on command

areflexia: Complete loss of *myotatic* reflexes

astereognosis: Tactile agnosia; the inability to recognize objects by touch even though tactile, thermal, and proprioceptive functions remain intact

asthenia: Generalized weakness

ataxia: Lack of coordination

athetosis: Slow, irregular, twisting movements, especially of the hands and fingers

atrophy: Wasting of muscle

Babinski reflex: Results in the dorsiflexion of the big toe on stimulation of the sole of the foot

Babinski's sign: The actual loss or lessening of the Babinski reflex; commonly seen in patients with upper motor neuron lesions

balance: The state of physical equilibrium

balance dysfunction: The inability to maintain the body's center of gravity over its base of support

baroreceptors: Receptors located in the carotid sinus that are sensitive to changes in blood pressure

biomechanical substitution: An alternative movement strategy in which abnormal movement patterns are substituted for normal patterns due to the person's inability to move normally

blocked practice: Occurs when the learner practices one task or activity before moving on to the next activity

bony block: Excess bone growth within a joint that restricts motion

bradykinesia: Slowness of movement

bridging: A position that requires a patient in hook-lying posture to fully extend the hips and thereby lift the trunk off the resting surface

chorea: A condition marked by rapid, irregular, and flowing involuntary muscular twitching

closed chain activities: Performed with the distal part of an extremity in a weight-bearing position

collateral: That which accompanies or functions as an accessory, as in side branches of nerves

contraction: A shortening or tightening, as of a muscle
    concentric: Those that produce limb movement with shortening of the muscle
    eccentric: Lengthening rather than shortening of tensed muscle
    isometric: Muscle contraction that produces high levels of tension in the absence of limb movement
    isotonic: Produce equal levels of tension throughout the range of limb movement
    tetanic: Sustained and generally induced by stimulation

convergence: Both eyes moving together to scan the environment or track an object

cupula: Gelatinous cap at the apex of the cochlea and spiral canal of the ear, in which the hair cells are embedded

cutaneous receptors: Receptors in the skin that are sensitive to touch

deafferented: Devoid of afferent nerve input

deconditioning: A process by which the body loses strength and cardiovascular endurance as a result of long-term disuse associated with illness, hospitalization, or chronic neurological conditions

decussate: To cross over to the contralateral side

denervation: Lack of normal innervation

disability: Any limitation in functional mobility; the *inability* to perform a task

disease: Any pathology that occurs at the level of the organ

divergence: The opposite of convergence; the eyes do not move together—an abnormal condition

dorsal rhizotomy: Surgical transection of spinal nerve rootlettes that results in diminished abilities in the sensory modalities of proprioception, discriminative touch, pain and temperature sensation, as well as the loss of reflexes mediated at those levels

dysdiadochokinesia: Inability to perform rapid alternating movements

dyskinesia: Defect of movement

dysmetria: Overshooting or reaching beyond the target; past-pointing

dystonia: Abnormal tone or postures

effector organs: Muscles or glands that contract or secrete in response to nerve impulses

efferent fibers: Those that carry messages from the CNS to the periphery

electromyographic activity: Graphic recording of muscle contraction brought on by electrical stimulation

epicritic: Concerned with acute sensibility; refers to the phylogenetically newer portion of the somatosensory system, which deals with the fine discrimination between degrees of touch or temperature

flaccid paralysis: Loss or impairment of motor function due, in part, to decreased or absent muscular tone

flexor reflex afferents: The cumulation of afferent fibers entering the spinal cord from a variety of muscle spindle receptors

folia: The many transversely oriented folds in the cortex

foramen (plural, *foramina*): Openings or passageways

functional limitations: The inability to accomplish any of the tasks of functional mobility

functional mobility: The ability to perform a functional task (see *functional task*)

functional tasks: The common movements needed for daily activity; the list includes, but is not limited to, bed mobility (eg, rolling from side to side); moving from the supine to a sitting posture; moving from sitting to a standing posture; transferring from one surface to another (eg, moving from a bed to a wheelchair); ambulating; and climbing stairs

genu recurvatum: Buckling of the involved limbs as the weight is shifted onto the extremity; hyperextension of the knee

Golgi tendon organs (GTOs): Receptors that are sensitive to changes in the length and tension in a muscle

gravity-eliminated planes: Planes, or surfaces, that serve to support a body part so that it can move free of the force of gravity

gross motor patterns: Movement generated in proximal joints

habituation exercises: Those that require that the patient be repeatedly positioned so that symptoms are elicited for purposes of CNS accommodation

handicap: A societal limitation placed on a person with an impairment or disability

handling: A process whereby therapists put their hands on the patient in specific regions (*key points of control*) to facilitate targeted movements and inhibit other, unwanted movements

head thrust: A move performed by a therapist, who quickly and gently moves the patient's head to neutral (or center position) from a starting position of 30° off center

hemiballismus: Unilateral chorea; rapid and irregular movements

hemiplegia: Paralysis of one side of the body

high-functioning patients: Those who are capable of performing functional tasks, though their movement strategies may be inefficient, unsafe, or both

homonymous hemianopsia: Loss of vision on one side of the visual field

homunculus, motor: A word *(homonculus)* which actually means "little man," and is used to refer to a hypothetical creature that controls the human being

hook-lying position: A position in which the patient lies supine with the knees flexed so that both feet can be positioned flat on the surface on which he or she is lying

hypertonia: Excessive tone of skeletal muscle

hypotonia: Diminished tone of skeletal muscle

impairment: A problem or symptom that a patient presents as a result of abnormal structure or function of organs or tissues. Pain, edema, and weakness are all examples of common impairments.

incoordination: Inability to produce smooth, rhythmic motion that is not due to weakness

intention tremor: Shaking or tremor activity during an active movement

internal biofeedback: Information received from joint receptors, muscle spindles, GTOs, etc., regarding the location of joints and muscle length

internal capsule: A collection of myelinated fibers composed of sensory axons traveling from the thalamus to the cortex, and motor fibers originating in cortical regions and projecting to the brainstem and spinal cord

joint compression: The application of pressure to a joint

key points of control: Anatomic points or areas at which therapists handle patients

kinesthesia: The sense by which position, weight, and movement are perceived

knowledge of results: Feedback or information about how a task was performed. This information is useful when provided after the skill has been completed; it is not particularly helpful when communicated during the activity.

labyrinth: The bony portion of the inner ear

low-functioning patients: Patients who require manual assistance to perform functional movement. They may benefit from the application of selected facilitation techniques to promote motor activity in a posture or during a functional movement.

mass movement patterns: The patterns of motion used in proprioceptive neuromuscular facilitation (PNF), which are characteristic of normal motor activity. These patterns are *spiral* and *diagonal,* in keeping with the spiral and rotary characteristics of skeletal muscle, and closely resemble the movements used in sports and work activities.

mechanoreceptors: Receptors that surround joints and provide information on joint position

metamorphosia: The visual distortion of objects, such that things appear much larger or smaller than their actual sizes

midline: Referring to the midsagittal plane of the body

motor cortex: That portion of the cerebral cortex located at the posterior portion of the frontal cortex; the center of activity for all voluntary movement; Brodman's area 4

movement decomposition: Breakdown of movements between multiple joints (eg, the movements between shoulder, elbow, wrist, and hand move in segments not as one fluid movement)

muscle spindles: Receptors sensitive to length of muscle

muscle tension: Generated as a result of muscle contraction and varies depending on the type of contraction; also known as muscle force

myelin: Insulating sheath produced by Schwann cells that surrounds axons

myosin: A muscle protein found on the A band of the sarcomere

myotatic: Pertaining to the proprioceptive sense of muscles or monosynaptic component of afferent and efferent fibers

myotatic reflexes: Monosynaptic reflexes with skeletal muscle responses

neural encoding: A process by which the neural signal produced by the initial stimulation causes an action potential in the receptor that is then transmitted to the axon of the peripheral nerve that relays information about the stimulus (eg, intensity and duration)

neuraxis: The CNS, sometimes specifically referred to as the brain stem and spinal cord

nociceptors: Receptors that detect pain and have either free nerve endings or a minimal number of capsules

nystagmus: Involuntary rapid movement of the eyeball

otoconia: Calcium carbonate crystals that provide the membrane overlying the hair cells in the inner ear receptors (saccule) with a specific gravity

overflow phenomenon: The process by which activity is detected in an unexercised muscle during excitation of a muscle in another part of the body

paralysis: A temporary or permanent loss of function

paresis: Slight or incomplete loss of motor function; weakness

peduncles: Bands of fibers that connect parts of the brain

pelvic obliquity: An inclination or slanting of the pelvis

phasic: Pertaining to movement

posterolateral: Referring to posterior and lateral positions

predictive deficits (also *feedforward deficits*): Inability to anticipate movement patterns needed for a task resulting in spontaneous or reactive movement versus planned movement; frequently seen with damage to the cerebellum

presynaptic inhibition: Inhibition of neurotransmitter release due to the depolarization of the nerve terminal by a second neural input

program generators: Neuronal circuitry that is capable of activating patterned movements such as locomotion, respiration, chewing, at all levels of the neuraxis

prosopagnosia: The inability to recognize familiar faces or distinctive characteristics of unfamiliar faces

protopathic: Primitive, phylogenetically older portion of the somatosensory system; this systems fails to discriminate between sensations in terms of sensing and localizing pain

random practice: Occurs when tasks or activities to be learned are practiced together

range of motion: Range of a joint's movement

reflex inhibiting patterns (RIPs), dynamic: A specific handling technique used to produce inhibition of excessive tone

reciprocal: All connections within the cortex are *reciprocal* (ie, information transmitted from the sensory cortex to the motor cortex is then relayed back to the sensory cortex via association fibers)

When referring to movement, *reciprocal* refers to complementary movements such as supination and pronation or flexion and extension.

recruitment overflow: An abnormal increase in the recruitment of motor units

reflexive movement: The purest example of the reflex stimulus model; a stimulus is provided and movement occurs without the mediation of conscious thought

reinnervation: The process of reintroducing nervous innervation after a period of denervation

reverberating circuits: Axon collaterals re-excite the same neuron through excitatory interneurons

rigidity: Abnormal muscle tone characterized by relatively uniform resistance to passive movement, not velocity dependent

saccades: Sequenced, rapid eye movements; used to localize specific, typically stationary, stimuli

segmental programs: Program generators that are located at various levels of the neuraxis

simultanognosia: The decreased ability to perceive and interpret stimuli as a whole

smooth pursuit: The ability to track an object with the eyes while the head remains stationary

somatognosia: The lack of awareness of body structure and the inability to recognize one's own body parts and their relationships to each other

somatosensation: Body sense

somatotopic: System of organization in the brain that shows the correspondence between a given area of the brain and a specific part of the body

spasticity: Hypertonicity

stereognosis: Ability to recognize objects by touch

stimulus transduction: Depolarization or hyperpolarization of cell membranes on stimulation

strength: The measure of the force output of contracting muscle; directly related to the amount of tension produced in contracting muscle

subluxation: Partial or incomplete dislocation of joints

synapse: The junction at which the axon of one neuron comes into contact with the body of another cell, or its dendrites, for the purpose of communicating neurochemical messages

synergistic: Muscles that work together to produce motion; at times, may contract to compensate for weakness in the primary muscle that performs the joint movement

tapping: A technique in which the therapist taps on weak muscles for the express purpose of forcing volitional contraction. Tapping on the muscle belly facilitates muscle activation by eliciting quick stretches of muscle spindles.

tonic: Holding contraction, stationary

touch: The ability to sense the texture and movement of objects across the skin

twitch contractions: Simple, spasmodic contractions that occur independent of stimulation

unilateral neglect: Failure to respond or orient to stimuli presented contralateral to the side of a brain lesion, usually seen with lesions in the right hemisphere

ventral posteromedial nucleus (VPM): A portion of the thalamus which receives sensory information from the face

ventral posterolateral (VPL) nucleus: A portion of the thalamus which receives sensory information from the body

vermis: Median portion of the cerebellum

vertigo: Sense of rotation or movement of one's person or one's surroundings

vestibular apparatus: Composed of receptors in the inner ear and their connections with nuclei, and concerned with equilibrium

vestibular ocular reflex: Assessed when the patient focuses on a stationary object while actively moving the head from side to side or up and down

viscoelasticity: A property that allows muscle to resist movement and return to resting lengths after being lengthened

visual scanning: The ability to gaze up, down, and laterally

visual spatial agnosia: Deficits in spatial relations and spatial position

volitional movement: Conscious, or deliberate, movement

weakness: The inability to generate normal levels of tension in muscle

INDEX

Page numbers followed by *f* indicate figures; those followed by *t* indicate tables.

A

Abnormal postural reflexes
  neurodevelopmental treatment for, 72, 73
Abnormal tone. *See also* Normal tone
  assessment of, 63, 64t
  with lesions of movement pathway, 33
  treatment of
    strengthening programs in, 89
Acetylcholine
  in muscle contractions, 89, 90f
Actin
  in muscle contractions, 89, 90f
Action potentials, 26
  in muscle contractions, 89, 90f
Active assistive exercise (AAE)
  for flaccidity, 112
  for muscle strengthening, 118
Active range of motion (AROM)
  in assessment of muscle weakness, 101–102
    in patients with spasticity, 101
  with free weight
    for muscle strengthening, 118
  synergy with hip flexion during, 105, 106f
  of upper extremities, 106, 107f
Active resistive exercise (ARE)
  for muscle strengthening, 115
Afferent connections
  in prefrontal association cortex, 20
Afferent nerves, 24
Agency for Health Care Policy and Research (AHCPR)
  stroke rehabilitation guidelines, 54
Agnosia(s)
  definition of, 147
  evaluation of, 148
  sensory and perceptual dysfunction in, 136
  tactile, 149
  visual object, 148
  visual spatial, 143
Akinesia, 24
Alpha motor neuron
  in integration of sensory information, 30
Alpha motor neuron axons
  in muscle contractions, 89, 90
Ambulation, 48. *See also* Gait cycle
  balance assessment during, 188–189
  balance dysfunction in
    alternative movement strategies for, 188–189
  in balance training, 213–214
  as controlled falling, 188
  gait cycle in, 48–51
  ideational ataxia and, 138
  in incoordination, 164
  position deficits and, 151

in sensory and perceptual dysfunction
    case study of, 140
  spatial relations deficits and, 138, 151
  in weakness of lower extremities, 96–99
Amyotrophic lateral sclerosis (ALS)
  motor unit decrease in, 91
Antalgic gait, 51
Aphasia, 58
Approximation, 70
  in facilitation, 71
Apraxia
  causes of, 147
  constructional, 145–146
    block design tests of, 146
    graphic tasks in evaluation of, 145f–146, 145–146
  definition of, 145
  dressing, 146
  effect on functional mobility tasks, 136
  ideational
    definition of, 147
    evaluation of, 147
  ideomotor, 147
    definition of, 147
    evaluation of, 147
  components of, 53
  rationale for, 54
Assessment model for disabilities and impairments
  steps in, 53, 56
    community mobility assessment, 64–65
    observation, 58–59
    reobservation, 63–64
    testing for disabilities, 53, 59–61
    testing for impairments, 61–63
Assistive devices
  observation of
    in disability assessment, 59
Association cortices, 16t, 19. *See also* Motor cortex
  limbic, 20
  parietal-temporal-occipital, 20
  prefrontal, 20
Astereognosis, 148
Asthenia
  from cerebellar lesions, 160
Asymmetry
  in sit-to-stand maneuver, 94f-95f
  in weight-bearing
    pelvic obliquity from, 94–95
Asynergy, 160
Ataxia(s)
  cerebellar, 164
  Fregly and Graybiel Quantitative Ataxia Test Battery for, 197, 199f, 199–200, 200f
  ideational, 137
  from somatosensory loss, 190
  spinal, 164
Athetosis, 24
Ayres Figure-Ground Test
  for figure-ground deficit, 142

B

Babinski reflex, 18
  primary motor cortex and, 18
Babinski's sign
  in upper motor neuron lesions, 25
Balance. *See also* Balance dysfunction
  in adaptation to environment, 185
  anatomy in, 185–186
  challenges to
    motor responses to, 186
  definitions of, 182
  general tests of
    Berg Balance Scale, 200–201
    clinical balance assessment, 201–202
    Clinical Test for Sensory Interaction Imbalance, 197, 198f
    Fregly and Graybiel Quantitative Ataxia Test Battery, 197, 199f, 199–200, 200f
    Fukuda Stepping Test, 203
    functional reach, 202
    "get up and go" test, 201
    postural stress test, 204
    Romberg test, 196
    timed "up and go" test, 201
    Tinnetti tests, 202–203
  impairment of
    causes of, 182
  interaction of neuromuscular and musculoskeletal systems in, 182–183
  laboratory tests of
    caloric tests, 205
    platform perturbation tests, 204–205
    rotational tests, 205
  maintenance of
    constraints to, 182
    integration of sensory information with muscle coordination for, 185
  movement strategies for
    ankle, 183, 184f
    hip, 183–184
    stepping, 183, 184, 184f
    suspensory, 183, 184, 185f
  sensory component of
    somatosensation in, 185
    vestibular information in, 184–185
    visual input in, 185
  sensory systems in
    proprioception, 185–186
    vestibular, 185, 186
    visual, 186
Balance dysfunction
  assessment of
    motor system in, 192
    sensory system in, 192–194
  disability assessment in, 186–191
    ambulation, 188–189
    climbing stairs, 189
    rolling, 187
    sit-to-stand maneuver, 187–188
    stable sitting posture, 187
    stable standing posture, 188